Reflections in an
Orphan's Eye

Reflections in an Orphan's Eye

A Decade at Oxford 1947-1957

ALTON L. PROVOST

To order additional copies of this book, contact:
Xlibris Corporation
1-888-795-4274
www.Xlibris.com
Orders@Xlibris.com
27338

CONTENTS

Foreword 11

Introduction 13

Prologue 15

1. Leaving Home 21
2. My Arrival 89
3. The College that Became an Orphanage 111
4. The Dentist 120
5. The Shoe Shop 127
6. The Industrial Building 132
7. The Baby Cottage 142
8. My First Day at School 163
9. The "How Are You. Fine I Hope" Letter 173
10. The Picture Show 177
11. I Nearly Drown and See My First Naked Girl 180
12. End of the First Year-1947 187
13. Out of the Frying Pan and into the Walker Building 197
14. The Watering Hole 217
15. Mr. Gray's List 223
16. I Meet the "Big Boys" 240
17. The Toy 247
18. The Errand Boy 254
19. The Ink Book 261
20. The Tonsil Clinic 266
21. The Year 1950 270
22. My Move From Walker Building to 1-B 275
23. The Korean War 282
24. The Dairy and Bob Davis 287
25. Bringing in the Cows 297

26. World Champion Cow-Caller 301
27. Mules, The Milk Run, Bridling Bell 304
28. And What is This Knob Marked "V-HOLD" For? 313
29. The Manure Wagon 318
30. Little Orphan Al's Revenge.. 321
31. Heat, Birthing, and the Mummy 329
32. The Balloon Boys 337
33. Ace's Show 342
34. Whipping and Old Ace 347
35. Cornsilk Fags 353
36. Dabs 355
37. The Blue Flame.. 363
38. The Return of the Balloon Boys 368
39. Mr. Walker's Firewater 373
40. Hog Killing 378
41. The Disappearance of Wun Hung Lo 386
42. Sick Call and the Dreaded Polio 391
43. Why We Talk Funny 398
44. Mountain Oyster Hunting With Red Ryder...................... 408
45. Birthdays and Friendship.. 412
46. The Bell.. 415
47. Orphans' All-Time Favorites Peanut Butter and Ice Cream 420
48. Snow, Snow Cream, Sledding and Frozen Tits 425
49. Tom Adams 431
50. Colored Farm Workers 436
51. The "Bonecrushers".. 439
52. The Four Visions and the Famed Middle Distance 442
53. Concerning Pseudo-Saints and Other Unwanted And
    Wearisome Theological Flotsam 449
54. Puberty.. 455
55. Melda 459
56. My Angel Benefactors 474
57. On Pecans, Salt, Tomatoes and Strawberries 479
58. Musky Dines 486
59. The Tale of Butch's Pig in a Poke 497
60. The Ditchbank Crew 504

61. My Seemingly Eternal Search for Identity 506
62. Chicken Farming 511
63. Time and Unforeseen Occurrences 516
64. The Crossroads of My Life 531
65. "Pig" Talton-My Second Test of Resolve 546
66. Why I Didn't Fumble the Football 558
67. The Secret of the "Red Bread" 566
68. Hot Buttered Popcorn and Its Influence on Segregation
    in the South 572
69. "Come Here, Football!" 577
70. But We Really Weren't Running Away 584
71. Life Becomes a Little Easier 595
72. "Pupils Who Left for Other Reasons" 601
73. On the Occasion of My Departure from
    "This Damned Place" 606

Epilogue: Life After Oxford 615

Dedication

This book is dedicated to orphans everywhere, with special love and understanding to 'sylum dogs of Oxford Orphanage. Orphans know. Orphans understand.

Orphans never forget.

FOREWORD

Time and distance are wonderful healers. Experiences of youth are compressed and sometimes extinguished by the responsibilities and complexities of adult life. I first became acutely aware of my own mortality at about the age of fifty-five, when in the short span of eighteen months, three of my older brothers died. In the ensuing years, I have endeavored, consciously and deliberately, to delve into my preconscious, to review again the events of my youth, and to record my reactions to these events and how they shaped my life. I realize whatever morals, character, and personality I possess as an adult were molded and influenced to a great degree by the aggregate of my reactions to the experiences and situations encountered during my childhood.

This work is an account of my life from birth in 1939, to 1957, at which time I left Oxford Orphanage at the age of seventeen. In the span of forty-odd supervening years, I have earned an undergraduate degree in Physics and Mathematics, and post-graduate doctorates in Optometry and Law. I have practiced Optometry and Law for thirty years, and along the way, my wife and I managed to raise four wonderful and talented children.

On a cold, rain-swept early morning in February 1947, at the quite innocent and equally guileless age of seven, I was taken from my home in Kinston, North Carolina to historic Oxford Orphanage by E. T. Regan, assistant superintendent of the orphanage, and Eunice Broadwell, the orphanage case worker, in a 1946 black Ford sedan.

As we drove slowly through the Main Gate, along the long, wide oak-lined Main Road to the gothic Victorian Main Building, then turned left for a short distance and swung right onto the semicircular driveway in front of the imposing Manderley known as Hicks Memorial Hospital, I sensed with great foreboding that I did not belong in this place, and consciously hoped that my stay indeed would be a brief one.

Exactly ten years later, on yet a similar cold, rain-swept early morning of February 15, 1957, I walked resolutely from the Main Building, back up the Main Road beneath sprawling oaks ten years taller, and through the Main Gate, pausing for one last reflective look at my life.

I quite distinctly recall thinking that, although my ten years at Oxford Orphanage had not been happy ones, certainly they had been memorable, and I vowed that some day I would record my ten-year odyssey, omitting nothing.

I invite you to come along with me as I chronicle this decade's worth of *Reflections in An Orphan's Eye*.

INTRODUCTION

Got a couple of hours to kill? Good. Then let me tell you about an interesting thing that happened to me on my way to growing up. Thought for awhile there I wouldn't get to do it. Grow up, that is. But here I am. I'm okay now. Honest. Or, at least I believe I'm okay. I'll let you decide, since you've been so kind as to stay with me awhile. Thanks. Company's good.

And don't get me wrong. I'm not bucking for sympathy or anything. Road kill doesn't need sympathy; it just wishes the horrible event never had occurred. That some big old eighteen wheeler, that in my youth we just called a transfer truck, had passed by two seconds earlier, or later, or had taken another route entirely.

And pardon me if I tend to wander too far afield, or ramble on for a moment or so. I always thought "shell shock" happened only to soldiers in wars. But that isn't entirely true. Sometimes it happens to small children.

> "It's strange that in great moments of crisis, the mind whips back to childhood."
>
> Phillip Ashley, in
> *My Cousin Rachel*

PROLOGUE

I sat quietly in the center of the padded back seat of the big black Ford sedan, my spindly white legs dangling over the edge, not touching the floorboard, fidgeting nervously with my second grade report card, occasionally glancing up while keeping my head down, focusing alternately between the two unsmiling foreigners seated in front of me, the driver, a sandy-haired, stern-faced man of about fifty, whose cold blue eyes seemed never to blink through white-gold rimless spectacles and who, since meeting him (not being formally introduced, mind you) a few minutes earlier I had sensed to be an adult-to-avoid-forever, and his pleasant-enough looking companion, a gray-streaked, dark-haired woman dressed in black, of about his same age, who was to speak very little during our four-hour journey.

Not yet having cause to be fearful for my safety (and my life), I figured that if these two (still unsmiling) grownups (which is what youngsters called adults back then) were mama's friends, they would shortly begin remarking about how tall I was or how much I had grown, which all grownups of that era were wont to do when in the presence of small children and searching for words to fill the conversation void, because in Kinston, North Carolina in 1947 what was there really in our innocent world to talk about anyway? Obviously, this was a very dull period in Southern American life.

At that moment, subconsciously I began to mix with my neophyte worldly (in)experience a generous dose of healthy skepticism born solely of the nagging apprehension and doubt as to the direction of my immediate future. Sitting alone on the back seat of the black Ford sedan,

I felt a sudden surge of depression. My daddy's car was just like this one, and my mind raced fleetingly to the laughter and carefree lives we children led before my daddy's death; of weekend trips in the family car to granddaddy's cabin in Swansboro; of rides through the countryside during the war, even though gasoline was rationed so severely. The awful incongruity of the symbolism I attached to a black Ford sedan would, by the end of that rainy, cold February day, be indelibly impressed into my memory forever. Even in later years, when I saw this car in picture shows or magazines, the contradictory meaning my experiences attached to the vehicle would rise up to haunt me yet again.

When I awoke on the cold and rainy morning of February 15, 1947, little did I know that within twenty-four hours my secure seven-year-old world would be shattered, replaced by one of doubt, fear and distrust. My sister Eoline had been gone for several months, but mama never had explained to me where my sister had been taken. My sister and I, despite her totally unfounded lack of appreciation of me during our pre-orphanage days, for which with passing time I have decided to forgive her, have been close. Years later, Eoline disclosed to me that she never was informed she was being taken to the orphanage. Often I have imagined how frightened my nine-year-old sister became when she discovered late on her day of departure from home that she would not be returning for a very long time.

On that fateful day, mama had accompanied Eoline on her trip to the orphanage with Miss Broadwell, the orphanage caseworker. Mama had bade a tearful goodbye to Eoline in Miss Broadwell's office in the Main Building, telling my sister she would see her, as Eoline remembered, "real soon," with more emphasis on the "real," that translates (at least to a frightened child) into a period of time totaling a few hours. It was, however, nine long months before my sister was to see our mother again.

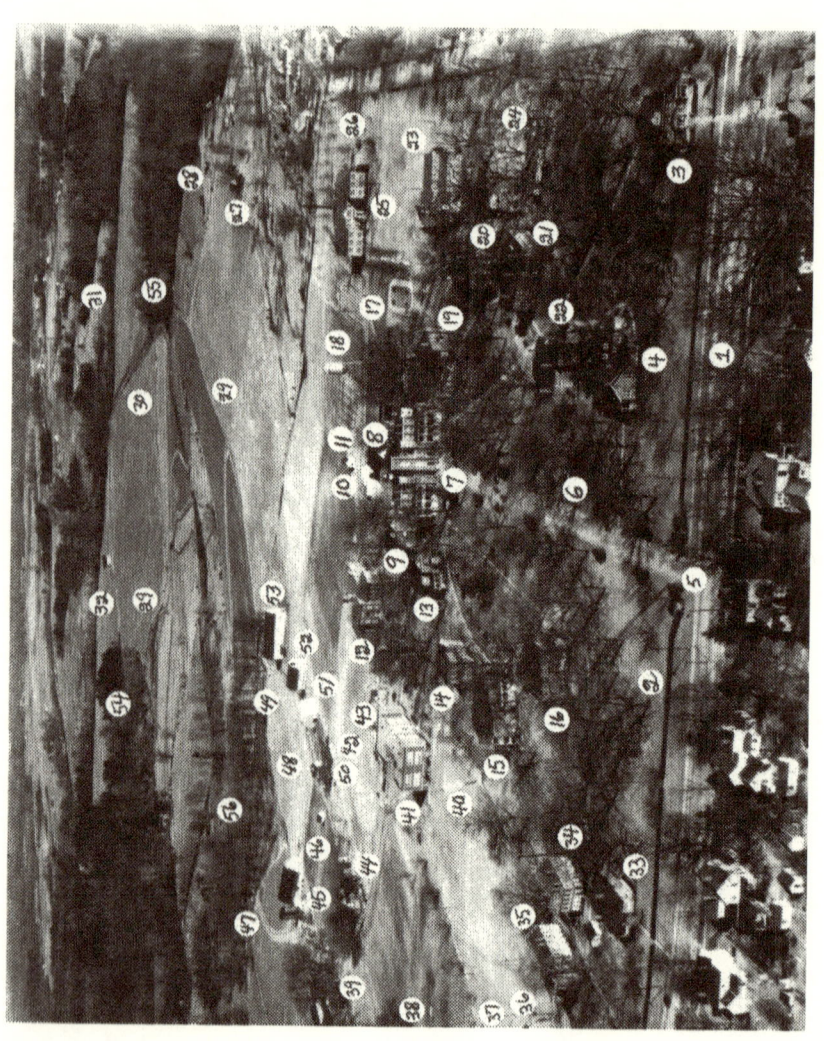

Oxford Orphanage 1951 Place Locator

1. College Street
2. Eyes-high Hedges
3. Superintendent Gray's residence
4. Annex (Royster Building)
5. Main Gate
6. Main Road
7. Main Building
8. Kitchen and Dining Rooms (Behind Main Building)
9. Business Office (with Mr. Gray's office inside)
10. Swimming Pool and Bath House
11. Musky dine (muscadine) patch
12. Hicks Memorial Hospital
13. 1-B
14. 2-B
15. 3-B
16. 4-B
17. Skating Rink
18. Water Tower
19. 1-G
20. 2-G
21. 3-G
22. 4-G
23. Baby Cottage (Dunn Building)
24. York Rite Chapel (Beginning of construction)
25. Industrial Building
26. Peach/Apple Orchard
27. Beef Cattle Barn and Pasture
28. Hog Pens and Sheds
29. Farm Road
30. Railroad Track
31. "Balloon" Patch
32. Farmer's Barn
33. E. T. Regan's House
34. Shoe Shop

35. Printing Shop
36. Electrical Shop
37. Football Field and Bleachers (Daniel Memorial Field)
38. Tom Adams' House
39. Snug House/Potato House/Outhouse
40. "Dabs" (Marbles) Battleground
41. John Nichols School
42. Baseball Field
43. Masters Cottage (under construction)
44. Walker Building
45. Dairy/Little Dairy/Silos
46. Strawberry Patch
47. Bull Pens and Barn
48. Valley of the Shadow of the Mummy
49. Calf Weaning Stalls (Home of the Mummy)
50. Tool Shed/Corn Crib
51. Mule Barn
52. Green Barn (Home of cats)
53. Long Barn
54. Thousand Dollar Spring (in woods)
55. Trash Dump
56. Main Cow Pasture

CHAPTER 1

Leaving Home

At around seven o'clock on that dreary February morning, a black Ford sedan parked on the street in front of our house, and I heard a sharp knock on the front door. Mama opened the door and welcomed inside a woman dressed in black, about fifty years old, and a slim, fiftyish bespectacled man dressed in a gray woolen suit. They were not smiling. Mama talked quietly with the couple for just a few minutes, then knelt and hugged me tightly. She looked into my eyes, told me she would see me "real soon," with emphasis on the "real," and I noticed her eyes were red as though she had been crying. Which she had been.

At that very moment this did not seem strange to me, because many nights following my daddy's death I could hear mama crying, and often she would remain in the front room, which we had always called simply the "store," long after she had bathed Pete and me and put us to bed for the night. I was aware that Eoline was no longer with us, and mama certainly kept my sister's whereabouts from me. Pete and I were the only children remaining at home after Eoline left in July 1946, and since then I had spent most of my free time helping entertain three-year-old Pete, while Mama minded the store.

I recall vividly my sense of apprehension in the presence of these two early morning visitors; they neither smiled nor spoke to me, and appeared eager to make their visit a brief one. The rain had begun falling harder, and with his umbrella held over me, the man quickly walked me to the black sedan, opened the rear door, and I climbed inside. Without a word, the man closed the door, then hurried back inside the house to collect the woman in black.

As the car pulled away from the curb in front of our house, mama stood on the front porch with Pete by her side, waving goodbye. She was not smiling. I rarely saw mama smile after that day.

I had as much indication of what lay ahead as would a small puppy, being placed (likewise) without comment (likewise) on the back seat of (likewise) a large black Ford sedan, not knowing why it had been placed in this big metal box, where it was being taken, how long would be the journey, and if and when it would be returned to the comfort and safety of its home.

Mama had awakened me earlier than usual on that cold, rainy morning of February 15, 1947, washed my face and helped me get dressed, and I sat quietly alone in my daddy's heavy wooden high-backed chair at the head of the large oilcloth-covered kitchen table while she fixed me scrambled eggs, grits and bacon that I ate with the large buttermilk biscuits mama still prepared from scratch every morning, a year and a week after my daddy had been taken from me. That chair, claimed quietly without interference or objection as my own for the past year, would remain mostly unoccupied for a very long time after that day.

I had started second grade at Lewis Elementary School the previous August, and each morning mama fixed me eggs and biscuits and bacon, and I sat quietly in my daddy's big wooden chair at the head of the table, watching mama feed baby Pete, and after breakfast I trudged off to school seven city blocks away, quite alone and just as lonely. There is a difference; I was both.

Each afternoon I returned via those same long seven city blocks to a home without laughter or joy, and late in the day I would walk alone the two blocks up East Bright Street to where, until earlier that year, I had met my daddy when he got out of the car at the corner of Queen and East Bright Street, expecting that any moment a car would stop, my daddy would get out, and my life would continue as it was supposed to.

My daddy's place was at the "head" of the large, rectangular wooden "supper" table that stood in the middle of the kitchen. Although the family ate all its meals at this table, we still referred to the table as the "supper" table, as is the custom in the South.

Often I sat at the opposite end of the supper table, and occasionally during mealtime my daddy would laugh and say, "Okay, Cottontop, just so you understand, *this* (and he would point his thumb at himself) is the *head* of the table." I would look embarrassed and mama and the other kids would laugh. The joke, of course, was that his was the important seat at the supper table, from which sprang undisputed control of the family, while, although seated at one "end" of the large table, my influence in family life bordered a spittoon's distance away from the insignificant.

You noticed, did you, that I spoke of my daddy. *My* daddy. A lifetime later, I still call him not just "daddy," but *my* daddy. Is there attached to this emphasis on the possessive, some sort of deep-seated Freudian significance, as though wanting to hold onto him? Or, if I referred to him as *my* daddy, would this somehow bring him back to me?

My daddy. My buddy. My protector. My best playmate. My cherished memory. Gone forever. Taken tragically and needlessly from me on a gray February 9, 1946, when at the young age of six, we shared an unspoken promise that he would protect me for as long as we lived, which was supposed to be forever. Mortality was not even a consideration in our relationship.

And here I was a year later, at age seven and, after breakfast, found myself sitting on mama's lap (not *my* mama, just mama) while she cried softly. Not saying a word-just sobbing quietly while holding me close to her. Had there occurred yet another tragedy in our now-abbreviated family? Mentally I took a head count, but fell far short of a full family.

Mama's emotions, and my quiet puzzlement-she had cried a lot during the past year-were interrupted shortly by the aforementioned not loud but businesslike knock on the front door. Sliding me gently off her lap, mama retrieved from her apron pocket a tear-stained, off-white rumpled handkerchief, dabbed her eyes, replaced the soiled cloth in her apron pocket, and opened the front door to reveal the two foreigners standing silently in our doorway.

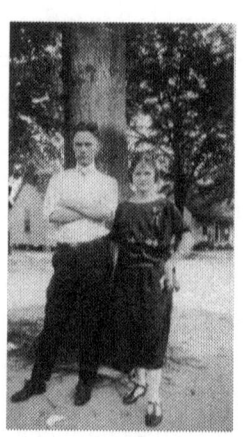 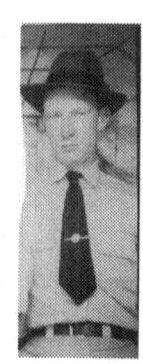 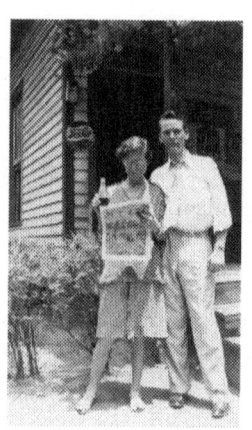

Left photo: 1926. Bennie and Pearl's wedding day.
Center photo: November 1945. My daddy, three months before
　　his death in February 1946.
Right photo: 1949. My brother Doc, with Mama at 208 East
　　Bright Street.

Introductions all around? Hardly. Their stay was quite brief; the Harsh Man said they had a long trip ahead and that they had better be off. The Subservient Woman in Black made no comment, as though she performed this routine daily. Mama knelt before me, still crying softly, suddenly unable to restrain her emotions. She hugged my slim shoulders tightly, and kissed my cheek, while I stood before her, unmoving, embarrassed by the two unfriendly (and to me quite unwelcome) strangers in our home so early in the morning, not having the slightest comprehension of the meaning of the unfolding play of which (I began to sense) I was the central and quite tragic character.

Mama held me once again firmly by my shoulders, looked into my totally unknowing eyes, and said very softly, "Now, you go with these people, Alton. I'll see you real soon." To a seven-year-old child who had never been separated from his mother for even one night of his life, "real soon" was a unit of time measuring, at its outer limit, two hours and fifteen minutes. I read mentally the opening of the front door by the Harsh Man as a silent cue, and stepped through the doorway of my home, leaving behind my first life forever.

Clutching tightly my second grade report card, I darted through the freezing February rain toward the large black Ford sedan, parked on the hatchet-chipped curb in front of 208 East Bright Street; the Harsh Man opened the back door and I scrambled onto the back seat.

Sitting pliantly alone in the back of the big black car, little did I realize that during the next six years I would suffer more than fifteen separate episodes of inhumane physical abuse at the hands of no less than seven uncaring, loathsome adults, that I would out of contempt and utter desperation strike back and threaten two of these seven, and that one of these two malicious bastards was as that time sitting at the wheel of the big black Ford.

Four of the fifteen physical assaults would be administered by hard slaps across my face, one by a tobacco stick across my back, one with a leather belt, and nine by wooden slats across my back, butt, and legs. The most severe and humiliating physical trauma would come at the hands of the driver of the big black car, who was to strike me a total of sixty-one times with a wooden slat while holding me down by means of a vise grip on my neck to prevent me from moving. The physical abuse would begin that same night, and my daddy would not be there to protect me.

We rode for several hours, never stopping, and neither Harsh nor Subservient ever spoke to me. The two grownups occasionally chatted quietly, mainly about the steady rain that fell the entire trip. I was in the second grade, and mama had handed me my report card just before I walked out our front door. So during the entire trip I sat in the middle of the back seat, remaining absolutely quiet, clutching my report card as a baby would its security blanket. Not having been informed otherwise, I assumed naturally that upon completion of this short trip, I would be returning later that day to the security of my home. Which made mama's crying even all the more puzzling.

Just as a room is always larger, a man always taller and a road always wider the first time we see them, the trip to I-didn't-know-where seemed an inordinately long journey. My four-hour travel from Kinston to Oxford at age seven was somewhat akin to Dickens' trip to Camden Town at age ten, ". . . solitude and dreariness, and it rained hard all the way, and I thought life sloppier than I had expected to find it."

Recalling the experiences of that day in the ensuing years, it was as though I were becoming the central character in a Shakespearean play, a dream if you will. Before the day was out, however, the "dream" would segue into a frightening, surreal nightmare.

How I Fell Into this Bucket of Grief

Allow me to pause for a moment somewhere along this postwar North Carolina two-lane macadam between Goldsboro and Raleigh, to explain just how I ended up in this big black car whose destination was to me a mystery.

Wasn't my fault. But I have decided not to fault anyone. I'll be brief, but it's an interesting view of life in an average wartime sleepy Southern town. We'll be back on the road again shortly.

The darkest days in Southern United States history occurred during The Reconstruction (1867-1877), that period following the Civil War that was rampant with political, social, and economic turmoil occasioned by the trauma of readmission to the Union of eleven Confederate states that had seceded at or before the Civil War. It was in the midst of this debasing humiliation and repression that the first children were admitted to the Oxford Orphan Asylum in 1873. I arrived seventy-four years later.

Newly created state governments, including that of North Carolina, were controlled during this period by a coalition of Negroes, carpetbaggers, and scalawags, and it was not until 1877 that the last federal troops were withdrawn from Southern soil. Into this interval of Northern corruption, vindictiveness, and economic domination were born four persons who were to play important roles in my life.

In 1873, the year the first children were admitted to the Oxford Orphan Asylum, William Henry Thomas was born in the small town of Sanford, located in Lee County, southwest of Raleigh. The following year, on August 1, 1874, Pete Daniel Provost was born in Onslow County, a coastal county located northeast of Wilmington. Two years later, on May 31, 1876, Agnes Kellum was born in Onslow County, and in 1879, Maud Britton was born in Sanford.

William Henry Thomas became a brickmason by trade. In 1899, "Will," as he was known to his friends, met Maud Britton at a church social in Sanford. A year later, Will, age 27, married the twenty-one-year-old Maud, and two years later, the couple moved to Kinston.

Pete Daniel Provost became a successful tobacco farmer and carpenter in northern Onslow County. At the age of twenty-four, Pete purchased two acres of land, and with the help of friends constructed a three-room cabin on the beach at Swansboro. Two years later, in 1900, Pete met Agnes Kellum, and in 1902, Pete and Agnes married and set up housekeeping in Maysville, retaining the cabin at Swansboro as a retreat.

The marriage of Pete and Agnes produced four children. My daddy, Benjamin Daniel, was born in Maysville, Onslow County on August 24, 1905. The name "Provost" is generally pronounced with the "t" silent, rendering the phonetic "Provo" or, as was the case then (and still is) more common in coastal North Carolina, "Provow." In point of fact, even as the twenty-first century began, occasionally a "Provost" in that area will change his name to "Provow." Strange people, those Provosts. Or Provows.

Today, the six persons most central to my life lie at a much-deserved rest in Maplewood Cemetery, on the corner of Shine Street and Davis Street, only a block from where I was born; Pete and Agnes Provost, Will and Maud Thomas, Bennie and Pearl Provow. Carved into my granddaddy's headstone is the name "Pete Provost," into my grandmama's, "Agnes Kellum Provost." These carvings were ordered as such by my daddy. However, carved into my daddy's headstone is "Bennie D. Provow," and into my mama's, "Nina Pearl Provow."

"Bennie," as all his friends knew my daddy, was the oldest of four children born to Agnes and Pete; Gilbert, Lilly, and Georgia came soon thereafter. When Bennie was nine years old, the family moved to Kinston, at the edge of a region geologists call the "coastal plain," but which is referred to by the locals as "tobacco," or "scrub pine" country.

"Scrub pine" is a scraggly pine tree with prickly cones and drooping or spreading branches, in contrast to the glorious longleaf pine of western North Carolina, a quite statuesque tree with long needles in bundles of three and long cones.

For decades, large billboards along the highway leading into town championed Kinston as "The World's Foremost Tobacco Center." Seeing these larger-than-life-and-then-some signs as a child, I assumed quite naturally that "foremost" must mean the best, and I was really proud that I lived in such an important town that was recognized throughout the world as a famous tobacco center. As a child, my infallible logic reasoned that if a message was displayed on as large a sign as a billboard, it had to be true. And some beliefs die hard.

In 1914, Pete and Agnes moved their growing family to Kinston, purchasing a small wood frame house. The backyard contained a large orchard. The family retained its cabin on the coast at Swansboro.

The 1899 marriage of Will Thomas and Maud Britton produced seven children. Nina Pearl, my mama, was born in Sanford, North Carolina on March 6, 1907. In addition to "Pearl," as everyone knew mama, Will and Maud had two sons, Sam and Perry, and four more girls, Nan, Clyde, Kate, and Ruth. In 1917, when Pearl was ten years old, Will moved his large family to Kinston, where he continued his trade as a brickmason.

My uncle Gilbert and aunt Lilly told me that as a young boy growing up in Maysville, their brother Bennie, a quite handsome, quite serious, and quite determined fellow, was always tinkering with anything mechanical, be it a car or radio or farm implement, until he could take it apart and put it back together, and that he was very proud of his abilities.

Following graduation from high school in 1922, Bennie Provow attended a trade school in Raleigh to study what was at that time called the "cooling" trade, the rudiments of what we now call refrigeration systems. Upon earning his diploma and the impressive title of "refrigeration engineer," Bennie became first a worker and soon thereafter the manager of the only "ice plant" in Kinston. Today, I still possess my daddy's personal, well-worn ice pick that for years rested atop the icebox in our kitchen. A few years later, Bennie hired his younger brother Gilbert as his assistant manager.

In 1925, Bennie Provow met Pearl Thomas at a social in Kinston, and according to my uncle Sam Thomas, Pearl fell in love with the tall, good-looking "iceman." Daddy always referred to mama as his "beautiful Pearl." Following their wedding in 1926, Bennie and Pearl moved into a four-room, square-shaped wood frame house in Kinston. John Benjamin ("J.B."), the first of six sons, was born on March 9, 1927. In 1931 came Norwood, whom I never knew by any other name except "Doc," then Bill (1932), and Kenneth ("Kenny"-1933). The couple's only daughter, Eoline, was born in 1937.

The year following the birth of Eoline, the growing family moved to a larger wood frame house at 208 East Bright Street, just a block and a half from Queen Street, Kinston's main street. The house proper consisted of three large rooms. The first room, the living room, extended the width of the house, and was about fifteen feet deep. In the center of this room stood a large, pot-bellied stove, seated in a deep, square-shaped metal pan, that was used to prevent hot coals or burning wood chips from spilling out onto the wooden floor.

From the living room, a door opened into the front bedroom, and behind this room was what we called the back bedroom, extending the width of the house. If one walked out the rear door of the back bedroom, he was then standing on what was called the "dog trot," an open-air walkway about fifteen feet long, that connected the back bedroom with the separate part of the house that included the kitchen, bathroom, and later J.B. and Doc's bedroom.

At the immediate far end of the dog trot, a door opened to the right into the kitchen. Actually, there were two doors, an outer screen door, and an inner wooden door. During the warmer months, the wooden inner door was opened all the way to the wall, and only the screen door was used.

Dog trots connecting the house proper to a detached kitchen were quite common in the South throughout the first half of the twentieth century. This design was not based on considerations of aesthetics; rather, the configuration served two quite practical purposes. Since "air conditioning" had not been invented, the detached kitchen kept the heat out of the house proper during the hot Summer months. Secondly, the average house was constructed of highly-combustible wood. With a detached kitchen, there was of course less chance of the main house burning to the ground should a fire start in the wood- or coal-burning kitchen stove.

To the right along the kitchen wall stood a large sink, above which was a window that faced onto the front of the house. On either side of the kitchen sink were counters with cabinets above, attached to the wall. Along the wall facing the kitchen door stood a large oven supported by four curved iron legs, on top of which sat a four-burner stove. The "icebox" stood along the left wall upon entering the kitchen, and in the middle of the room was a rectangular solid oak table, large enough to seat comfortably six persons. There were six sturdy oak chairs around the "supper" table; only one chair, larger than the others, had armrests. This chair, of course, was my daddy's chair, and nobody else sat in the chair, even when my daddy was not at home.

The dining room table, that we and everybody in the South called the "supper" table, regardless of what meal was being served, was covered with a tablecloth, made of "oilcloth," a fabric treated with clay, linseed oil and pigments to make it waterproof, and which was the standard material of which tablecloths were made at the time. The Wonderful Age of Plastics had not yet arrived.

Our meals were called breakfast, dinner (the noon meal), and supper, the evening meal. Twice each day, even on the weekends, mama made biscuits from scratch, using buttermilk. Leftovers from the meal were placed in bowls in the center of the supper table, and covered with a smaller oilcloth.

Buttermilk is strong-tasting and just as strong-smelling stuff, but my daddy drank nothing else with his meals, breakfast, dinner, or supper. Sour whole milk yields a distasteful-looking gunk called "clabber." When this clabber is churned, it yields both sweet butter and a lumping residue called "buttermilk." Left alone and allowed to warm, this milk soon turns sour and curdles. This awful (to me) tasting, awful smelling stuff is what we just called "clabber." We kids would clutch our throats and feign gagging when daddy tried to get us to taste the sour liquid.

A washboard, with a corrugated metal surface, hung on the far wall of the kitchen near the stove and oven. When the weather was warm, mama washed our clothes in a large sink located on the dog trot just outside the kitchen door, and hung the clothes to dry on clotheslines stretched along the full length of the dog trot. During cold weather, mama washed the clothes in the large kitchen sink. Mama spent most of her waking hours in the kitchen.

During the early 1940's, we did not enjoy the comforts of air conditioning in our home. But neither did anyone else. The term "air conditioning" was not coined until 1906, and it was not until the mid-1930's that air conditioned picture shows became a reality in the United States. Even then, air conditioning remained for the most part a luxurious oddity until after World War II. And the relatively inexpensive, though questionably efficient window air conditioning unit did not appear until 1951, when I was twelve years old.

Two other luxuries did not appear until 1939, the year I was born; the automatic dishwasher, that remained out of reach of the average homeowner for another twenty years, and the first automobile air conditioner, introduced by Packard. Again, twenty years later, this was still an add-on luxury.

Transoms were quite common features in office buildings, hotels, and schools during the nineteenth and first half of the twentieth centuries in the United States. These small, hinged windows above doors allowed for cross ventilation when doors were closed for privacy or to control noise levels. During Winter months, the transom could be closed to retain heat in a room. Even after the first window air conditioners became available in 1951, transoms remained in common use for many years, until the advent of central air conditioning in the early sixties.

Our house faced west, fronting onto East Bright Street. On the north side of the house a dirt driveway led from the sidewalk alongside the house to a large one-car garage, enclosed, and roofed in corrugated metal. Because both my daddy and his father were mechanically-minded, they enclosed the open doorway and converted the garage into a carpentry workshop.

The property had a large backyard that bordered the Episcopal Church property; the two properties being separated by a wire fence supported by pine log fence posts. Large yellow roses grew all along the fence separating the properties.

The Great Depression did not spare Kinston, North Carolina. The young couple's second son, "Doc," was born in 1931, and two years later, in an effort to provide his growing family with inexpensive food, my daddy transplanted fruit trees from my granddaddy's large orchard, and these trees soon yielded apples, peaches, pears, and muscadines, that I called "Musky Dines," distinctly a two-word fruit in my fledgling mind.

By 1937 the family was supplementing my daddy's income from his job as manager of Kinston's still sole "ice plant" as they were called at the time, by selling fruit produced in the family orchard. In 1939, the year I was born, my daddy converted the fifteen-foot deep by twenty-foot wide family room into a small neighborhood store, selling cigarettes, candy, soft drinks, some canned goods and cereals, and fruit grown in our small but productive orchard.

The income from the store and my daddy's salary from the ice plant enabled the family to purchase a new black Ford sedan. By the time Bennie and Pearl's fifth child and only daughter, Eoline, was born in 1937, the family was running out of space. Daddy built another room onto the kitchen and bathroom at the rear of the dog trot, making a bedroom for twelve-year-old J.B. and eight-year-old Doc. The baby

Eoline slept in the front bedroom with mama and daddy, and the younger boys, Bill and Kenny, occupied the back bedroom.

Given that the nation was in the midst of a depression, the growing family fared quite well. My daddy's foresight in planting the orchard and transforming the front room of the house into what today we would call a "convenience" store, enabled the family to afford its new automobile.

Because Bennie's brother Gilbert was daddy's assistant manager at the ice plant, Bennie was able to spend more time with his growing family, and by the time I was born on April 30, 1939, the Provost family, when measured by the economic yardstick of the times, was certainly prospering. Bennie and Pearl were Episcopalians; the family attended church regularly, and each child maintained what we referred to as a "miter box." A "mite" is a very small contribution or amount of money. The children deposited coins earned for work around the house and in the orchard, into these small pasteboard miter boxes. Every year on Easter Sunday, the kids turned in the miter boxes as an offering at church.

As a small child, I had difficulty grasping the logic involved in saving money, presumably for myself, because mama told me it was "my" miter box, only to give away to somebody else what for an entire year I had saved for myself. However, I followed the lead of other family members and did what my daddy told me to do. Made living in the Provost household a whole lot easier.

The Year 1939

The year of my birth was one of the most memorable of the twentieth century in the United States. That year Ted Williams, my childhood hero, played his first game with the Boston Red Sox, Joe DiMaggio won the American League batting title with a .381 average, and that awesome steamroller known as the New York Yankees swept the Cincinnati Reds 4-0 in the World Series.

In that same year, the infant called "television," formally introduced at the 1939 World's Fair, broadcast the first baseball game ever, between the Brooklyn Dodgers and the Cincinnati Reds, and Igor Sikorsky, a fifty-year-old Russian-born American, designed, constructed, and flew successfully the first American "helicopter."

In 1939 Florey and Chain concentrated "penicillin" and tested it with success, and Paul Miller developed that toxic contact insecticide known as "DDT." Also that year, *Gone With the Wind* opened to rave reviews in Atlanta, John Steinbeck won the Pulitzer Prize for his heart-wrenching tale of the Great Depression, *The Grapes of Wrath*, and the most feared gangster in American history, Al Capone, was released from federal prison, his body racked with third-stage syphilis.

In mid-March 1939 Hitler's armies overran Czechoslovakia; on September 1, 1939 the Nazis struck Poland, and World War II officially got under way two days later when Great Britain and France declared war on Germany. Back in the United States, President Roosevelt declared to a nation at peace, in a "fireside chat," that "This nation will remain a neutral nation . . ."

However, when on October 11, 1939 world-renowned physicist Albert Einstein, a Jewish refugee from the Nazis, warned President Roosevelt that the Germans were working on the problem of harnessing atomic energy into a bomb, FDR conferred privately with key congressional leaders, and together they started the "Manhattan Project," the best-kept secret of World War II, whose sole purpose was the development of an "atomic bomb."

Of greater concern to the average American in 1939 was the fact that the nation was still in the grips of The Great Depression; eight million Americans were unemployed, and the average worker earned sixty-two cents per hour, or about twenty-three dollars per week.

As of the date of my birth, the only hand-held writing instruments in common usage were the rudimentary mechanical lead pencil, the wooden "lead" pencil and the fountain pen. The "ballpoint" pen was not invented (by Hungarian brothers Ladislao and Georg Biro) until 1938. Likewise, the only commonplace general usage copier for schools and businesses was the wet-copier mimeograph machine. The patent for the first "dry" copier, called the "xerograph" (Latin for "dry writing") was filed by American Chester Carlson on April 4, 1939, twenty-six days before my birth. Through high school, I never used a "ballpoint" pen, nor did I ever read material copied on a xerograph.

The properties of Teflon, a substance unaffected by acids or solvents, and corrosive-proof, used today in many household kitchens, was not discovered until 1938, and was not available commercially until 1948, when I was nine years old. The first synthetic fiber in widespread use, the superpolymer called "nylon," was made from coal, air, and water. Its initial commercial use was in the making of ladies' sheer nylon hosiery that went on sale in Wilmington, Delaware in 1939.

The first "funny" book, aptly titled "Famous Funnies," debuted in 1934, and in June 1938 Action Comics introduced the character "Superman" to America's youth. The following year, 1939, the year of my birth, Detective Comics unveiled "the Bat-Man," who over the years was surpassed in funny book popularity only by Superman.

The automatic dishwasher finally became a reality in 1939, and the first automobile company (Packard) began installing air conditioners in its cars as an added luxury.

Such was the world into which I was born, at home, at 4:20 a.m. on April 30, 1939, as Bennie and Pearl's sixth child. In addition to me, the children at that time included J.B., age 13, Doc, age 9, Bill, age 7, Kenny, age 6, and two-year-old Eoline. My parents named me Alton Lee, and called me Alton until I was two years old, after which my daddy dubbed me "Cottontop" because my hair was so blond it was nearly white. This is the name I answered to for the ensuing five years. However, my older brothers claimed that daddy also referred to me as "that white-headed little pissant."

There was little dispute among my older siblings that I quickly became my daddy's favorite. We received our sense of humor from our father. Early on, he taught us to laugh at ourselves, and more often than not, daddy was the "butt-end" of his own jokes. We children referred to our father as "daddy," and to our mother as "mama."

The earliest recollection I have of my daddy was of me sitting on his knee, and him pushing his balled-up fist under the crotch of my pants. He then quickly pulled out his fist and, with his thumb pushed between his index and middle fingers, wiggled his thumb and asked me, "Look, Cotton, what have I got here?" His satisfaction was in seeing the embarrassed look on my face, especially if other persons were present.

Daddy was proud of his family. The earliest photographs I have of me involved his work. The first photo, taken when I was about eighteen months old, shows my sister Eoline, my brother Bill and me sitting in the sun at the edge of the Kinston ice plant's large "cooling pond." The second photo, taken when I was about two years old, shows all of us kids sitting in the seat and footwell of a large white ice wagon, used by the ice house route men to deliver ice to the customers in town.

My earliest recollection of mama was of her bathing me while I stood naked in the shallow pan before the radiating heat of the large pot-bellied stove on a Winter night. She would heat a large pitcher of water, then pour it into the pan. When it was the proper temperature, she would pick me up and stand me in the pan of water. Then she soaped the "washrag" and washed my face, ears, and hair. Then I instinctively held out first one arm and then the other. After washing my hands and arms, she washed my body. Next, I held onto mama's shoulders and extended one foot and then the other, for her to wash.

After bathing me, mama poured several small pans of warm water on my head, each successive pan of water rinsing off a lower part of my body. Then she wrapped a towel around me, lifted me out of the pan of dirty water, and dried me off. Daddy referred to these rituals as "little whores' baths;" whatever that meant at the time whizzed right past me.

During the Summer months, I became so dirty playing in the yard and orchard that this bathing routine was performed at the large open-air sink located on the dog trot just outside the kitchen.

Mama was a petite woman of five "foot" six to Southerners, five "feet" six to everyone outside the South, with thin auburn hair and an easy walk. She was quite pretty, soft-spoken and was blessed with a constant twinkle in her eye and a ready smile. Mama's greatest loves were, in order, her family, her piano, and her poetry. By the time I turned three, she was reading me stories of Br'er Rabbit and Uncle Remus at bedtime, and she and I enjoyed the funnies in the Kinston *Daily Free Press* from before the time I could read. She and I would sit together at the supper table, and she would spread out the funnies section of the paper. She would read the "balloons" to me, and when she laughed, I would laugh along with her. If mama thought it was funny, it must have been funny.

For a period of four years, until my brother Benjie Pete was born on April 25, 1943, I was the baby of the family. After Pete was born, I became known as the "knee baby," an apparent neologism meaning the next to the last child born. You'll not find this expression in any dictionary.

We referred to the cabin on the coast at Swansboro as "granddaddy's cabin." During the Summer months, the family would pile into daddy's big black four-door Ford sedan and head off for a weekend at the beach. As soon as we arrived, the other kids would put on their "swim trunks" and race across the stretch of beach between the cabin and the water.

The older children knew that I would not follow them to the beach because I was petrified at the sight of the dozens of fiddler crabs, that were called "sand fiddlers," that made their homes by burrowing into the sand near the water. The horrible little creatures seemed literally to spring from their holes in the sand. I quickly panicked at the sight of what my brothers called the "daddy" fiddler because the male sand fiddler had one greatly enlarged claw and another smaller claw, the disparity in the size of the claws causing the ugly things to appear even more menacing, and the moveable eyestalks protruding from atop the crab and twitching from side to side only added to my apprehension of venturing alone onto the beach.

My fear of the horrible little devils was only intensified by the dire warnings of my older brothers during the family outings to Swansboro. Bill and Kenny would amuse themselves on the two-hour car trip by describing to me in gruesome detail how giant sand fiddlers as big as my daddy devoured little three-year-old boys. By the time we arrived at granddaddy's cabin, daddy or mama had to carry me across the sand and deposit me at water's edge. Seemed like everybody picked on me.

Coastal Onslow County has always been known for its delicious and plentiful supply of oysters. On Sunday afternoon, as we packed for the return trip to Kinston, daddy always purchased several "tow" sacks (as we called burlap bags) full of oysters. Daddy had constructed a brick cooking pit with a metal grate over it, in our side yard at home. He would start a fire in the pit, then dump out the oysters and spread them over the grating. Next daddy would soak the now-empty tow sacks in water and spread them over the heap of oysters, wetting the tow sacks occasionally, thereby steaming the oysters until the shells popped open.

In the '30's and '40's oysters were plentiful and cheap along the coast of North Carolina, and my parents invited the neighbors to these Sunday night "spreads" of steamed oysters and Schlitz beer. Years later, when Doc and I reminisced about our childhood, he told me our father should have been a psychologist because he seemed to understand human nature so well, and was a master at the art of persuasion. The Sunday night oyster feasts usually drew upwards to thirty of the neighbors, and Kinston cops were always welcome. At some point during the festivities, daddy would ask for quiet, at which time he would thank all those present for their friendship and goodwill. As Doc explained it, the money daddy spent on oysters and beer for the neighbors each week was a small price to pay for the continued patronage of the family store that, as the United States entered World War II, was to become an important means of support for our large family.

Granddaddy Pete had purchased some land outside Kinston, on which grew mainly yellow pine trees. Ever the entrepreneur, daddy periodically felled a few of these yellow pines, then cut the felled trees into sections approximately twelve to eighteen inches in length. Daddy had fashioned two chopping blocks from a hardwood tree, each about three feet high. Using one of the ice plant's trucks, daddy transported the pine tree sections to our backyard, where after school Doc and J.B., using hatchets, chopped away at the outer parts of the sections, that left remaining what daddy called the "heart" of the pine. The boys then cut these center parts of the tree sections into small strips, gathered about two dozen of these richly resinous, highly-combustible strips, bunched them together, and tied the bundles with string.

These bundles of pine strips, or "kindling," were taken to the family store, stacked in the corner, and sold as "lighterd" (as kindling was referred to in that area) that was used as a "lighter," or fire starter, for coal stoves, for five cents a bundle.

Like most Southern women during the thirties and forties, mama cooked with lard, that is the end product of melting the fatty tissue of hogs. Lard is an excellent cooking and baking fat, and also acts as a quick soothing salve for burns occasionally suffered while cooking. Because more hogs are raised and more pork consumed in the South than in any other region of the country, lard was cheap and readily available.

Daddy enjoyed "souse" along with his buttermilk. Souse, better known to some as pickled pigs' feet, is pickled in a solution of brine or vinegar, and daddy kept a small jar of this Southern delicacy on a sideboard in the kitchen. We kids viewed souse with the same cautious sideways glances as we did buttermilk, and like the sour-tasting milk, quickly declined daddy's offer for us to taste the small animal's feet.

In addition to fresh-baked, mouth-watering biscuits, mama prepared what we called "cornpone," or cornbread, by mixing a batter of cornmeal, water and lard, pressing the mixture into small patties and setting them to bake. They were tasty and filling, hot or cold.

Mama also prepared my favorite, delicious cracklin cornbread. When hog fat is cooked to produce lard, the by-product yields "cracklings" ("cracklins" to us Southerners), small bits of chewy, crispy rendered hog fat and skin. Mama would sprinkle a few handfuls of cracklins into the cornpone, mix and bake the patties to produce an appetizing food, complete with mama's patented finger indentations, and bake them in the large square oven.

Neither of my parents smoked cigarettes. Instead, like thousands of Southerners of their generation, they "dipped" snuff. When harvested, green tobacco leaves are hung in barns in bundles straddling long tobacco sticks. The green tobacco is "dried," or "cured" using heat from furnaces with metal flues. Thus the term "flue-cured" tobacco. This flue-cured "bright leaf" tobacco harvested in that region was crushed and ground into a fine powder called "dry snuff." Using a small curved piece of paper that remained in the snuff can, mama and daddy would scoop out a "pinch" of snuff, pour it in the side of their mouth between the gums and wall of the jaw. The nicotine is released through the gums. A tin can served as a spittoon. Mama's favorite brand of snuff was "Tube Rose," daddy preferred "Society."

The family used Vick's Inhaler for stopped-up noses, Luden's Cough Drops for coughs and sore throats, and Ex-Lax for constipation, all of which mama sold in the family store. She sold a lot of Beech Nut

Chewing Gum, and we kids chewed gum until our jaws ached. I grew up believing that Southerners' all-time favorite sport was not baseball, but chewing gum.

Mama sold two kinds of teeth-cleaning products. The original Colgate Tooth Powder came in a plain white tin oval container, and the red printing simply read "Colgate Tooth Powder." To use it, you simply dumped a small mound of white powder into the cupped palm of one hand, wet the toothbrush and dipped it into the mound, then brushed your teeth. Mama also sold Colgate Dental Cream, "cream" being what we today call tooth "paste."

Lined up neatly on a shelf in the store were boxes of toothpicks. A dining table was improperly set if it lacked a box of toothpicks alongside the salt and pepper shakers. Toothpicks had two uses. Parents used them to "pick" lodged food from between their teeth after meals. Kids used them to "pick" the meat from inside crushed black walnuts. We never heard the term "dental floss."

According to mama's later account of events, in late 1939 or early 1940 a rift developed in the close relationship between daddy and his younger brother Gilbert, the cause of which mama never revealed. The upshot of the brothers' disagreement, however, was that daddy resigned his management position at Kinston's ice plant, and two days later accepted a job as an assistant engineer for the railway.

The railway station in Kinston was not far from our home, and because the ice plant also served the rudimentary "refrigeration" needs of the railway passenger cars, daddy had many friends who worked for the railway.

The railroad tracks were only a "stone's throw" from our house. The reason I know this to be a fact is because my older brothers, in the idleness of youth, used to throw stones at the passing trains. Our parents frowned on such sport, however, and this activity ceased immediately upon the beginning of my daddy's employment with the railway. Eoline and my older brothers knew the train schedules well, and during the Summer months the kids would run down to the tracks and wave to daddy as he passed by on the train. Daddy's fellow railway workers-daddy certainly would not have enlightened them-probably never figured out why these little snot-faced kids who for months had pelted them with rocks, were now smiling and waving and calling them "daddy."

On December 7, 1941, the Japanese launched their surprise attack, hitting Pearl Harbor, the Philippines, Malaya, and Thailand. The following day the Anglo-Americans declared war on Japan. In early 1942, the U.S. government greatly expanded its food and materiel storage facility at what is today the Cherry Point Marine Air Station. In May 1942, daddy quit his job as assistant engineer for the railway, and began working as a civil service employee at Cherry Point, with the job description of "refrigeration engineer."

I turned eighteen on April 30, 1957, and on that day mama informed me that I was to go to the First National Bank in Kinston the following day. Upon my arrival at the bank, the bank manager informed me that in July 1942, when I was three years old, my daddy had opened a savings account for each of his six children, and had instructed the bank to inform each child of the existence of the account only after the child's eighteenth birthday. I used this money to pay my first two years' college tuition, just as I knew my daddy must have intended. I loved my daddy very much. Still do.

Each civilian employee at Cherry Point was issued an identification badge on which was pasted the employee's photograph. Due to the wartime threat of sabotage along the eastern coast of the United States, base employees were required to wear their identification badges at all times, and the Military Police checked the photographs against the employees' faces upon both entering and departing the government facility.

U.S. government employees at Cherry Point wore tan uniforms, with a dark tie. As was the style during the thirties and forties, my daddy wore a fedora. These soft felt hats were creased lengthwise, and the brim could be turned up for regular wear, and down when it was raining. Daddy always left for work in the morning with his fedora and necktie in place. And he always returned from work late in the day from the two-hour ride from Cherry Point, with his tie untied and his fedora cocked back on his head, looking tired but always in a good mood.

Four or five other Kinston residents worked at Cherry Point, and the men started their own car pool. The meeting place was the

intersection of Bright Street and Queen Street, which is Kinston's main
street, and was about two blocks from our home. The car transporting
the men usually arrived at the drop-off point at around 6:30 p.m. each
day, and because our home was closest to the meeting point, on the
days daddy did not drive, he just walked the two blocks home. I used to
run to the meeting point and wait for daddy to arrive. He would scoop
me up into his arms, give me a big hug, and holding his metal lunch
box in one hand, he would make a fist with his other hand and bend his
forearm until it was parallel to the ground. Then, interlocking the fingers
of both my hands over his forearm, daddy would carry me swinging the
two blocks home, raising and lowering his forearm in an attempt to
make me lose my grip, both of us laughing all the way home. My daddy's
return home to me was always the highlight of my day.

Daddy's one steadfast rule at home was that, regardless of what
his children were doing at the time, we all had to be home ready for
supper when he arrived from work. Period. My sister Eoline recalls
that she knew she was late for supper when she saw daddy coming
down the sidewalk waving three or four birch switches in his hand. He
never called us to supper-it was our responsibility to be waiting at
home when he arrived.

Several months after beginning work at Cherry Point, daddy and
the employees began to notice that the military guards at the entrance
checkpoint were looking at the employees' faces and just waving them
through. Ever the practical joker, daddy decided to test the base's security.
He cut out a picture of a chimpanzee from a magazine, and pasted it
over his identification photograph. After entering the facility the next
day unchecked and wearing the picture of the chimp unchallenged all
day, daddy and the other men decided to expand the test of security.

Daddy convinced the other members of his car pool to paste pictures
of chimps over their identification photos, and for several days, the men
passed through the checkpoint and worked on the base unnoticed. Finally,
an officer noticed one of the chimp badges, and all five or six of the
"chimp" employees were ordered to report to the base commander. Much
to the men's surprise-they thought they would be fired-the base
commander, after learning that the men had carried on their pretense

for several days before being discovered, applauded them for uncovering the base's lax security. That same day, the military guards were changed at the checkpoints and security was heightened at the base.

As in many large families, the youngest child must make himself heard or is more often than not ignored by busy parents. I can recall at ages three and four sitting at the kitchen table while mama was cooking supper, yelling at her "Answer me! Answer me!" when she failed to respond to my neverending questions and demands for all her attention.

At that young age my sister did not want me following her and her six-year-old girlfriends all over the neighborhood, and she would turn and kick me in the shins in an attempt to dissuade me from joining her group. More often than not it worked.

My parents brooked no profanity from us kids, and an inadvertent "hell" or "damn" would have as its certain consequence a belting or switching, depending on the gender of the transgressor.

In the Summer of 1942, just after my third birthday, the U.S. government instituted rationing and price controls throughout the nation. These measures were considered equitable because they prevented those with the financial means to do so, from scooping up those goods and materials for which the war effort created shortages. Since the Army required sufficient amounts of cotton and wool to clothe its soldiers (including 64 million flannel shirts, 165 million coats, and 229 million pairs of trousers), the shortage of cloth available to civilians led to shorter skirts, rising several inches above the knees, and to the creation of a new two-piece bathing suit.

Each man, woman, and child in the United States was issued a book of ration stamps monthly, and each essential item in short supply was assigned a price in "points." The stamps in the ration book, which was worth forty-eight points each month, could be spent on any combination of goods, including meat, butter, canned vegetables, sugar, and shoes.

At the end of December 1941, the federal government issued an order forbidding the sale of new tires anywhere in the country. And on May 15, 1942, gasoline rationing began, not so much because gasoline was in short supply, but gas rationing would save rubber used in the manufacture of tires. And in 1942, the War Production Board (WPB) prohibited the further manufacture of automobiles for private use, and the same year drastically restricted the construction of new private homes. Such was the state of the nation during my early years.

Daddy not only earned a good wage as a federal government employee, overtime was readily available. To support his large family (the seventh child, Pete, was born on April 25, 1943) daddy worked often on weekends. In order to counter the institution of food rationing in 1942, Americans planted Victory Gardens in their backyards. Our large backyard orchard produced peaches, apples, corn, muscadines, peanuts, and artichokes.

Throughout the war, our family enjoyed these fruits and vegetables, and mama sold the produce in our family store. I can still recall vividly my utter amazement the first time Doc told me to "pull on that vine" laying on top of the ground, and when I did so, peanuts began popping out of the ground. We put the pulled vines on the ground in the sun, and about a week later, after the peanuts had dried, we pulled the peanuts off the vines, bagged them and set the bags of peanuts on a shelf in mama's store, ready for sale.

Artichokes were popular vegetables at the time and did not stay long on the store shelves. Same for peaches, apples, and corn. When these fresh foods were in season, the family derived more income from the family store than from daddy's job as a refrigeration engineer working for the U.S. Government.

One morning I was attempting to join Eoline and her friends, and as usual not wanting the "pest" around, she made the really BIG mistake of yelling at me, "Damn you, go away!"

"If you don't let me go with you, I'm gonna tell mama you said a cuss word."

Gotcha! It worked like a charm. She let me follow after them, for awhile anyway. After the blackmail incident, I would follow Eoline and her friends around, listening intently for an errant "hell" or "damn." Sometimes I got lucky.

Because I was the baby of the family for four years, I became mama's shadow. To keep me in the kitchen with her while she was cooking or washing clothes, mama often mixed flour with water to make a pasty glue, and gave me a pair of scissors and an old Collier's magazine. I could occupy hours of my time by cutting pictures from the magazine and pasting them along the kitchen walls.

In their superbly insightful book, *Generations*, authors William Strauss and Neil Howe discuss the "Silent Generation," which includes that generation of Americans born between 1925 and 1942. As a product of that generation, I remember well the Second World War from my childhood. My generation boasts "the twentieth century's lowest rate of crime, suicide, illegitimate births and teen unemployment." In addition, "the Silents have produced nearly every major figure in the modern civil rights movement."

Stuck between the G.I. Generation and the self-absorbed Baby Boomers, I have always associated myself with the former, while being somewhat disdainful of the excesses of the latter. Another writer has dubbed my generation the "In-Betweeners," for somewhat the same reasons as Strauss and Howe placed us in our historical niche.

In 1944 at the age of five, I was well aware there was a war going on. Each day mama and I would read the funnies in the Kinston *Daily Free Press*, and I could see the headlines and the battle maps of the European and Pacific theaters of war. Mama explained to me what was going on, and assured me our family would always be safe, that the war was far away.

At night, the stillness was sometimes pierced suddenly by the strident wailing of a siren, and daddy would quickly pull down the blackout shades and turn out all the lights. When this occurred we knew a blackout drill had begun in Kinston. These exercises were ordered periodically by Civil Defense officials, simulating conditions required in the event of attack by the German Luftwaffe.

Peering around the blackout shade, I could hear the sound of the civil defense inspection car as it moved slowly down the street, two pale yellow horizontal slits of light where the headlights should be, straining in vain to illuminate the way, the officials stopping periodically to issue warnings to violators of the blackout.

Civil defense air raid warnings were serious business during the war. The threat of saboteurs arriving by rubber raft from Nazi submarines off the coast of North Carolina was very real, and security was a primary concern along the state's coastal plain.

At night we would gather around our parents' dresser in the front bedroom and listen to the old Philco Baby Grand table model radio, warmed by the heat from the glass vacuum tubes, the squawk, crackle and static from weak airwave signals carrying throughout the wood frame house. Just as today people watch television, back then we "watched" the radio because this is from where the sound emanated. Except that the radio allowed us kids to use our imaginations. Aside from The Fat Man, who was described as such by the narrator, we mentally assigned our own childish, imagined descriptions to these fascinating radio drama characters.

Til Then remains today my favorite song of all time. It tells the story of hope of loved ones separated by the war and promises that "One day, I know we'll be back again." The Mills Brothers really did this timeless classic proud.

Ranking alongside this beautiful tune were the equally heart-wrenching *I'll Be Seeing You*, another love song demonstrating the heartbreak of loved ones separated for an indeterminate time by war, and the unforgettable 1943 hit parade favorite *You'll Never Know*. By the age of six, I could sing these songs with mama as she played them on her piano.

It was during this period that mama wrote many of her songs and set them to music. Her favorite, and mine, was *Just a Handful of Memories,* that she wrote and played for us in 1945, but due to intervening years of grief and trauma was not recorded and copyrighted until 1950. The song was published by Oak Music Publishing Company of Whitakers, North Carolina.

In the center of Kinston, on the southeast corner of Caswell Street and Queen Street, still stands today the two-story square-shaped red brick Standard Drug Store, with its main entrance on the corner and a side entrance fronting on Caswell Street. A six-foot wide overhang still extends along the front and side of the drugstore to keep customers dry during rainy weather. It hasn't changed in over sixty years since my youth.

Upon entering the drugstore's front door, along the left wall stood a large array of magazines, funny books, and newspapers. A soda fountain, complete with the standard Formica-covered countertop lined with red-covered swivel stools common to most drugstores of that era, occupied most of the space along the right wall. The area between the soda fountain and reading materials was filled with round Formica-covered tables, each of which was adorned by two well-worn "ice cream" chairs, those small, flimsy armless wire chairs with round seats prevalent in ice cream parlors all across the United States at the time.

The high wooden prescription counter at the rear of the drugstore separated the pharmacy from the rest of the drugstore.

My brother J.B. was twelve years older than I, and Doc was four years younger than J.B. On a particularly sweltering day in the Summer of 1943, after I had just turned four, Doc, who at that time was twelve, told me and my sister to come with him, but he didn't say where we were going. Barefooted, we followed him, hopping along like a couple of agitated bunny rabbits on the hot sidewalk along East Bright Street, then turned right onto Queen Street and hopped for another three blocks. Stopping at the corner of Queen and Caswell, Doc told us to wait there, whereupon he entered the Standard Drug Store and spoke briefly with the teenage soda jerk behind the counter.

As the two boys were talking, Doc suddenly pointed to Eoline and me standing at the entrance of the drugstore, and placed some money on the counter. The teenage soda jerk, obviously a friend of Doc's, slid the coins off the counter into his open hand, slipped the money into his trousers pocket, smiled at us and waved. We returned both.

Doc rejoined us, and we hopped along after him down Queen Street, our hopping finally ending two blocks later in front of the Paramount picture show. The old picture show, a landmark in town, was located in the middle of the block, with signs reading *"Paramount"* perched atop each end of the broad marquee facing east and west along Queen Street.

The large signboard on the face of the marquee projecting over the entrance of the theatre proclaimed, in large black hand-mounted letters, that Bob Steele presently was starring in such-and-such Western picture show. Oversized black-and-white pictures emblazoned at angles along the outer theatre wall inside the lobby depicted the Western hero in various action scenes, heightening further my puerile anticipation at witnessing the five-and-a-half-foot tall Steele outfight, outride and outgun numerous nefarious no-goods. And on the screen, my hero was eight feet tall.

Doc stepped up to the glassed-in ticket window, flashed the popular wartime two-finger "V for Victory" sign, and said "Three, Sweetie," to the smiling blond about thirty years old perched on a high barstool inside the ticket booth. The pretty blond replied, "Twenty-seven cents," and Doc slid three dimes through the mousehole at the base of the glass partition. The ticket lady, still beaming, tore three blue stubs from a roll of tickets and pushed three pennies change with the stubs through the mousehole.

Pocketing the pennies, Doc said, "Thanks, Sweetie," and ushered my sister and me through the large swinging doors and into the pitch-dark picture show. At the age of twelve, my brother Doc addressed all females, except mama and his teachers, as "Sweetie," and I never saw one of them not break out in a smile upon being so addressed by my brother.

I always admired my brother Doc and, had I known the meaning of the word at the age of four, most assuredly I would have called him "cool." The teenage girls in the neighborhood referred to him as "handsome," he seemed to be friends with everyone in town, and people always wanted to do him favors. My daddy and my brother Doc were probably the original "networkers." Years later, Doc confided in me that as a young boy he observed that daddy went out of his way to help people, regardless of their station in life, and that people in turn always wanted to do things for daddy and our family.

Doc was at home with his popularity. Even at age twelve he exuded a quiet confidence that manifested itself outwardly as an attitude of nonchalance. My sister and I looked up to Doc and trusted him implicitly. And he appeared to have that effect on everyone.

The inside lobby of the Paramount emitted a distinctive aroma of hot buttered popcorn and a sense of welcome and comfort. For ten cents, Doc bought Eoline and me each a large box of hot buttered popcorn, and we cautiously walked into the pitch-black theatre, stood still for awhile waiting for our eyes to adjust to the darkness, and Doc found us three empty seats.

Following a span of just a few minutes, during which time Eoline and I quickly cleaned out our popcorn boxes, the "Prevues of Coming Attractions" appeared on the large screen before us, giving the audience tantalizing glimpses of dramatic action scenes of upcoming picture shows. Next, the Movietone News of the Day appeared, and the deep, authoritative voiceover of Lowell Thomas informed us of U.S. Army victories over the Italians and Nazis in Italy as we viewed large cannons firing, supposedly at the hated Nazi positions.

Following the inspiring "News of the Day," we were treated to an installment of a "serial" featuring Buster Crabbe as Flash Gordon. First, we sat on the edge of our seats as Flash escaped miraculously from the clutches of futuristically-clothed villains, only at the end of which our hero again found himself in a perilous position of seemingly inescapable demise. I couldn't wait to come back the following week.

Our picture show culminated in the main feature, that found our wrongly-accused, two-fisted, pint-sized hero plotting with another prisoner to break out of a prison fortress located in a desolate part of the Wild West. After tricking the hapless guard and effecting his ingenious escape, Bob Steele kept me literally on the edge of my seat for the next thirty minutes as he tracked down and brought to justice those pesky, black-hearted villains who were responsible for Bob's unjust imprisonment. A lesson learned that day-nobody messes with Bob Steele.

Walking out into the blazing sunlight of that Saturday afternoon, squinting my eyes from the glare, I sensed a depression that comes only from seeing a good time end, and I knew at that time I had found my home away from home—the Paramount picture show. Hot sidewalks or not, I could not wait to return next Saturday.

Hands down, the best bargain for a kid in wartime Kinston was the Saturday matinee at the Paramount. For nine cents I could become enshrouded for a few hours in the escapism of a cowboy picture show, an exciting weekly serial, a March of Time, or an RKO Pathe News newsreel to keep abreast of America's rout of the Japs and Krauts, prevues of coming attractions and several Looney Tunes cartoons. For the extra nickel of the fifteen cents mama gave me, I had my choice of a big Baby Ruth candy bar, a large soft drink, or a tasty box of hot buttered popcorn, chock full of enough salt to cure a small ham and make my lips shrivel up like prunes.

In my impressionable young mind, I rode hell-bent for leather, sitting tall in the saddle alongside my heroes The Durango Kid, Hopalong Cassidy, Sunset Carson, Bob Steele, Johnny Mack Brown and numerous other fearless and intrepid champions of the Old West, as they outsmarted, outfought, and eventually shot the guns out of the hands of various and sundry no-good riff-raff, usually without losing their white ten-gallon hats in the fisticuffs.

Following a few standard setbacks, good eventually triumphed over evil, nary a drop of blood was spilled, and comic relief was provided invariably by that trio of inimitable sidekicks, Smiley Burnette, Gabby Hays, and Fuzzy St. John. Those were the days. Proof that in some instances the "good old days" were exactly that, and half a century later, I still cherish those golden memories.

Often small children learn best by example, not having much of a reference point, and my ethics and morals were molded in large degree during those Saturday afternoon picture show outings. Good was universally represented by the white ten-gallon hat and outfit, the golden palomino horse, and the polite and clean-shaven hero, who always rode tall in the saddle. Bad was invariably depicted by the opposite. Evil doers of evil deeds were eventually called to task for their malefactions, and in my mind indelible lines were drawn between acceptable and unacceptable conduct.

Among the lessons impressed on me during those lazy, idyllic Saturday afternoons were, don't rustle cattle, don't rob banks, don't run defenseless settlers off their land, and don't ever even think twice about insulting or threatening physical harm to a beautiful, twenty-year-old blond cowgirl with big tits. The oft-repeated moral that righteousness and honesty always triumphed over perfidious and unprincipled misconduct was the common thread that coursed throughout these endearing Saturday afternoon black-and-white B-westerns. But these simple lessons of morality, shown often not by words but by actions, were indelible indeed-they have fortunately lasted a lifetime.

Following the picture show that first Saturday afternoon, my sister and I skipped along the wide, scorching concrete Queen Street sidewalk alongside Doc, retracing our hops to the Standard Drug Store. Once inside we waved recognition to the young soda jerk, and Doc sat us at one of the small Formica-covered ice cream tables. Presently, two large soda fountain drinks were placed in front of my sister and me, and Doc introduced us to his teenage friend and classmate at school, "Dave."

After shaking hands with each of us (Doc taught us to always stick out our hands when we first met a grownup, as we respectfully referred to adults in that era-Doc said the grownup would like us better if we shook hands with him or her), Dave asked,

"Do you kids like funny books?" Dave must also have been a mind reader.

"Yes," we replied in unison, our little faces beaming with delight.

"Okay," said Dave, "You all go take a look at all the funny books, and each of you can have one to take home."

We scooted off our rickety wire high chairs, heading for the vast array of multi-colored funny books lining the far wall.

"Hold on just a minute, you two," called Doc. "What do you kids say to Dave?"

"Thanks, Dave," I said sheepishly, and quickly turned and scurried back to the plethora of funny books. Doc taught us to always thank anyone who did something for us. Another of my older brother's lifelong Lessons in Successful Networking.

I knew exactly what I wanted. The first funny book I had ever seen was an Action Comics my brother Bill had read to me. It featured Superman, who had the ability to fly through the air. Intriguing concept, that fly-through-the-air-unassisted thingy. Thanks to mama, by the age of four and a half I was well acquainted with Red Ryder, the red-headed cowboy, and his resourceful ten-year-old Navajo sidekick, the pidgin-English speaking Little Beaver, and how the two of them constantly protected the common folk of Rimrock, Colorado from being terrorized by lawless desperados.

Through Al Capp's Li'l Abner I was introduced to social satire at its finest. Capp presented Abner as a stupid, lazy, naïve, gullible hillbilly, and lampooned most of the other characters in the funny papers equally. Li'l Abner was constantly evading the marrying clutches of the quite innocent, equally voluptuous Daisy Mae Scragg, and the lovable Shmoos were instant favorites of mine when they showed up later in the strip.

Another of my heroes was The Phantom; though I was too young to fathom the ongoing sultry romance between The Ghost Who Walks and Diana Palmer, I enjoyed the Masked Man's unrelenting war against crime and his defense of justice and right. My youthful introduction to the future was supplied by Flash Gordon, who stimulated my interest with stories of spacecraft, unknown worlds, and beautiful, sexy women. On Sundays, I could hardly wait to journey through space with Flash as he battled a plethora of intergalactic bad guys. As I grew into a teenager and developed a twitch in my groin, it came to me one day why funny book characters like Daisy Mae Scragg, Diana Palmer, and the voluptuous females in Flash Gordon were created. The producers of those funny books were after the adult readers as much as they were after the audience of children.

The antithesis of Flash Gordon was that dumber-than-life duo Mutt and Jeff, who were as apt to talk to the artist and the reader as to one another. The short, feeble-minded Jeff, in the top hat and highly successful with the women, matched well with Mutt, tall and intelligent, whose exasperation with his stubby partner led often to Jeff receiving a black eye for his smart-aleck comments.

Through The Lone Ranger, I learned the importance of staunchly defending truth and justice, and I rode excitedly beside my masked hero on his beautiful horse Silver, with his faithful Indian partner Tonto, as we fought stagecoach and bank robbers, and cattle rustlers, and defended defrauded old widows and pretty young victimized girls alike. Though because of his mask, The Lone Ranger was accused of crimes he had not committed, I rode along with him as he fought to clear his name, and like many other youngsters of my time, I carried in my pants pocket a "coveted" silver bullet (that they sold by the dozens at the local five-and-dime).

In the Katzenjammer Kids I saw my brothers Bill and Kenny as personifications of the blond Fritz and the dark-haired Hans, pranksters who without letup played tricks on the maid, the neighbors, and even on small animals, just for the sheer fun of it; their grandfather's spankings were to no avail.

And I followed the unaging eleven-year-old Little Orphan Annie (what was an "orphan," I wondered) through her seemingly endless misadventures, admiring her courage, good nature, and toughness. Annie had to take care of herself in her continuing search for moral justice, aided by her loyal dog Sandy ("Arf") and her elderly benefactor Daddy Warbucks.

Another funny paper strip that had begun to define in my puerile mind the distinction between good and evil was Dick Tracy. This violent, bloody funny book, with characters like Mumbles, Cueball, and B.O. Plenty, demonstrated that justice, in the form of my fearless police detective, always triumphed over perfidity.

Studying the vast selection of funny books that hot Summer afternoon in the Standard Drug Store, I had difficulty deciding between the Action Comics' Superman and the Whiz Comics' Captain Marvel. I suppose my empathy for the poor and disadvantaged crept into my psyche from an early age. When the baby Kal-El was propelled from the dying planet Krypton, and was found near Smallville (what a hokey name for a town, I thought, even at that early age) by Jonathan and Martha Kent, they had at first taken him to an "orphanage" (whatever that was).

However, tugging equally at my heartstrings that day was Captain Marvel, who as young paperboy Billy Batson, when he uttered the word "*Shazam*," acquired instant strength, wisdom, courage and speed, transforming into a full-grown adult. Talk about a crime-fighter! Equally impressive was Marvel's young friend, the crippled Freddy Freeman, who was endowed with super strength, but remained the same age. Together, this dashing duo fought for truth, justice, and The American Way. My kind of guys!

I cannot recall whether that afternoon I chose Superman or Captain Marvel, but Doc told me soon afterwards, when mama started allowing me to go to the Saturday Paramount matinees alone, that I would stop (or hop, depending on the season) by the Standard Drug Store, and if Dave were working behind the soda fountain, Dave would "take care" of me. And he did. Dave always gave me the big fountain drink of my choice, and one funny book, absolutely free. Outside my family, Dave became, hands down, my very best friend in the whole wide world. And I always shook hands with Dave when I met him, and gave him a big "Thanks, Dave," when I left. Friendship.

In wartime small Southern towns, folks were friendly, but also minded their own business, and in 1944, a child could walk down to the Standard Drug Store late at night and feel as safe as if it were high noon.

On Halloween night, 1944, when I was five, Bill and Kenny asked me to go over to the Episcopal Church with them. I felt honored that my big brothers wanted to include me in their company. Stupid kid! Innocently, I walked with my two older brothers around the block, up the marble steps and into the church. I followed the boys up to the altar, where Bill told me to wait. My brother Bill was what the police authorities would call the "ringleader." He said he and Kenny had to go to the house to "get something," and that they would be "right back."

Waiting there in the darkness of the cavernous church, I was jolted by the sudden loud pealing of the church bell. Becoming frightened, and not seeing my brothers through the darkness, I quickly made my way to the front door of the church, reached for the large brass handle, and pushed hard. The heavy door didn't even budge. Not an inch. Frantically, I pushed with all my might on the door, but to no avail. Suddenly, I heard footsteps behind me.

"Who's there?" asked the tall man dressed in black coming toward me down the darkened aisle. It was the pastor.

"I can't get out," I said with an equal mixture of embarrassment and fear. The pastor tried to open the door, but the massive oak would not budge.

"It's stuck," said the pastor, then added, "By the way, Alton, what are you doing here at night all by yourself?"

"I'm not by myself," I replied, then quickly added, "Bill and Kenny are with me. They said they had to go get something and they'd be right back." Stupid, stupid kid. I still hadn't caught on. But I could not see Bill or Kenny in the darkness of the church. Neither could the pastor.

"Let's go around to the front and see why we can't open the door," suggested the pastor, somewhat puzzled. Walking through the side door of the church and around to the front, the curious pastor tried to open the church door. Nothing. Then, feeling with his hand along the bottom edge of the massive door, he exclaimed,

"This is why we couldn't get out." Looking down, I saw a wedge of pinewood stuck between the bottom of the large oak door and the concrete floor.

"Appears your brothers played a trick on you," said the pastor, with a smile.

"Come on, I'll walk you back to your house. You'd better watch out for those brothers of yours. They're a couple of experienced pranksters."

Bill and Kenny had fooled me once more. Luring me into the church, they had rung the church bell knowing it would summon the pastor. Then they locked me in the church, knowing the pastor would scare the daylights out of me in the darkness. And I learned the meaning of a new word, "prankster." A prankster is a big brother who locks you in the Episcopal Church on Halloween night-and teases you about it for the next month. The plural of "prankster" is two big brothers named Bill and Kenny.

Because the family store provided a considerable part of our income, our parents were determined not to allow us to eat up all the profits. Despite this obviously necessary economic restriction (seven kids loose in a candy store in their own home), mama occasionally offered us a special treat, and each of us was given a choice of a soft drink or a candy bar.

Because of this availability of sweets, I fell in love with Moon Pies, Dr. Pepper, salted peanuts and RC Colas at an early age. A Moon Pie is a marshmallow patty sandwiched between two round, four-inch diameter, chocolate-covered cookies. I was eating Moon Pies and drinking RC Colas nearly ten years before the 1950's recording by Lonzo and Oscar of the hit song *Give Me an RC Cola and a Moon Pie*.

In the 1940's, Dr. Pepper contained enough caffeine and carbonation to give us kids a cheap "high." I was addicted to the stuff, and mama kept an ample supply in our soft drink cooler.

"Mama, can I have a Dr. Pepper? And when I finish it, can I have another one?" May as well get both orders in, in the same breath. We Southerners love our carbonation and caffeine so much, that if the (damn) Yankees ever wanted to (again) subjugate the South, they need only flood the South with boxcar loads of free Dr. Pepper. The stuff turns us almost instantly into blithering, docile children. But better send along a packet of Tom's Peanuts to pour into each Dr. Pepper. We Southerners invented peanuts. I still have a photograph of mama standing in front of our home, reading the Sunday funnies while holding in her other hand a Dr. Pepper.

In the center of our store stood a soft drink cooler of the type more prevalent during the forties and fifties. It had two insulated doors that opened to the top, with insulated sides. A drainage tube extended from the bottom of the cooler at one end. Initially, soft drinks were placed standing to fill the cooler. Two twenty-five pound blocks of ice were placed atop the cooler, and mama chipped away at the ice with an icepick, the ice chips falling over and between the standing soft drinks that, of course, at that time, were all in glass bottles. Then the two insulated top-opening doors were closed, keeping the soft drinks quite cold for several days.

As the ice melted, the cold water settled around the drinks. The trick was to open the insulated door quickly, remove the desired drink, then quickly close the door, thereby keeping the warm air from entering the cooler. After a few days, the drinks (except during the cold Winter months) became too warm, at which time mama drained the water by way of the rubber hose at the bottom of the cooler, and refilled the bottom of the cooler with ice.

The Tobacco Auction

During tobacco harvesting season in the 1940's, the large, shallow and quite cumbersome pallets of flue-cured "Bright Leaf" tobacco were loaded onto open-sided flatbed trucks for delivery to the massive tobacco storage and auction center just off Caswell Street in Kinston.

Tobacco trucks entering town from the west were prohibited from taking the more direct and convenient Queen Street route to the auction warehouse; rather, the truck drivers were required to cross Queen onto East Bright Street, turn left onto McLewean Street at the first intersection, travel north for several city blocks, turn left onto Caswell Street, then re-cross Queen Street to get to the sprawling auction facility several blocks away.

Even years before my time "on the corner," as we kids referred to the practice, neighborhood children, including my four older brothers, had learned to time their mad dash across the intersection for the express purpose of forcing the always-in-a-hurry truck drivers to suddenly brake the always-overloaded lumbering vehicles as they negotiated the sharp left turn at East Bright and McLewean.

It was nigh onto impossible for a tobacco truck to make that perilous, sharp left turn without the inertial effect of the heavy load hurling loose stalks of tobacco, and occasionally, if we were really lucky, an entire pallet or two of the precious cargo, off the truck bed, and any errant stalk of the "Bright Leaf" hitting the pavement bounced up and was transformed instantly into an American monetary denomination better known to us kids as a "dime," once redeemed at the tobacco auction warehouse, and used by the lucky "finders" to gain instant admission into the Saturday afternoon Western matinee at the Paramount, along with hot-buttered popcorn and ice-cold soft drinks, and our favorite funny books at the Standard Drug Store on the corner of Caswell and Queen.

During tobacco harvesting season mama didn't have to look far to find us kids; we were always stationed "on the corner." What a life! The Bowery Boys would have been proud of us.

The Twins and Seeing Spot Run

When I finally reached about age thirty, I caught on that Bill and Kenny were not always telling me the truth. So at age six I was considered fair game to these two jokers.

In the three hundred block of East Bright Street lived two young girls about Eoline's age. The girls were named Betty Jean Hall and Betty Jean Garner, and, oddly, didn't look a bit alike. I say "oddly" because until I went to the orphanage at age seven, I believed what Bill and Kenny told me, that because the girls were both named Betty Jean, they must be sisters, you know, same name and all.

What really blew my fragile, unassuming mind, though, was that the two "sisters" didn't even live in the same house, but on opposite sides of East Bright Street. Early on I must have had a problem with logic. Sometimes I think my parents kept me around to provide comic relief entertainment for the Provost family. Or, perhaps the family had already seen the latest picture show playing at the Paramount, and did not have anything to do for entertainment on a Saturday night.

One day when I was about five years old, I was reading about Dick and Jane in my sister's first grade reader, when Bill and Kenny told me that Dick and Jane had recently moved to Kinston, and the family lived on Independence Street, about a city block away from our house.

Knowing what the textbook kids looked like, and being only five years old and quite impressionable (some might call stupid), pretty soon I began pacing up and down Independence Street, stopping to peer in all the front windows of each house, hoping the always pleasant, always immaculately-dressed, ultra-polite children would notice me and come out to play. They never did, and I was quite disappointed, because I believe I had developed a "crush" on Jane. And I never got to see Spot run, either.

The Big Red Indian

One Summer afternoon in 1944, I was playing on the dogtrot with my sister, when our game was suddenly interrupted by the deafening rumble of an unmuffled engine reverberating between our house and the corrugated metal garage-turned-workshop. I looked up in surprise, and there sat my daddy astride a monstrous, frightful Indian motorcycle, gunning the engine and grinning at me.

"C'mere, Cotton," his voice strained, motioning to me with his open hand. With great trepidation I approached the huge, rumbling metal monster.

Daddy reached down, put his arm around me, and swung me up onto the steel horse behind him. I ended up with my skinny white legs astride two black leather saddlebags situated atop the rear wheel of the motorcycle.

"Hang on, Cotton," daddy yelled above the roar of his constant revving of the powerful engine. My heart rate instantly matched that of the big machine, and I clutched desperately at the sides of daddy's shirt as he tilted the cycle to the left, making a sharp turn, and we were out of the driveway and heading south on East Bright Street.

My maternal grandparents Will and Maude Thomas lived in the Simon Bright apartments about six blocks from our home. Just before these apartments, the railroad tracks intersected East Bright Street, angling to the right in the middle of the block.

"We're gonna turn, son," daddy yelled over his shoulder, and about that time he swerved sharply off the street and headed the big Indian down the middle of the railroad ties. Scared out of my wits, I hung on for dear life, feeling the rippling of the motorcycle's tires across the wooden crossties. What a ride! And what's a "motorcycle helmet," anyway?

That was the day I fell in love with motorcycles, and memories of that first exciting ride, hanging on to my daddy's shirt, remain with me half a century later. Following that first ride, anticipation quickly replaced apprehension, and I eagerly looked forward to daddy's familiar invitation, "Wanna go for a ride, Cotton?"

The red monster was a 1939 Indian Chief "74." It was big. It was loud. It was downright scary. It was painted "Indian Red," had oversized tires, and a chrome-plated handlebar crossbar that was to become my open-air seat from which to view the streets of Kinston and the surrounding countryside. The big machine sported regulation Indian saddlebags, cost $450.00 when new, and daddy purchased it in 1943 for $270.00. With its powerful Bonneville Special motor, it could take off from a standing start like a scalded dog, and was but a blur of red as it passed you on the highway.

Not until well into adulthood was I able to see the Indian for what it meant to daddy. It was in reality his one escape from the strains and worries incident to raising seven children in a post-Depression, wartime economy in a small Southern town.

And I was his riding buddy, someone he loved and with whom he wanted to share his joy. Sitting on the handlebar crossbar, my spindly white legs dangling on each side of the front tire, daddy taught me how to "lean into the turn" so as not to fall off, and to do likewise if I were sitting behind him straddling the saddlebags. Soon I grew to enjoy the thrill of the ride, and daddy relished in my delight. Indeed, I lived in a seemingly never-ending Norman Rockwellian world. Those were truly the halcyon days of my life.

In early Summer of 1944, I was my second month into my fifth year, and daddy, who could not serve in the military because he had seven children, followed the progress of the war on a daily basis. My oldest brother J.B. was sixteen at the time, and had informed daddy that he was going to enlist in the Navy as soon as he was of age.

At bedtime one night, my parents were huddled so close to the old Philco one would have thought they were going to eat it, and daddy was laughing and joking that it was all over for the "Krauts," as he called the Germans. Of course daddy was brought closer to the war because of his government job at Cherry Point Marine Air Station, where he came in daily contact with the military.

That day in memory was D-Day, June 6, 1944.

The Ice Plant

The icebox in our kitchen stood in the corner on four stout wooden legs. A block of ice was placed in a separate compartment on top of the icebox proper. This block of ice rested on wood slats, with a pan to catch the melted icewater beneath the block of ice. Insulation was the key to having an efficient cooling system. Our icebox worked quite well.

During the late 1930's and early 1940's, the large blocks of ice were loaded onto horse-drawn or mule-drawn white ice wagons at the ice plant. The ice produced at the ice plant came down the ice chute in hundred pound blocks. The iceman slowly drove the ice wagon up and down the city streets, and customers in need of ice came out to the sidewalk and told the iceman how much ice they needed. In 1941 a 25-pound block of ice, designed to fit into the top compartment of the standard icebox, cost twenty cents.

The iceman deftly and quickly used his ice pick to chip a 25-pound block from the larger hundred-pound block of ice. During the hot

Summers of the North Carolina coastal plain we kids would follow behind the ice wagon, marveling at the expertise of the iceman with his ice pick, and begging for loose ice chips resulting from his chipping away the 25-pound blocks.

Ice plants were referred to also as "ammonia plants" because compressed ammonia was used as the refrigerant. Water was poured into the large rectangular vats, the sides of which consisted of tubing filled with compressed ammonia. The ammonia absorbed the heat from the water, which dropped the water temperature, turning the water to ice. The water closest to the sides of the vat quickly formed ice more rapidly than did the water at the center. This resulted in the center of the hundred-pound block of ice having a whitish, or milky appearance.

Heat absorbed by the ammonia being compressed in the pipes was dissipated by water surrounding the outside coils. Therefore the ice plant at Kinston, just as other ice plants, kept a large pond of water beside the plant, known as the "cooling pond," that was usually filled with water lilies, or what we kids called "pond" lilies.

The Pocket Watch

From an early age I was fascinated by my daddy's watch and fob, that he allowed me to play with anytime I wanted to. Rather than wear wristwatches, men of my daddy's generation wore pocket watches in a small vest pocket or pants waist pocket. Thus, the name "pocket" watch. The watch "fob" is a short chain attached to the pocket watch and worn hanging in front of the vest or waist.

However, so few pocket watches are used today that although one can still find "pocketbook" and "pocketknife" in the dictionary, many dictionaries have deleted the word "pocket watch." Daddy would calmly and quite seriously sit at the supper table, take out his pocket watch from his waist pocket, twirl the round gold watch by the fob, open the cover to expose the face of the watch, look at me with a serious face and then look at his watch and remark, "Well, it's just about time to spank Cotton," or "Well, it's just about time to lock Cotton in the garage for the night." And in a few minutes he would have all us kids laughing at what "time" daddy had.

Coloreds

In my youth we kids grew up on chock-full-of-carbonation Dr. Pepper, greasy, salty Tom's peanuts, Chattanooga Moon Pies, the fast-acting and ultra-reliable Ex-Lax, and something else I could not even pronounce at the time. As certain as spit mixed with a chawtabacca begets the search for a cuspidor, the natural order of my Southern world was segregation, the separation of the racial groups that hung on to the South like a pesky tag on the coat of Progress. Only we didn't recognize segregation for what it really was because it was the natural order of our society. I believe Southerners invented the "status quo." A true Southerner will let you mess with his gun before he'll let you mess with his status quo.

In 1940's small town North Carolina, we called blacks "colored folks," at that time a term of respect. My daddy and mama deplored the use of the word "nigger," and many of their friends were colored. Kizzy, a pert, slim colored woman who worked for mama in our store and helped cook and supervise us children during the day, was an integral part of our family and our lives. We had to mind Kizzy just like we minded mama. When I was taken to the orphanage in February 1947 at age seven, I missed Kizzy as I missed mama. She was a part of our family.

Mama died in February 1962 while I was aboard a troopship in the Sea of Japan on the way to my first of two tours of duty in Korea, compliments of Uncle Sam's Army. At mama's funeral, that I did not attend, Kizzy stood silently between Doc and J.B., unable to contain her sorrow. Mama and Kizzy were the same age and were as close as sisters.

The use of the word "nigger" held two meanings, quite confusing to "whites" (whose usage, by the way, gave way to "Caucasian," that is also a misnomer, many would argue). Say the word "Negro" aloud fast twenty times, and somewhere around the fifteenth repetition it starts coming out "nigra," then "nigger," that gave way to the use of "nigger" as a derogatory expression. Many whites (er, Caucasians) are sensitive to this, and tend not to use the (quite respectful) word Negro for fear of being misunderstood, or worse yet, labeled "racist."

What seemed to confuse us whites is that the colored males who lived across East Bright Street from us spoke among themselves as "nigger," but the word was used mainly as a term of recognition and endearment. At the same time, I discovered, coloreds were astute enough to poke fun at themselves.

It was not until the latter half of the twentieth century that coloreds and Negroes began referring to themselves as "blacks." I believe the use of "African-American" begs the issue. A colored person, or black person, proud of his heritage, will not desire to cover his pride, or attempt to be something he is not.

Mama wrote poetry and songs, and played the piano quite well. East Bright Street in Kinston was the dividing line between the whites and coloreds on the west side of town. With Kizzy's help, mama had quality time to devote to her poetry and music. Several of her songs were recorded. The most popular was *Just a Handful of Memories*, a lamentation of unrequited love, written shortly after my daddy's tragic death, that was recorded and began being sold in stores in 1950.

One Summer night in 1950 when Eoline was in 1-G (the first girls' cottage after "moving up" from the Annex), the girls were listening to a call-in request program on Oxford's only radio station, WOXF, when Eoline heard mama's song being played. When the other girls in 1-G learned that our mother was a songwriter, Eoline became an instant celebrity, and all the young girls wanted to meet mama when she came for her monthly visits. For me, mama's talents in the field of music and poetry have been always a source of pride and inspiration, yet tempered with a tinge of regret as to what might have been.

The coloreds in our neighborhood frequented our "convenience" store, although that word was not in vogue at the time. They were major purchasers of cigarettes and "lighterd," the resinous firestarter strips my brothers chopped from the heart of the yellow pine. When daddy brought back bushels of oysters from our weekend trips to granddaddy's cabin in Swansboro, the colored folks from the neighborhood were just as welcome as were whites to the steamed oyster feasts.

We children played with Kizzie's kids in our yard, and they enjoyed peaches and apples from our backyard orchard. We childishly called them "coal lumps," and they returned the puerile banter by calling us "soda crackers," but it was all good-natured fun. However, I do recall that we always refused to play "hide-and-go-seek" with the colored kids after dark, for fear we would not be able to find them. And that's a fact.

Daddy always carried a snub-nosed .38-cal. revolver in his right hip pocket, and anyone who lived nearby was familiar with the gun's pearl handle dangling in full view outside his hip pocket. More than once a frightened, battered colored woman showed up in our front room store on a Saturday night, seeking daddy's protection from a violent, abusive, drunken husband or boyfriend. These women were always welcome, and daddy would always keep them safe and call the police.

Daddy jokingly told us it was good for business, but both my parents were possessed with an abiding empathy for those less fortunate than our family. I always felt safe with my daddy; he never looked for trouble, but neither did he back down from any man.

I must take issue with the Usage Panel of the American Heritage Dictionary of the English Language, Third Edition, that defines "colored" as "offensive, of or belonging to a racial group not regarded as white." First, the National Association for the Advancement of Colored People (N.A.A.C.P.) was founded in June 1909, and as we enter the twenty-first century, this well-respected and influential organization has not elected to delete the word "colored" from its title. Second, this definition would appear to include Asians and Hispanics, which I have never heard referred to as "colored."

Third, the Monday evening, February 11, 1946 issue of the Kinston *Daily Free Press* ran the widely-read newspaper's regularly appearing column entitled "News of Interest to Our Colored Readers." The column noted that Mr. and Mrs. John W. Shaw announce the birth of their son weighing eight pounds on February 8, 1946, that the junior choir of St. John's Baptist Church was entertained Friday night at the church, that chicken salad was served to seventeen members of the choir, and that the Adkin High School boys and girls basketball teams won games recently over Darden High School in Wilson. Certainly, the Kinston *Daily Free Press* was not using "offensive" language in 1946; rather, the word "colored" was one of time-honored respect in an era of widespread segregation in the South.

The colored kids who played with us in our front yard and in the streets of Kinston called us "soda crackers," in reference to our pale white skin, but we never were offended by the term, and its usage was certainly not intended by the coloreds to be derogatory. My four older brothers played stickball with the colored teenagers along East Bright Street in the late 1930's and early 1940's, and all these pickup games I witnessed consisted of mixed races on each team. Occasionally during this period, I saw white teenagers fighting whites and black teenagers fighting blacks, but never experienced a white boy and a black boy so much as argue. Such conduct was simply not acceptable, and would not have been tolerated by parents of either race.

Finally, colored workers at Oxford Orphanage were listed alongside the orphanage Superintendent and other teachers and workers in the list of "Staff of Workers" section of the Oxford Orphanage Annual Reports, disseminated to literally thousands of Masons throughout North Carolina each year. The Seventy-Ninth Annual Report, for the year 1951, contained a photograph of F.M. Pinnix, manager of the orphanage printing department from 1927 to 1950, who had died on November 20, 1951. The next page contained a photograph of Ira Smith, a "highly respected and faithful employee of Oxford Orphanage for 31 years" who had died on April 28, 1951. Ira Smith was colored.

In today's world, some may believe the word "colored" to be offensive. However, in the segregated South of my youth, this simply was not true. However, I did learn the difference between colored and white at an early age. It started out as a childish prank.

"Whites Only"—"Colored Only"

In August 1945, two significant events occurred of interest to me. The first event changed the world, and in the second, I learned a valuable lesson about the world in which I lived.

Just before dawn on August 6, 1945, the *Enola Gay*, an American B-29 bomber, took off from Tinian Island in the Marianas. It arrived over Hiroshima, Japan, at 8:15 a.m., where it released its solitary atomic bomb. In a blinding flash, 80,000 people died, and most of the city ceased to exist. On August 14, 1945, Japan surrendered. World War II had at long last ended.

A week after Japan surrendered, I started first grade. Finally, I had grown up; I was going to school each morning with my big brothers and sister. I was one proud kid. Mama knelt and gave me a kiss the first day of school. Undoubtedly, she was happy for me. Or, perhaps she was simply happy to rid herself of the little human leech.

My brother Bill was the town's greatest practical joker. And he was not disinclined to play a trick on his own daddy. Everyone was fair game to Bill. And daddy was usually good-natured about his son's fun because he appreciated Bill's humor.

Except the Summer night when Bill hid daddy's black belt that went with his tan work uniform, and for two days daddy went to work at Cherry Point beltless. Not funny. Not to daddy, anyway. Or the time two days before Christmas when daddy came to the breakfast table to discover a pickled pig's foot floating in the wide-mouthed quart of his favorite buttermilk. Bad timing for Bill. Two days before Christmas? The dumbass.

Daddy just smiled good-naturedly, and asked Bill what was the unluckiest number he could think of. Bill thought for a moment, then replied "thirteen." "Okay," said daddy. Two mornings later, on Christmas day, we all awoke early and excitedly gathered at the front bedroom wall where "Santa Claus" always hung each of us kids a large stocking filled with goodies.

Bill's stocking looked kinda . . . well, kinda . . . empty? Reaching deep down into his stocking, Bill pulled out a long piece of adhesive tape, to which was stuck . . . well, yes . . . exactly thirteen pennies. Daddy told Bill they were special pennies, called "pickled pigs' feet pennies." My brother Bill wasn't too keen on the concept of timing.

Anyway, on the way to school that first morning, we approached Kinston's bus station, whereupon Bill announced he had to pee, really bad.

"Come on, Alton," he said, "We'll both do pee." I was proud that my older brother had invited me to do pee with him, so I followed him into the bus station, already crowded with passengers waiting to board the bus to Raleigh and points north.

As we entered the door to the bus terminal, Bill whispered to me, "Now, Alton, there are two toilets in here, and we're in a hurry. You take that one," he said, pushing me toward a dingy, well-worn wooden door that years before had received about a half a coat of quickly-faded light green paint.

So, in I walked and immediately became acutely aware that mine was the only white peepee in the restroom. Two old colored men were waiting in line at the toilet, and a third was washing his hands at the scrungy-looking sink. The entire room smelled of . . . well, of . . . dried peepee?

One of the old colored men turned to me, and remarked, "Can't wait, sonny boy?" Then, pushing the other colored man back with his hand, he said, "Go ahead, sonny, we's ain't in no hurry." And the two men moved away from the toilet.

"Thank you, sir," I replied, and stepped up to the toilet, quickly bled my little weed, buttoned up my pants and walked out into the (comparatively speaking) fresh air. Bill, Kenny, and Doc were standing outside the bus station with my sister Eoline, laughing and pointing at me as I walked out.

"Come on, little colored boy," said Bill, laughing, and we continued on to school. I trotted on down the sidewalk, and when I could, I asked Doc, "Doc, why did Bill call me a 'colored boy?'"

"I'll show you later," replied Doc. Later that afternoon, as we approached the bus station on the way back home from school, Doc said, "Come on, Alton, and I'll show you what Bill meant." I followed Doc into the bus station. "Bill was just tricking you, Alton, same way J.B. tricked him on his first day at school years ago." Pointing to the door Bill had led me into, Doc explained. "See that sign on the door?" I looked, and there printed about two-thirds of the way up from the floor were the words "*Colored Only.*"

"That toilet is for the colored people," he said. "Now see that door next to it? What does it say?" I looked up. At the same spot on the adjacent door was printed "*Whites Only.*"

"Will I get into trouble?" I asked with great concern.

"Certainly not," replied Doc. "Now, if a colored person goes into the 'Whites Only' toilet, the Kinston cops can arrest him and put him in jail."

"But can the cops put me in jail?" I asked, quite puzzled.

"No, Alton," said Doc. "It don't work both ways."

At the innocent young age of six, on my very first day of school, I had been taught my first lesson in both discrimination and segregation. But like Doc said, in a small Southern town in 1945, "It don't work both ways." Even at such an early age, my innocent mind could not comprehend why a white person could use a "Colored Only" toilet, but a colored person could not use a "Whites Only" toilet. If that's the way it was, I supposed, there had to be some logic behind it.

Miss Wellbuilt

By the time the Japs finally threw in the bloody towel in August 1945, I was already four months into my sixth year of annoying my daddy and mama and laying solemn claim of ownership over any stray dog or mangy cat that wandered within a hundred yard radius of our garage, and, already having elevated my rapidly expanding young mind to polysyllabic heights, I entered first grade, only to become living proof that we do find love in the strangest places.

I cannot recall my first grade teacher's name, but I certainly remember how heavy-shirted she was, and I eagerly awaited the part of each school day when Miss Wellbuilt would bend deftly at her slim waist over my desk in order to impart some tidbit of educational utility, wondering all the while when one or both of her overripe lollapaloozas might slip out of their cloth traps and plop gently onto my first grade reader.

I do recall that as I peered up from my Dick and Jane stuff and nonsense, I had great difficulty looking the pretty woman in the eye because of these well-formed intervening jugs, the apex of which appeared to be adorned with a protruding "button" of some sort, the size and shape of these buttons seeming to change with her mood. If you look forward to seeing a woman each day, does that mean you are in love? Or, if I might word my question another way, if I had not been in love, would I have looked forward to seeing her each day? If I wasn't in love, I certainly was in a heckuva lot of curiosity and wonderment, because my beautiful teacher had a deadbolt lock on the Department of Bosoms and Buttons.

Sixguns

My favorite Western stars of the 1940's appeared to compete with each other as to who would sport the largest gun belt with the shiniest silver baubles. And if one sixgun was good, it logically followed (to me, at least) that *two* blazing Colt .45's surely would double my prestige and influence among my siblings and friends. Certainly convinced my highly-impressionable young mind, anyway. Mama gave me a choice of how to spend my fifteen cents on Saturday afternoon, either the Western matinee at my second home, the Paramount, or an hour or so reading funny books and annoying all the other customers by slurping shamelessly my large fountain drink at the Standard Drugstore.

And this choice of how to spend my fifteen cents was determined simply by glancing into the Standard Drugstore on my way to the Paramount. If my very best friend in the whole wide world, Dave, was the soda jerk du jour, my afternoon's schedule was set. Only if Doc's classmate was not working was I forced to decide between Western action and popcorn, or slurping sodas while reading funny books.

Thanks to mama's saintly patience and interest in my learning, by the age of five I could read my sister's first grade reader. And because for a year or so mama had been reading the funny papers and funny books to me, I grew to enjoy the drugstore funny books almost as much as the picture shows.

One Saturday afternoon in the Fall of 1945, when I was six, I was sitting in the Standard Drugstore, slurping air through a straw from a long since depleted soda cup, when a silver glint in a glass-enclosed counter situated in front of the store pharmacy captured my full attention. I blinked rapidly, unable to believe my eyes. No, it couldn't be! Not here, in the Standard Drugstore in the sleepy little Southern town of Kinston, North Carolina. Jumping Jehosophat!

Slowly, I slid forward in my chair until my toes touched the floor, pushed the rickety wire chair back with my skinny butt, and like a moth to a flame, drew myself to the still-glinting object that, the closer I edged, became *two* shiny metal objects. Ohmigod! Sixguns!

I drew near to the glass case with the same reverence I would approach the Episcopal Church altar with a miter box chock full of pennies on Easter Sunday. There they lay before me, as real to my eyes as were the sixguns of Lash LaRue or The Lone Ranger, fitting snugly in (to me, at least) two authentic holsters attached to a no-nonsense studded gunbelt.

I was suddenly mesmerized. With all the reverence I could muster, I knelt before the glass display case, pressed my open palms and nose flush against the pane, and gazed absolutely unflinchingly for what seemed an eternity, at the first thing for which my young heart had really and truly longed. To the other customers in the drugstore, it must have appeared as though I were praying to the God of Glass-Encased Sixguns. And I was.

After a long time, my concentration was broken by a presence behind me. Looking over my shoulder, I saw Dave admiring *my* silver, engraved pearl-handled prizes.

"Sure are pretty, aren't they?" smiled Dave.

"Yeah, they sure are," I replied longingly, turning my dream-filled eyes back toward *my* treasures.

That night at bedtime, mama, as was her routine, sat on the edge of the bed while I said my prayers. I asked God to bless daddy and mama and my brothers and Eoline; then made a special petition to my very best friend, the Lord, who had suddenly edged out Dave, to intercede with mama and daddy to convince them to buy me two special presents for Christmas. And I was quite specific as to what those special gifts were to be. And just to make His job easier, and to avoid any misunderstanding, I even told God where mama and daddy could find these objects of my desire. And it was also okay with me if mama heard me praying to God. I felt confident the two of them could and would work out the details and would Do the Right Thing.

Just for effect, I repeated my prayer nearly every night until Christmas Eve. When mama tucked me in bed for the night, I noticed she was wearing her patented Mona Lisa half-smile, that made it hard to tell whether she had a gas pain, or knew something I didn't, and didn't want to tell me. I could read my daddy like a book, he never hid his feelings. At six foot one he didn't have to hide anything. What you saw in daddy was what you got. But mama's true thoughts were at times a little difficult for my young mind to fathom. But then again, at age five I didn't really have a lot of experience in reading my parents' intentions. I wasn't exactly the main cog in the Provost family wheel.

I fell asleep that night with visions of two pearl-handled revolvers and invitations from an array of my favorite B-western stars to join them in their next Saturday afternoon matinee dancing through my head. Upon awakening early Christmas morning, I went out into the front room of the house, where I saw our Christmas tree now surrounded with brightly colored gifts. My eyes quickly scanned the presents for size, the shape of the box that stored my present having been memorized from the glass-encased vault at the Standard Drugstore.

But I found no matches under the Christmas tree. Not even close. After the family had gathered around the tree, mama reached into the pile of presents, and smiling, handed me a large gift. Quickly tearing off the multi-colored wrapping paper, I opened the box to find not two, but one pearl-handled six-shooter. But I was delighted. The one beautiful gun was nearly twice the size of those I had admired in the drugstore display case. And it held a huge roll of caps.

I was a happy kid. For the next hour, nobody and nothing got out alive. I shot the door, the walls, the cat about sixty times, mama, daddy, and every one of my siblings at least a dozen times each. I practiced my quick-draw technique on Bill and Kenny, winning each time because they had only their index fingers to shoot with, and a blazing sixgun will out-duel an index finger any day under God's bright sun.

I fell asleep Christmas night with my cooled-off revolver at my side, under the covers so nary a nogood varmint would steal it from me and render me gunless and impotent. That was my very best Christmas ever.

And I believe part of this distinction was that my daddy and mama really enjoyed giving me a gift that brought me so much joy.

My daddy died six weeks later.

My Daddy's Death

I have been unable to determine from conversations with my brothers exactly when my daddy began to change. We do know daddy had always loved his children, even though he would not hesitate to keep us in line with stern lectures, and maybe a switching or two to my sister. It is possible that daddy began to feel the financial pressures incident to supporting a wife and seven children in the midst of a war. My brothers could recall no families they knew at the time that had more than three children.

As of the telling of this story, only three of us children are still living—Eoline, two years my senior, Pete, four years younger than I, and I. Over the years we have speculated-though admittedly less frequently with the passing of time and the complexities of our own lives-as to how our lives, and the lives of our parents and four older brothers, would have differed had daddy not died.

We all loved our daddy. He was a kind, caring, intelligent person, who attended church regularly with his family, gave part of his earnings to the church, readily extended credit to the less well to do customers of the family's small convenience store, and worked long hours at Cherry Point for the U.S. government to ensure our well-being. Even today, more than fifty years after his death, we three children talk about him and wonder . . . what if? None of us has ever placed any blame on daddy because of the circumstances in which we found ourselves as a result of his untimely death. We prefer instead to describe the tragedy as "unfortunate."

According to my brother Doc, daddy began to change sometime in late 1944 or early 1945, while he was working at Cherry Point. Daddy and his brother Gilbert had always been close, but now daddy would not even speak to his brother. Their relationship was further strained by the fact that their father died on January 20, 1938, whereupon their mother had moved in to live with Gilbert and his wife Evelyn, and the mother tended to side with Gilbert in any family disagreements.

When I turned six, daddy gave me my own personal hatchet, and assigned to me a drawer in his heavy wooden workbench in the garage, in which to store this most prized possession when not in use. Expressly, he told me, that hatchet was to be used to help Bill and Kenny chop up the heart of those yellow pine trees into lighterd, and, feeling the great weight of responsibility, I proceeded dutifully to do my part of mainly getting in everybody's way.

However, I did not stop with lighterd; rather, I chopped anything outside the house that I determined needed chopping, a category that to me included anything not human or animal, until eventually I made the mistake of chopping the large, heavy wooden legs that supported daddy's large, heavy wooden workbench. But daddy didn't get angry with me-he never got upset with me. Years later, my older brothers told me they never once remembered daddy whipping me, or even speaking harshly to me.

In order to avoid further damage to his property, however, daddy politely banished me from his garage workshop, and I had to ask one of my older brothers to fetch my trusty hatchet whenever I needed it for important chopping tasks.

All little boys need challenges-that's how they become responsible young men. By means of that tried and true method of determining such things, known universally as "trial and error," I discovered that, although the metal hatchet did not fare well against other metal objects, the concrete sidewalk running alongside East Bright Street presented a not insurmountable challenge, and thus I attacked it with my hatchet on a fairly regular basis.

The only other transgression I committed with my ubiquitous hatchet involved the fence that separated our backyard orchard from the Episcopal Church's property. Just so happened that the mainly ornamental wooden fenceposts holding up the four strands of wire were made of pine.

Pine trees are the source of kindling, or as we called it, lighterd, so one day when I didn't have anything else better to do, I began chipping away at those fenceposts, dutifully and admittedly quite proud of myself, cutting them into small strips of lighterd.

And just to prove my worth to the family, I even got some string and bundled the strips, took them up to the house and gave them to mama to sell in the store, cocksure of the praise that would be heaped upon my industrious little shoulders for a job well done.

"Where'd you get those from, Alton?" mama asked, opening the back door for me.

"From out back," I responded with pride, and added "Out in the orchard."

Now, mama was well aware that Bill and Kenny did not cut the lighterd "out in the orchard." The chopping block always stayed behind the garage.

"Come and show me," said mama, with just a tinge of concern in her soft voice. So I did.

Coming through the peach trees into a small clearing, mama looked ahead, where she observed just enough left on two pine fenceposts to barely hold the nails to which was attached the wire fence.

"Oh!" exclaimed mama, still in her soft voice, mixed now with a bit of surprise.

"Daddy's not gonna like this, Alton," she said, looking down at me, still clutching my trusty hatchet. She thought for a moment, then finally said, "Let's not say anything. I'll fix it. Now, you go put your hatchet back in the garage, and get ready for supper."

Sensing that perhaps what I had done, I should not have done, it was several days before I got up the nerve to venture to that part of the yard. And when I finally arrived at the scene of the crime, there they were, two fenceposts that looked a lot newer than the others holding up the fence. Doc told me years later that mama had told him and Kenny, and the two boys had taken the wood saw, and had one of Doc's high school buddies drive them to the country to relieve some unsuspecting farmer of a young pine tree.

Late afternoon on a dreary, cold Saturday, February 9, 1946 found me in my warm woolen coat and red woolen toboggan, as we called those caps in that era, kneeling on the sidewalk in front of our house, flailing away determinedly at the edge of the concrete sidewalk with my favorite hatchet. Mama had just fed me some hot buttered biscuits she had made but a few minutes earlier, bundled me up and let me out to play while she took care of baby Pete, preparing his bath in front of the pot-bellied coal stove in the front bedroom.

The stillness of that late afternoon, my concentration on the task at hand-indeed my life as I knew and enjoyed it-was shattered forever by three rapid shots of gunfire. Being unable to localize the sounds, and assuming it did not concern me, I had just raised my hatchet for another determined strike at the pesky concrete sidewalk, when mama's piercing, hysterical screams burst from the front bedroom of our house.

Youthful curiosity segued into concern for mama, and, still clutching my hatchet, I walked around the house to the dogtrot, up the four well-worn wooden steps, and carefully opened the door leading to the back bedroom.

There on the opposite side of the room lay my daddy, sprawled grotesquely across the bed, his expressionless face turned toward me, blood flowing from a small hole in his forehead and from the corner of his mouth. Immediately a knot of apprehension gripped my throat; I tried to swallow but was unable to do so. The scene momentarily numbed my senses.

Desperately, my infantile mind sought to splice together into some sense of logic, my motorcycle buddy, my entire life's stabilizing force, with the same being lying motionless on the bed in the semidarkness.

When pint-sized Bob Steele shot Black Bart at the Saturday matinee, the gunshot was more muffled than the three sounds I had just heard, and Black Bart did not bleed. However, here before my eyes was blood, appearing bright red even in the fading afternoon light streaming into the bedroom window.

Being unacquainted with death, I stood transfixed in the doorway, listening to mama's convulsive sobs, grasping firmly my hatchet handle, staring into my daddy's unblinking eyes. Suddenly, my frail chest tightened, tears welled up in my confused eyes and I could not stay the flow of emotion. Finally Doc, who had been trying unsuccessfully to calm my frenetic mother, appeared in the doorway before me, holding my daddy's pearl-handled revolver down by his side.

Defensively, I raised my hatchet, pointing the sharp cutting edge at my older brother. For the first time in my life, I experienced fear. I was six years old. But Doc, who was himself only fourteen years old, lay the revolver on the floor beside him, calmly knelt before me, slowly took the hatchet from my tight grasp, and said,

"It's okay now son, everything's going to work out for us." And my older brother held me close, both of us sobbing uncontrollably at our loss. From that day forward, until he died in 1993 at the age of 62, Doc always called me "son." Whatever his reason for referring to me as "son" and not "Al," Doc confided to me two months before his death that my daddy undoubtedly accepted me as his favorite among his seven children. My daddy died on February 9, 1946. My brother Doc, ironically, died on the same date in 1993.

The front page of the Monday, February 11, 1946 issue of the Kinston *Daily Free Press* devoted equal space to three news stories. The headline of the leftmost article read "Firing Squad to Execute Homma," referring to the military courts martial death sentence of the Japanese general who, in the early days of World War II, had led his forces in the capture of Corregidor. A United States military commission's verdict held General Homma directly responsible for the murder and torture of more than eighty thousand U.S. and Philippine war prisoners.

The center headline announced, "Stalin is Unanimously Elected Soviet Leader." The article noted that "Premier (Joseph) Stalin was elected unanimously to the Supreme Soviet," but added also that "Voters had no choice of candidates." In a pre-election campaign rally held in Moscow, Stalin blamed World War II on the excesses of capitalism, while disclosing the formation of a new five-year plan which included giant increases in production and improved living conditions."

The rightmost of the three articles announced, "Youth is Held in Local Slaying," and related how fourteen-year-old Norwood Provost had slain his father Benjamin, "a local merchant and civil service employee," at their home, 208 East Bright Street, on February 9, 1946.

The article went on to relate that funeral services for my daddy would be held that day at 2:00 p.m., and that a coroner's inquest would be held at City Hall at 7:30 p.m. Tuesday, February 12, 1946. The story added that my daddy had been a refrigeration engineer at Cherry Point, and that Norwood was a student at Grainger High School in Kinston.

Wheeler Kennedy, a Kinston policeman and friend of the family, arrested Doc shortly after Daddy was killed, but the police released my brother into mama's care later that same day.

At 2:00 p.m. on Monday, February 11, 1946, more than a hundred mourners gathered at Maplewood Cemetery in Kinston to pay their respects to my daddy. I stood silently with Doc and mama as the Episcopal pastor delivered a heartfelt eulogy, praising my daddy for his overall devotion to his family, his kindness shown to others less fortunate than our family, and the prayer that our large family could remain intact.

I loved my daddy so very much, and at the age of six could not even begin to come to terms with the fact that I never would see him after that day. Mama held up during most of the graveside service, but had to be helped to the car by Doc and J.B. She dearly loved my daddy, and until her death sixteen years later continued to speak lovingly of the life she had shared with "Bennie."

I found myself in a state of mild shock, overwhelmed by the solemnity of the ceremony, the stillness of the cloudy, cold February afternoon as I stood silently between Doc and mama, watching as my daddy's casket was lowered slowly into the ground. My innocent mind was assailed by the permanence of the closing of the casket, the finality of the ceremony. I had lost my daddy, my protector, my very best friend. I would grow up without his love, without his laughter; no more motorcycle rides through the streets of Kinston, no more weekend trips to granddaddy's cabin in Swansboro, no more greeting him with laughter and recognition as we met on the East Bright Street sidewalk on his return from Cherry Point after work each day. It was a tragic day for a young child of six.

On that awful day, I was overwhelmed by the foreignness of the hushed voices around me. My fragile mind was assailed by the significance of the closed casket. At age six I was most unfamiliar with death. Half a century later, still I am not familiar with death. My daddy's funeral was the first, and last, such morbid ceremony I have ever attended.

Mama, J.B., Doc, Bill and Kenny have all passed away since that day, and I have been unable to bring myself to suffer the unbearable depression occasioned by witnessing, at age six, my daddy's casket being swallowed up forever by the cold, damp earth. And I have requested in writing that my children not attend my funeral.

Guy Elliott, an attorney, mayor of Kinston and a close family friend, became Doc's attorney. At the inquest held the day after my daddy's funeral, testimony from neighbors and policemen who knew our family well, testified that on occasion my daddy, when intoxicated, had become threatening and abusive to mama. The general feeling was that Doc had acted in the defense of mama, but the findings of the inquest were inconclusive, and a disposition of the case was suspended pending additional testimony.

Initially there appeared to be sufficient evidence to support a finding of justifiable homicide. However, my daddy's sister Georgia was a registered nurse, living in Wilson, North Carolina and working at a local hospital, at the time of my daddy's death. Georgia and my daddy had been very close since childhood, and Georgia had taken my daddy's side in his squabbles with their brother Gilbert.

Incensed at what she believed to be an affront to her deceased brother's character and memory, Georgia hired a local attorney, who pressed the District Attorney to indict Doc for daddy's murder. Aunt Georgia's attorney was successful in convincing the Lenoir County grand jury to indict Doc for murder, and trial was set for June 25, 1946 in Lenoir County Superior Court.

An article on the front page of the Wednesday, June 26, 1946 Kinston *Daily Free Press* announced "Provow Trial is Opened in Court." The article reported that "the morning session was taken up with the selection of the jury and hearing of defense witnesses." Defense witnesses "without exception attested to the good character of the defendant and to the violent nature and high temper of the deceased, especially when under the influence of alcoholic beverages."

The trial lasted two full days, and I sat silently with mama, Eoline and my brothers in a standing-room only packed courtroom, listening to the state's solicitor question many state's witnesses as to the good character and lack of violence on the part of my daddy, clearly refuting the testimony offered by witnesses for the defendant, my brother Doc.

And during these two long days of testimony I relived my six years of life with my daddy. To me he was the person the state's witnesses represented him to be. He was loving, and kind, and helpful to others. He was my very best friend, and I missed him terribly.

Sitting there in the cold, unfriendly courtroom, my young mind was bombarded with vignettes of life with my family, of moments of joy and togetherness. Yet the discrepancies between my daddy's relationship with me and the manner in which he was characterized at Doc's trial crept ominously into my consciousness, nagging doubts that refused to fade away, that refused to be locked away in the inaccessible recesses of my memory, wrenching at my past. My mind declined to winnow out the illogical; perhaps the logical was the truth?

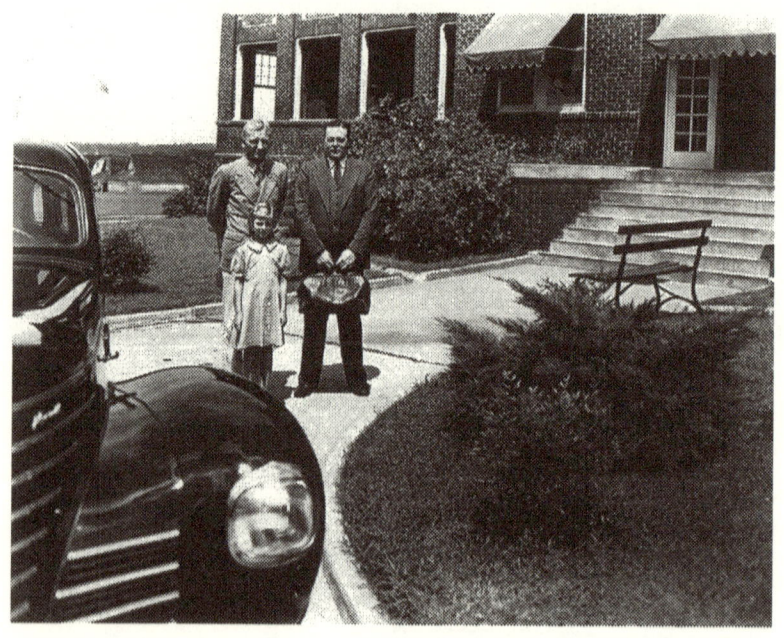

1947. Unidentified "new" girl upon her arrival at Hicks Memorial Hospital. On left Mr. Regan, on right Dr. Rives Taylor. The author's foiled escape attempt was made from the porch behind the two men.

The state's attorney had declined to charge Doc with First Degree Murder; but Doc had gone to trial on a charge of Second Degree Murder, to which Doc pled not guilty. After all the evidence had been heard before the twelve-man jury, neither Doc's attorney Guy Elliott, nor the state's attorney, felt certain of a verdict. There were as many witnesses attesting to my daddy's good character and love for his family as there were to his bad character. If the state had called little Cottontop to the witness stand, my brother would have gone to prison. Never in my six years had I ever seen my daddy strike mama, or yell at her or in any way mistreat any member of my family. It just did not happen.

In conference prior to the case going to the jury, Doc's attorney proposed that Doc plead "no contest" to the lesser charge of manslaughter, with the understanding that Judge Thompson would suspend the sentence and place Doc on probation, thus leaving Doc free to work and help take care of the family. The state's attorney accepted the plea bargain, the judge approved it, and the final judgment of the court was read aloud in open court by Judge Thompson:

> "*Judgment.* Let the defendant be imprisoned in the State's prison for a period of not less than seven (7) nor more than ten (10) years. Prison sentence suspended and defendant placed on probation for five years under the Supervision of the Welfare Board of Lenoir County until he arrives at the age of sixteen, and then the balance of his term of probation under the supervision of the Probation Department of the State, upon the terms and conditions set forth in the probation order."

I did not understand the words "suspended" or "probation," but did know the meaning of "prison" and "seven years" and "ten years," and upon hearing those words I began sobbing. But Judge Thompson had adjourned the court, and immediately Doc left the defense table, came over and knelt down in front of me and held me real close to him.

"I'm not going anywhere, son. I'm going to take care of you and mama. I'm sorry for what I did. But don't you worry about a thing." Then my brother took me by the hand and led me out of the courtroom. He was free.

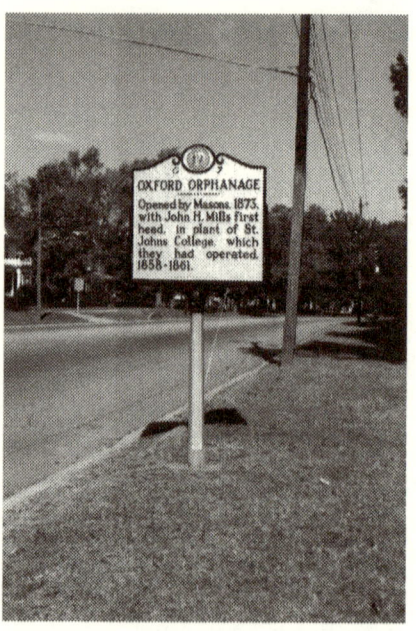

Oxford Orphanage historical marker, located on College Street near the orphanage Main Gate.

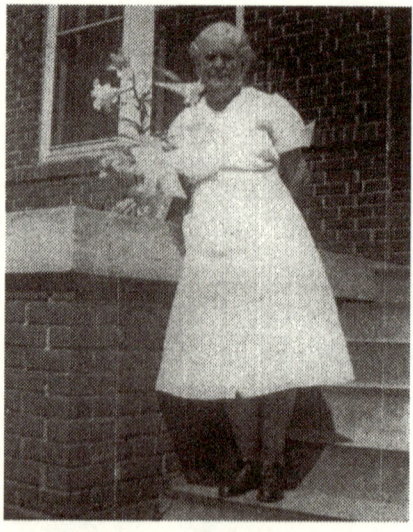

Mrs. Edith Scott Tomblin, Nurse, Hicks Memorial Hospital, 1942-1953

The June 27, 1946 headline in the Kinston *Daily Free Press* announced "Provow Draws a Suspended Term," thereby closing the chapter on the first, and happiest, part of my life.

But the Judgment itself was suspended without comment by Judge Thompson. Doc never spent one day of supervision. A month after the trial Guy Elliott, mama's close friend and advisor to the family, told Doc it would be best if Doc left town. Doc took his attorney at his word, left Kinston and moved to Washington, D.C. In 1943 my uncle Sam Thomas, mama's brother, had left Kinston for the nation's capitol, where he started Thomas Painting, Inc., a housepainting and wallpapering company. Doc realized his action in defending mama, resulting in daddy's death, was a stigma that would seriously limit his ability to earn enough money to support our family, so when Guy Elliott gave my brother the Southern version of the "get out of Dodge" message, uncle Sam Thomas offered Doc a job at Thomas Painting.

A year after Doc moved to Washington, D.C., uncle Sam offered Doc a full share of the business, and in 1947 the two formed Provost and Thomas, Inc. Doc and Sam operated their successful enterprise until 1964, at which time they sold the company and moved to West Palm Beach, Florida. Doc became a licensed Realtor, a profession he practiced until his death in 1993.

Beginning with his first paycheck from uncle Sam in 1946, Doc sent mama a portion of his earnings each week. He continued to bear the responsibility for mother's care until her death of a stroke on February 26, 1962.

So this is how I came to be riding through a freezing rain, on the road with my two jovial, boisterous, talkative and friendly traveling companions, Harsh and Subservient. Not really. Now, because I was coming from a famous town, and headed in the direction of another (slightly less) famous town, let me tell you how these two towns came to be.

A Tale of Two Towns

We could begin our story at any point along the time line that we desire. But let us choose as our beginning, the period before the birth of our nation, and before the founding of the two towns that influenced directly the first two decades of my life. It is often said among persons who profess to having expertise on the subject, that in reality, heaven is a place on earth called North Carolina, and that long before that lovely land was called "The Old North State" or "The Tarheel State," it was known as "God's Country." God bless North Carolina and its good people!

Extending into the eighteenth century, in that expansive wilderness of longleaf pine and native Indians, the custom/policy of English land grant proprietors was to allow formation of new counties as the slowly-expanding population would support the need for governing bodies. Thus large counties yielded their land to the emergence of new, smaller counties, which is how Granville County came into existence.

In 1663, King Charles II granted a charter to eight English gentlemen who had helped him regain the throne of England. These men of means were known as the "Eight Lord Proprietors." The territory over which they were given control was named Carolina in honor of Charles the First. Between 1663 and 1729, what is today North Carolina remained under the control of the Lord Proprietors and their descendants, one of whom was Sir George Carteret.

In 1729, seven of the Lord Proprietors sold their interests in North Carolina to the Crown, and North Carolina became a royal colony. The eighth proprietor, John Carteret (Lord Granville) retained economic interest and continued granting land in the northern half of North Carolina. Until 1775 all political functions were under the supervision of the Crown. On April 12, 1776, North Carolina authorized delegates to the Continental Congress to vote for independence from England. This was the first official action by a colony calling for independence. William Hooper, Joseph Hewes and John Penn were the delegates/terrorists from North Carolina who signed the Declaration of Independence.

On November 21, 1789 the State adopted the new Constitution, becoming the twelfth state to enter the federal union. North Carolina seceded from this union called the United States on May 20, 1861. During the Civil War North Carolina supplied more men and materiel to the Confederate cause than any other state. The state also suffered the largest number of losses than any other state during the War Against

Northern Aggression. It is best I let you know just where my sympathies lie, from the beginning.

Like most of North Carolina, in the seventeenth and eighteenth centuries and before, the land that is now Granville County was populated by Indian tribes, mainly the Tuscarora. Following the Tuscarora War of 1711, settlers from Virginia began to move into that area, drawn by the fertile land and plentiful water supply.

Most of the land in the northern half of North Carolina bordering Virginia was the proprietary domain of Lord John Carteret, whose title was Earl of Granville. In 1746 the local populace separated itself from western Edgecombe County and became the independent Granville county. The settlement called Oxford was made the county seat in 1811, and in 1816 the town was incorporated. In like manner, as time passed, and the population expanded, Granville County yielded land to form Orange (1752), Bute (1764) and Vance (1881) counties.

In 1761 Samuel Benton, Granville County's State Assembly representative, purchased a thousand acres of land and built a plantation, that he named "Oxford." In 1764 the State Assembly ordered that the area be known as the county seat, and Benton donated one acre of land for the construction of a county courthouse.

In 1811 the State Assembly authorized the county to purchase fifty acres around the courthouse from Thomas Littlejohn, and officials began laying out the town, selling lots at public auction in 1812. The town of Oxford was incorporated in 1816. Granville County produced several influential patriots/terrorists during colonial and revolutionary times. John Penn, a landowner in what is today Stovall, was elected in 1775 to be a member of the Continental Congress. He was one of North Carolina's three signers of the Declaration of Independence.

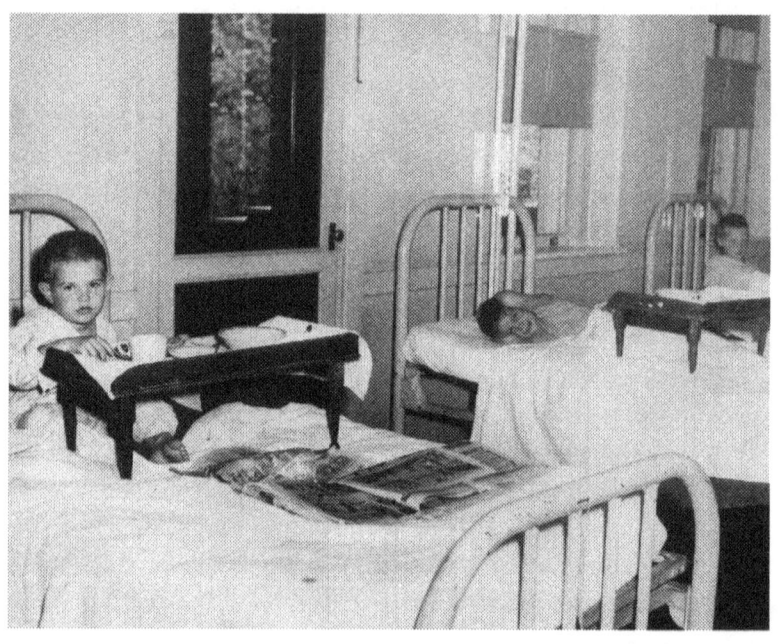

1947. Hospital first floor boys' ward. The author's midnight escape attempt was through these two doors, on February 15, 1947.

In Durham County in northeast-central North Carolina, the Flat and Eno rivers merge to form the broad and deep Neuse River. Named for the Neusiok Indians, the river meanders slowly for about three hundred miles in a southeasterly direction toward the Atlantic Ocean. The Neuse becomes navigable as it flows generally southeast past Kinston, the county seat of Lenoir County.

In 1740 William Heritage founded a planters' trading post on the Neuse River, and the fast-growing settlement was incorporated as Kingston in 1762. The town prospered and, following the Revolutionary War, zealous patriots, in a fitting show of disdain for their former English rulers and King George III in particular, reincorporated the town, dropping the "g" (and by now the despised King George III) to give us "Kinston."

Kinston's north-south main street was appropriately named Queen Street, and was bisected in the center of town by King Street. Richard Caswell, the first governor of North Carolina, lived in Kinston, and was one of the town's original trustees. He served two terms as governor, the first from 1776 to 1780, and again from 1784 to 1787.

The "Neuse," a Confederate ironclad gunboat better known as a "ram," was constructed in Kinston. The boat was sunk by its crew in 1865, as fierce fighting between Union and Confederate forces raged in and around Kinston. The Neuse's hull was raised in 1963, and the boat has been designated a state historic site.

Lenoir County was created in 1791 from the old Dobbs County. It was named in honor of William Lenoir, a hero of the Battle of Kings Mountain. When Kinston was established in 1762, it was still in Dobbs County. It became the county seat of Dobbs County in 1764, and when Lenoir County was formed in 1791, Kinston became the county seat of Lenoir County.

Several decisive Civil War battles were fought in and around Kinston, which was a strategic railway depot on the way to the important Confederate naval base at Wilmington. In December 1862 a Union Army force composed of 10,000 infantry, 640 Cavalry and 40 light artillery pieces under the command of Major General John G. Foster, defeated the Confederate forces at Kinston, and control of the city changed hands several times after that date. In March 1865, during the final Union Army assault on Wilmington, General William T. Sherman's army of 80,000 men defeated the forces of Confederate General Braxton Bragg and General Robert F. Hoke, forcing the Confederate forces to abandon Kinston.

Anyway, now you know where we came from and where we are headed. Didn't do too well against them Yankees, did we? Well, to get on with my glorious arrival. Sure wish it would stop raining, though.

CHAPTER 2

My Arrival

Ominous black clouds shadowed our black Ford sedan during the four-hour journey from Kinston, through Goldsboro, then Raleigh and Durham, and the little spit on the road called Creedmoor. The rain storm had intensified by the time we arrived at our destination in mid-afternoon. We passed through the center of a town somewhat smaller than Kinston, then along a residential area with wide streets, finally turning right between two square red brick columns.

We were now on what I learned later was called the Main Road, that ran for about a city block from the Main Gate to the Main Building, an imposing red brick four-story structure nearly a hundred years old at the time of my arrival at Oxford. Again without comment, bespectacled Harsh steered the big automobile to the left in front of the Main Building, then down a winding street past a small two-story red brick building on our right, coming to a stop in a semi-circular driveway in front of an equally imposing red brick four-story building.

Harsh braked the car on the driveway in front of steep concrete steps, at the top of which stood two large oak doors. Leaving Subservient Lady in Black seated in the car, Harsh addressed me for the only time during the trip.

"Come on, Alton, let's run for it."

I opened the car door, slammed it behind me, and skedaddled up the concrete steps still clutching my second grade report card. Upon entering the building, Mr. Harsh Man gestured with a wave of his hand toward a large white chair in the corner of the waiting room. I sat. I had finally arrived at the first challenge in my ten-year odyssey into Hell, the William J. Hicks Memorial Hospital.

"Wait here, Alton," he said, and walked through an open door into a small room just off the waiting room. The door closed behind him. I waited.

Sitting quietly alone on the soft-cushioned wing chair, my first pangs of misgivings began to creep into my consciousness. While not rising quite to the level of panic, my childish measurement of "real soon" as promised by mama had reached its outer limit about two hours after the big black Ford pulled away from the hatchet-chipped curb at 208 East Bright Street. During the entire three or so hour trip neither Harsh nor Subservient had spoken a word to me, nor had either of them smiled when they addressed one another. We could have been easily part of a Southern funeral procession. Perhaps we were. Little Alton's?

Suddenly I recalled how sad mama had appeared that morning; her red eyes announcing she had cried during the night. A lot. My puerile mind began to equate these signs with "ominous," though I couldn't even spell the word. And everything I noticed about the absolute quiet engulfing me was foreboding and inhospitable-the white walls, the white chairs, the white table on which rested a large white ceramic lamp, the white ceiling; everything was stark white and most unfriendly, and carried with it a repugnant odor of cleaning solvent that permeated the waiting room. Suddenly I wanted to go home. Right now. Immediately. Time's up. I want mama. End of outing. "Real soon" had arrived with great finality. Time to pick up my jacks and go home.

Presently the door through which Mr. Harsh Man had disappeared opened, and Harsh emerged, having grown no smile in his brief absence, and as he turned to his left just prior to exiting the front door of the hospital, met my innocent, steady, inquiring gaze with what I was able to characterize only as a look of absolute and total indifference. I would later describe his gaze as uncommunicative, and for all practical purposes, this most unfriendly of grownups just as well could have been looking through me as at me.

After a fleeting moment he broke off his stare, and departed the hospital. I felt as though he had intended to speak, then changed his mind. I did not like this unfriendly man. We would meet again. Our relationship would be fraught with fear, loathing and animosity.

My decision to end my little day-trip was halted abruptly when the door through which Harsh disappeared opened, and a stern-faced squat woman emerged.

Instinctively I arose as the large, thick-legged woman approached me, the "swish-swish . . . swish-swish" of the rubbing together of her white nylons announcing her presence in the small room. Here was that depressing "white" again. Scowl wore mostly white, with white stockings, a starched white dress, and a white cap perched atop totally white hair. Even her complexion was white. And she was not smiling. The third unsmiling grownup I had encountered that day. Not a positive sign.

As I was to painfully discover before the next day dawned, only two things about Mrs. Edith Scott Tomblin were black-her men's leather shoes, and her heart. Her snow-white, '20's style hairdo was cut short, with a permanent wave. She wore her all-white nurses' uniform mid-calf, and it was so starched it appeared as if she were surrounded from the waist down by a white teepee. She reminded me at once of a scowling cartoon vulture perched threateningly atop the limb of a rotting pine tree. Even her accusatory glare appeared as though her face had been starched and pressed simultaneously with her uniform.

Suddenly we had approached the "panic" stage in our little excursion. Perhaps I could cut short what was fast developing into a spiraling disagreeable situation. So, before the All-White Woman could speak, I looked up into her unfriendly eyes and blurted out,

"I want to go home now."

She stopped short, apparently taken aback at my boldness. Recovering quickly, she returned my stare and addressed me with an air of aloofness and finality.

"You can't go home."

"But my mama said I could go home anytime I want to," I lied.

"But you don't live with your mother anymore. You live in the orphanage now. This is your home from now on."

Suddenly I felt light-headed. I just stared up at her. My world crumbled around me. I could not comprehend what was happening to me. I began to cry softly.

During the year since my daddy's tragic death, mama had become my lighthouse, my port in any storm, my protector. Never had I been away from her at night. She had always been there for me. And when I left home that morning, she did not-and of course, thinking back on that horrible day years later, could not-tell me the truth, that is, that never again would I be under her care and protection. My first life was ending on a cold, rainy mid-afternoon in February 1947, without doubt the saddest day of my life.

Suddenly I did not like the Mean White Woman. Her threatening voice heightened my fear of the dispirited predicament into which I had been so rudely thrust. Suddenly and harshly, mama's shield against the uncertainties of my already disrupted young life had been cruelly ripped away, abruptly replaced by a child's confusing and immature doubts of a mother's love. It seemed to me in that moment of confusion and despair, that if mama really loved me, she would not have sent me to this awful place.

Embarrassed and humiliated, I stood consciously trembling before the White woman, my fragile psyche absorbing just the first of a series of assaults. More would soon follow. Many more.

Sensing another presence in the small waiting room, I turned toward the inner doorway. There stood a young girl, about sixteen years old, gazing silently down at me. Her understanding and empathy for my situation were at once apparent in the way she looked at me. She was not smiling. The look in her eyes conveyed at that very moment the message-I, too, once stood where you now stand, I understand your feelings of fear and utter despair, and I will help you get through this.

My sobbing was interrupted by the young girl's soft, comforting, almost imploring voice.

"Mrs. Tomblin, maybe if I took him to get something to eat . . ."

With a sense of relief apparent in her voice, the White Scary Lady who, I suddenly discovered, was not really named Mrs. White, or Mrs. Hateful, or Mrs. Idontlikeyou, but apparently "Mrs. Tomblin," stated,

"Okay, Ann, get him cleaned up, then get him a big bowl of custard from the kitchen."

Then, turning to look down at the pitiable sight before her, Mrs. Tomblin said,

"Alton, go with Ann and get yourself cleaned up. Maybe you'll feel better after some custard."

Yeah, whatever that is. Eat custard. Feel better. I could hardly wait. Like, like maybe I'll eat that stupid custard, and never want to go home again. Fat chance, lady.

Ann came over to me, gently placed her (warm) hand on my shoulder, and steered me from the (white) waiting room, and more importantly, out of the presence of the unpleasant White Lady called Mrs. Tomblin.

Turning left down a short hallway (with Ann still steering me with that very warm hand on my shoulder), we entered a spacious, long white-walled (yes, white) room with two rows of white metal-framed beds, covered by white cotton sheets and brown Army blankets, and pillows sheathed in white cotton pillow cases. All the beds were empty.

Ann steered me to the right and into a smaller white room in which was located a long white table around which stood two white wooden chairs, and a small recessed area used for hanging clothes. At the far end of the room a doorway opened into a small bathroom containing a large (white) porcelain-covered sink and bathtub.

Opening a cabinet above the sink, Ann took out a washrag and a towel, handing them to me. She sure was pretty. I hadn't seen my sister Eoline in a coon's age, and I had just been told that I might not see mama until halfway through the next millennium, and I suppose that at that moment of despair, I just needed some older female to comfort me. Suddenly I thought about asking Ann if she could be my sister. Maybe later.

"Come on. Let's find you a bed, and you can keep these for your bath tonight. I'll get you some pajamas after supper."

Back out in the large room of beds, Ann explained,

"This is the 'boys' ward. Across the hall is a room just like this called the 'girls' ward. Nobody is sick now, so you'll be by yourself tonight. Let's go down to the kitchen and Mrs. Londeree will get us some custard." There was that magical word "custard" again. But I was a smart seven-year-old kid. I knew when I was being bribed. I just couldn't figure out, though, how those biguns tricked me into this journey into Hell. So maybe I wasn't such a smart kid after all.

We exited the boys' ward, turned left at the main hallway, and followed the wide hallway covered with a black rubber runner, for nearly the length of the large hospital, where we turned left into a spacious kitchen, in the center of which was situated a large white table surrounded by six wooden chairs.

Upon entering the kitchen, a pleasant woman (not dressed in white, what a relief) turned from the stove where she was slowly stirring something in a large silver pot, smiled warmly at me and said,

"Who do we have here, Ann?"

Then she turned to me and said,

"I'm Mrs. Londeree. You must be the new boy, Alton. My, you look just like your sister."

Upon hearing the words "your sister," I was filled immediately with mixed feelings of elation and concern. Was my sister here in the hospital? Was Eoline presently being held against her will in the girls' ward? I knew only that I had not seen my sister for a long time. Unbeknownst to me, Eoline had been sent to the orphanage in July 1946, six months after my daddy died. With rising concern in my voice, I asked Mrs. Londeree,

"Where is my sister? Is she here? I want to see her now."

Dear, kind-hearted Mrs. Londeree. The surprised look on Ann's face told me that Mrs. Londeree had spoken out of turn. It was the policy of the orphanage administration to quarantine the "new" inmates for a period of one week, before releasing them to the general prison population. This restriction ensured that the "new" child did not have any communicable diseases such as chicken pox, mumps, measles, etc., that he or she might pass on to the other children. This amount of time was also required to administer to the child the required inoculations, undergo a thorough dental checkup, and be fitted with the appropriate clothing and shoes.

Quite a few children in the orphanage had several brothers and sisters with them. However, for the reasons enumerated just above, the orphanage supervisors could allow no contact, even with siblings, during this period of quarantine, and the general policy of the orphanage staff was to avoid any mention of siblings to the "new" children.

However, Mrs. Londeree had let the cat out of the bag, and when she did not respond to my questions, suddenly gripped by panic and with a hard lump forming in my throat, I turned to Ann.

"Where is she, Ann? Where is my sister? Why can't I see her now?"

I could not suppress the sudden surge of frustration and helplessness gripping me in that instant, and the rapid rush of tears filling my eyes blurred my vision. Never having experienced such emotional trauma, and enveloped suddenly in a cloud of mixed emotions, I just sat down on the floor of the kitchen and cried.

In the short span of four hours my protected, sheltered world, anchored by my mother's love, had been transformed beyond my control into a world of doubt, distrust and helplessness. In an instant, I had found myself under the control of seemingly cruel and uncaring adults whom I simultaneously disliked and feared.

Ann knelt down and helped me to my feet.

"Let's go to the playroom," she said quietly. I recall thinking at that moment, about forty tons of trauma dumped on me, and she wants to go to the *playroom*? I didn't want to *play* anything. I just wanted to get the hell out of this horrible place, and get back to 208 East Bright Street muy pronto.

Ann led me by the hand from the kitchen, where we turned right and walked along the wide hallway toward the front of the hospital. Shortly we turned left into a small room that contained a few toys and a Monopoly board game on a low coffee table in the middle of the room. Ann did not switch on the lights, and we sat on a large cloth-covered couch at one end of the room, in the ambient light of that cloudy, depressing Winter afternoon. Holding one of my trembling hands in her warm hands, she quietly and calmly explained to me that my sister was safe, that she knew Eoline quite well, and she tried to explain to me in a logical manner the reasons for me being kept separated from Eoline for awhile.

"Tell you what I'll do, Alton. If you promise to keep it our secret, in a few days I'll go get Eoline and bring her right outside here," she said, pointing to one of the large windows in the room.

"Just let me find the right time to get her here, and don't tell anybody about it. Can you do that?"

The huge lump in my throat, together with my sense of shame and embarrassment, would not allow me to voice a reply, so I slowly nodded in agreement thanks and understanding.

"It will soon be time for supper. Do you want to eat with us?"

I quickly shook my head. In that moment of utter despair and humiliation I did not relish the thought of sitting at a table in the presence of the dreaded White Monster, Mrs. Tomblin.

"I understand. If you want, you can stay here for awhile, and when it's supper time I'll bring you something to eat. Will you be okay?"

Still staring down at the floor, I nodded slowly. Perhaps I was not going to get that custard after all?

Ann departed, leaving me sitting alone in the semi-dark room, a virtual prisoner. For the first time in my young life, I was completely out of touch with my mother, with no one to turn to for comfort, solace or security. Mrs. Tomblin's earlier caustic rebuke continued to ring in my ears,

". . . You don't live with your mother anymore. You live in the orphanage now . . ."

I became emotionally overwhelmed with a foreboding, naked vulnerability, and my puerile mind was unable to assimilate the stark reality of my predicament. For in my despondency, it seemed as though the maw of hell had opened to devour me. In those moments of confusion, images of my family members flashed suddenly before me-daddy, Doc, J.B., mama, Eoline, Kenny, Bill, even baby Pete and my gray shorthaired cat that I had refused to name because I like the "ring" of the name "cat." I mentally scanned those closest to me-seeking out comfort and guidance. But none was forthcoming. I had not seen daddy for the longest time (he had died a year earlier), and my older brothers had all moved away from home. My mind's photograph of baby Pete showed mama carrying him in her arms. Certainly no help there. Through an agonizing mental process of elimination, my sister suddenly became my emotional savior, the wellspring of my continued sanity. She was nearby. She was family. She was contact with my past life.

Half a century later I still cannot find the words that adequately convey to a non-orphan the range of emotions that literally overwhelmed my fragile being on February 15, 1947. Orphans know. And every Oxford orphan carries with him or her throughout life the unique smell of the Hicks Memorial Hospital's black rubber hallway runners. They smelled like . . . well . . . like cleaning-solvent washed rubber, an odor that even to this day I associate with unpleasant times and equally uncaring people.

Left alone in the mid-afternoon quiet, I stood on the large couch and peered out the high window at the cold rain that had slowed from a driving, wind-swept downpour on my arrival to its present steady drizzle. The largest oak trees I had ever seen rose before me, their impressive twisted tentacles stretching as ominous sentinels guarding the sprawling orphanage campus. In the far distance I observed many lights on in a building that appeared to dwarf in size the building in which I presently was imprisoned.

The bleakness of that eerily serene Winter afternoon was punctuated occasionally by a child scurrying across my field of view on his or her way between the aforementioned multi-lighted monolith and small surrounding buildings. Presently there appeared to my far left a boy of about thirteen walking slowly beside a large brown rain-soaked mule, that was pulling a well-used wagon filled with tall, shiny metal containers.

Based on my limited childhood experience, I assumed this was the orphanage ice wagon, but wondered how they got the ice into the large shiny metal containers, or, for that matter, why someone would want to carry ice in this manner.

My gaze followed the slow-moving wagon along the slightly inclined, one-lane tar and gravel road, where it came to a halt at the base of a long gray stairway at the rear of the large building. After removing the wooden tailgate and placing it on the concrete, the boy lifted a container off the wagonbed and stood it on the ground. After he had placed another container on the concrete, the boy lifted the apparently heavy containers and trudged slowly up the long flight of stairs, stopping at a landing halfway up to set the containers down in order to get a better grip on the handles. The boy wasn't that stout, and the heavy cans (of ice) were giving him a time of it.

By then the boy and his cans (of ice) were out of sight, as the corner of the building blocked my view. However, the boy made five or six trips up the long gray stairway, each trip slower than the preceding one. After delivering the last of the metal cans (of ice), the tired boy replaced the wooden tailgate, led the mule by the bridle in a tight circle and, once he had pointed the mule and wagon in the direction from whence they had come, climbed onto the bed of the wagon and lay down. The driverless-appearing wagon soon disappeared from view as it passed the rear of the hospital.

While still standing on the couch peering out the window, unable to fathom why the boy had carried all that ice in metal containers up that long flight of stairs, and where the mule and wagon without a navigator finally would come to rest, the muffled sound of footsteps caused me to turn, and Ann entered the room carrying a white metal tray on which sat a small plate of food and a large bowl of what I learned was the much-heralded "custard."

Setting the tray of food on the rectangular wooden table in the center of the "playroom," as it was called, Ann looked at me and said,

"When is the last time you ate custard, Alton? I'll bet this will be the best custard you've ever tasted. I'll leave the tray here. Take your time, and I'll come back later."

I tried to eat my first meal in this strange, foreboding place, while sitting in the darkness of that depressingly cold February late afternoon. I nibbled at the food for a minute or so before concluding that whatever appetite I should have had was eclipsed by untold grief and disillusionment. I could not eat. Not even the custard.

Darkness finally fell on my first traumatic day at Oxford Orphanage State Prison, and at around eight o'clock Ann came into the darkened playroom to fetch me.

"It's time for bed, Alton," she said. Gathering up my tray of virtually untouched food, Ann exclaimed, "Oh, you hardly ate anything. You didn't like the food?"

"Not hungry," I explained, hoping she would not press the point about not eating. I just wanted to go home to mama, to leave this horrible nightmare, to make the awful "Mrs. Mean White" Tomblin go away. But that was not going to happen. Ann carried my tray of food into the kitchen and placed it on a counter beside a large sink. Then I followed her down the long hall and entered the boys' ward, at once turning right into the all-white room. The floor was constructed of small white square tiles, the chairs and table were of wood painted white, and the walls were painted an off-white gloss that age and harsh cleaning solvents had yellowed somewhat.

Ann opened the doors of a large white wooden cabinet attached to the wall at one end of the room, took out a white washrag and towel and what appeared to be a girl's nightgown, and handed the articles to me.

"The bathtub is in there," said Ann, pointing to a large white adjoining room. I could see in the room a flush toilet and a deep oblong glazed white tub. On the inside of one end of the tub was attached a short metal spout with a metal handle on each side. Noting that I made no movement toward the bathroom, Ann asked "Do you know how the handles on the tub work, Alton?"

"No," I answered tentatively. "Can you show me?"

The time was February 1947. World War II had ended just eighteen months before. Many children who arrived at Oxford Orphanage during the '30's and '40's never had experienced a bath in hot running water. This was at that time a luxury requiring the installation of a hot water heater, and during the period encompassing the Great Depression and World War II, such a lifestyle was well beyond the means of the average American family.

Thus most of the time while growing up at 208 East Bright Street, mama took me and my sister Eoline once each week to the Simon Bright Apartments where my grandma Thomas lived, and gave us a good bath in hot running water. It was the treat of the week. Aside from that, mama gave me one of those whatchamacallit baths in the large metal pan of hot water, heated from the stove and poured into the pan. No big deal, really. Sure saved on water, and I got just as good a bath as if she had bathed me at grandma's apartment.

Ann instructed me in the operation of bath preparation, advising me that after inserting the rubber stopper into the drain, I should be careful to slowly adjust the hot and cold water handles so as to keep from being scalded when I stepped into the tub. She helped me prepare the bath water, and as she turned to leave me in privacy, she asked, "By the way, Alton, how did you take a bath at home?"

"I had a bath like this once each week at my grandma's apartment, but usually mama gave me a little whore's bath in a big washbowl."

"A little *what?*" Ann asked, laughing, apparently not understanding my comment.

"All I remember is that my daddy or mama would call me at night for mama to give me a bath. She washed me and rinsed me off while I was standing in this big washbowl. Mama called it my bath, but my daddy called it a little whore's bath."

Ann laughed again, though at what I had no idea. Finally she said "From now on, let's just call it a bath. Is that a deal? Don't call it what you just said, because Mrs. Tomblin might get upset with you."

"It's a deal," I responded quizzically. I did not know what Ann meant, but I would do anything to avoid the wrath of the dreaded Hateful Woman in White. So, a "bath" it was. And Ann seemed to really care about me. All of a sudden I got this urge to ask Ann if she could be my sister.

Before my bath Ann asked me to sit on a small stool (white in color) in the middle of the bathroom. Pulling a (white) chair over and seating herself at my back, she draped a white towel over my frail shoulders.

"Before you take a bath, I have to comb out your head, Alton."

I noticed that Ann did not say "hair," but specifically said "head." I didn't understand-not only that, I didn't understand even enough to ask why she had to "comb out my head."

Suddenly I felt Ann pulling a fine-toothed black comb slowly through my hair. After each pass of the comb, she paused and wiped both sides of the comb on the white towel draped across my shoulders. I did not know the reason for this procedure, nor did Ann explain to me what she was doing, but I got the distinct impression she had performed this ritual many times before that night. And what was that white stuff she poured on my head?

Much later I learned that Ann had been combing for what kids called "cooties," and what is more commonly known as "head lice." Anyway, after her task was completed, Ann folded up the white towel and told me I could take my bath. After running the bath water, and without even touching the washrag or soap, I sat reflectively in the silence of the rapidly cooling tub water, desperately trying to come to terms with the strange social and physical environment into which I so rudely had been thrust, and with a ton of confusion, an emotion I could only describe many years later as that of rejection by mama.

Presently my thoughts of home were interrupted by a knock on the door, as Ann asked, "Are you all right in there, Alton?" I quickly dried off, pulled the rubber stopper from the bathtub drain, and put on the silly-looking what could only be described as a little girl's ankle-length cotton nightgown.

As I walked from the bathroom to the outer dressing area, I observed Ann pulling back the covers of the end bed at the far side of the boys' ward. Taking Ann's preparations as a cue that it was bedtime, I moved to the side of the bed closest to her, and she said,

"Okay, Alton, hop up here and I'll tuck you in." When she said "tuck you in" I thought I might instead ask Ann if she could be my mama instead of my sister, because my mama tucked me into bed each night. But I could decide later on that. Better not rush things.

The bed was the standard "hospital" bed of the times, the frame constructed of metal and painted white, and because it was Wintertime, a thick brown woolen "Army" blanket was folded at the foot of the bed. The height of the bed was made for grownups, so in order to get my skinny-assed seven-year-old frame onto the (very) high bed, I literally had to "hop" onto the bed by bending at the knees, then propelling myself upward, which, after hiking up the cumbersome (girl's) nightgown and making several attempts, I succeeded in accomplishing. Apparently Ann's instruction to "hop up here" was not a figure of speech.

The boys' ward contained fourteen hospital beds, seven to a side with a wide passageway between the two rows. The walls were painted off-white, or else age had rendered them thus, and the floors were stained hardwood. At the time of my arrival at the orphanage, heat was supplied to the hospital and some of the buildings on campus by means of steam radiators. During the Summer months "air conditioning" consisted of simply opening the windows to create a cross-breeze.

The brown woolen blankets were stamped "U.S." on one side in bold black letters. They were U.S. surplus from World War II, and the children referred to these very warm, very itchy blankets only as "Army" blankets. Once I was settled on the high bed, Ann fluffed the large pillow, I slipped under the top sheet and white cotton bedspread, and Ann pulled the Army blanket up to my chin.

"I'm going to study now," Ann said. "I'll look in on you later."

"You promise?"

"Yes, I promise. Now try to sleep."

But I couldn't. Fear of what misfortunes the next day might bring, coupled with my inability to comprehend mama's apparent acquiescence in allowing me to be sent to this frightful hell Mrs. Tomblin called the "orphanage," kept sleep at bay. Instead of experiencing a merciful sleep, in my state of despair I began to sob quietly into my pillow. Or at least I thought I was sobbing quietly. Perhaps not, however.

Suddenly I felt a large hand grip my shoulder, and turning abruptly I saw through tear-filled vision the blurred form of Mrs. Tomblin's body contrasted against the soft background glow of the light from the outer hallway. Certainly a devil masquerading as an angel.

"Young man," her stern, even voice began, never once loosening the iron grip on my frail shoulder. "You are not in your home now, and I'm not going to put up with your whining. Now go to sleep, or I'll give you the whipping of your life."

I held my breath, petrified with fear, not daring to move a muscle. And why did she call me "young man?"

After a few moments Mrs. Tomblin released her vise grip on my shoulder, and without another word, turned and walked out of the ward, the dissonant clicking of her heels hitting the polished hardwood floor and the swish-swish sound of her nylon hose covering her thick legs rubbing together, the clicking and swishing thankfully becoming fainter with each departing step.

I lay still, intimidated, fearing the awful Mrs. Tomblin would decide at any moment to return and carry out her announced threat. For the first seven years of my life I had been blessed with the love and care of my parents. The only time I could remember getting a "whipping," if one could really stretch the old imagination and elevate the incident to a whipping, was when, as a twerp of five years, I observed one day a stray dog in our front yard, coaxed the friendly mongrel into our garage, and secretly locked "my" dog in for the night.

An hour or so after bedtime, no doubt from hunger (It never occurred to me that you had to feed a pet), the unfortunate creature began barking incessantly. Upon discovering that it was I who had locked the poor thing in the garage, and being told defiantly that I had no intention of releasing "my" dog, mama effected a quick release of the hungry animal with a few strokes of a handful of birch switches across my bare legs. So much for "my" dog. They'll never make a picture show of that, thanks to mama.

The hospital seemed shrouded in a heavy February stillness. The huge building was such a lonely and ominous place, that only served to evoke further apprehension on my part.

The spaciousness of the boys' ward and the great height of the white-painted metal hospital bed with curved bedsteads, lent a Spartan atmosphere to the room. The sense that, even on such an expansive campus, I still felt as though being trapped in a small cage, was a feeling that was to remain with me for several years. The eerily tomblike atmosphere of the hospital, and the gagging smell of strong cleaning solvents on the rubber hallway runners only added to my depression that first day.

The only illumination of the cavernous boys' ward came from the incandescence emitted by the lone low-wattage streetlight being thrown softly through the bank of high front windows, casting odd-shaped moving shadows on the cream-colored wall opposite my bed, these dancing phantoms shifting with the change of direction of the wind in the cold outside.

There were no patients in the boys' ward with me on the day of my arrival, so Ann had assigned me the first bed closest to the entrance of the ward, on the side toward the front of the building. Between the first two beds, a door opened onto a large concrete-and-brick covered porch. Lying beneath the thick woolen Army blanket, sobbing quietly in twenty percent grief and heartache, and eighty percent outright fear for my life, I suddenly had the urge to get the hell out of this awful place, this prison, this cage, to flee from this hateful, threatening Old White Witch with the scowling face.

Because I was only seven years old and this escape thingy was not exactly everyday stuff for me, I had not planned the second stage of my Midnight Getaway from Hell-where to go after I made my successful escape from Hicks Memorial Hospital. But first things first-I'd work out the details as I went along. The first response to life-threatening danger is to run away, as fast as possible. This was my simple plan. Recalling the event years later, I am not certain whether I gave my escape plan much thought actually, but if I did, any debate on the subject must have been short-lived. Freedom and East Bright Street beckoned.

Noiselessly, I slipped from under the warm covers, and stealthily moved toward the bathroom, the creaking of the cold hardwood floor announcing my every step. In the bathroom I quickly and quietly put on my clothes, shoes and coat, then crept back across the creaking floor to the door situated between the two front beds.

I opened first the inner screen door, it in turn proclaiming my actions as though complaining. Either this served intentionally as a security alarm, or nobody ever oiled any hinges in this awful place. The outer door voiced similar objections, but at last I was standing on the cold concrete porch, my slim body rapidly becoming enshrouded in the freezing February night. The Old White Bitch's caustic admonition kept bouncing around in my head like an angry wasp in a closed tin can, "If you don't quiet down . . ."

For a moment I just stood silently on the cold porch, teeth already chattering, goose-bumps galore, freezing my skinny ass while sorting out the best approach to this spontaneous French leave.

Because of my (lack of) height, I was unable to see over the high shrubs located on the outside of the low brick wall, so I climbed up onto the wide brick ledge, and just stood there, gazing out into the cold, dark void of night, uncertain of my next move but determined I would not spend one night in this hell. Somehow I would find my way back to 208 East Bright Street, and safety.

I stood quietly on the brick porch ledge, shuddering from an equal dose of fear and the February night's cold temperature. Since that night I have always thought of fear as a "cold" emotion. An almost indefinable sense of fear of bodily harm shot through my head.

Suddenly I heard the creaking doors quickly open behind me, and turning I saw the White Hound from Hell aggressively waddling toward me across the porch like a two hundred pound enraged duck.

"What are you doing out here, young man?" she screamed, reaching up with her left hand, jerking me clean off the brick porch ledge and onto the floor. Her tone of voice spelled "vehemence" with a capital "V."

Although in my seven brief years I had never been struck in anger by any person, the manner in which the White Bitch angled her body to her left in order to store her bodily energy to gain momentum on the backhand, together with her harsh, threatening, demanding tone of voice, enabled me to anticipate the blow.

However, I would have fared better had I not anticipated her arm coming at my head out of the darkness, for having absolutely no experience at being brutally pummeled, somehow I stupidly turned my face *into* the blow of the flying backhand, and I distinctly heard the sickening *splat!* of the impact of the large hand on my nose.

I was sent sprawling backward, my body hit first the low brick wall of the porch ledge, and I crumpled, dazed and disoriented, onto the concrete floor of the porch. Even before I could cry out in fear and panic, I recall tasting something wet, sticky and slightly salty, that I discovered later was also colored red.

My previously sheltered world was rapidly expanding with new, strange and absolutely unsolicited sensations; I also had never tasted my own blood before that landmark evening.

The vehemence in the old bitch's voice startled me further. An eerie numbness crept through my frail body as I sat silently propped against the wall of the porch, looking up into the darkness at this irritated hulk of a woman. No argument from me. Absolutely. I give up. (For now, at least.) I looked up into her eyes and noticed what could only be described as emptiness, a seeming void of feeling one way or the other, as though this confrontation was but a play being rehearsed over and over again.

"You're not going anywhere, young man, not for a long time," she yelled at me, jerking me by my hair and pulling me to my feet. Then she pushed me back through the doorway and toward the bathroom. I was to discover that "a long time" in my case was ten long years.

"Now take off those clothes and give them to me. The shoes, too," she screamed.

"And wash that blood off your face!" Blood? *My* blood?

The hateful old bitch stood in the doorway of the bathroom, her face red with anger, her huge, beefy arms akimbo, while I quickly took off my clothes, washed the blood from my face in the large sink, and hurriedly put on my girl's nightgown.

"Now, get yourself to bed, young man!" And as I passed by her she slapped me across the face again. I found that is what evil adults call "for good measure," whatever that is supposed to mean. Crying and cowering like a wounded animal, I skedaddled across the ward, hopped onto the high hospital bed (in one try) and pulled the covers up close around my neck, fearing what was coming next. Instead, she gathered up my clothes and shoes and stalked out of the ward, apparently muttering (threats and bad words, I assumed) under her breath.

I lay under the covers, tears streaming down a face bruised and stinging from connecting with her large ham of a paw. Would tomorrow be a better day? Would I even be alive tomorrow? I wasn't sure. I lay quietly in the darkness of the cold ward, curled up in the fetal position under the brown Army blanket, alone in my misery.

Where was mama? Was she worried about me? Did she even know where I was? Facing the wide entrance of the silent ward, I poked as much (and as little) of my face as I thought safe, from beneath the scratchy woolen Army blanket, sobbing quietly in the gloom of both

Winter and My Life, fearing any moment that the Frowning-Demon-In-White would return to finish what she had started.

I lay alone in the cold February darkness, feeling tired, drained, dispirited. And stretched over all this grief and confusion was a suffocating cloak of desperation. And there was something else. It was hazy and diffuse, and difficult to focus on. Underlying this jumble of mixed emotions was a vague nebula of fear for my life.

This entire episode seemed strangely dreamlike-no, strangely nightmarish to me. I had awakened that morning to the voice of a mother who loved me dearly; tonight I had been put to bed three hundred miles away in a strange, gothically moribund place with a cruel slap across my face administered with gleeful malice by a She-Devil-In-White.

By the end of my two-week stint in "Tomblin's House of Horrors," this sadistic prison camp guard hiding in a nurse's uniform and I had developed a mutual feeling toward one another-loathing and contempt. The greatest difference between me and the other kids at the orphanage was, the other kids just "thought" they didn't belong there-I "knew" I didn't. When picturing this old grouch in my mind's eye, I surmised that either she had never learned to smile, or was so old she had long since forgotten. I got the feeling that if I could catch her smiling, I would have a secret known only by me.

Love. Care. Empathy. Understanding. These are qualities that come from a beneficent feeling toward those less fortunate than we. Mrs. Edith Tomblin came to Oxford Orphanage in May 1924, and retired thirty years later, on December 12, 1953, when I was fourteen years old. In the decades in which she was in charge of the orphanage hospital, Mrs. Tomblin was the first adult encountered by literally hundreds of intimidated and vulnerable six- and seven-year-old boys and girls. When abruptly separated from a parent or parents at such an early age, the natural reactions of such young children are fear and apprehension, commensurate with a sense of abandonment.

Only an insensitive, uncaring ass would believe that caustic chastisements such as "You don't live with your mother anymore!" and the equally heartless admonition that "If you don't stop crying, you'll get the whipping of your life!" can instill anything but fear and distrust of adults in the minds of small children. I avoided the heartless bitch more out of fear than of revulsion and loathing, but whether or not they can understand the latter two emotions, all small, frail and defenseless orphans are quite familiar with the word "'fraid."

I hated Mrs. Tomblin for her crass physical mistreatment of me and the other children, and for her Philistine and insensitive attitude to our vulnerability. I despised her for the entire time I knew her, just as did hundreds of frightened, vulnerable, displaced children who had the blameless misfortune to have encountered her their first day at the orphanage. She did not belong. Time will never heal such abuse.

And I was to fare no better as I left the hated Mrs. Tomblin and moved on to the Baby Cottage and later the Walker Building. My life had the same effect as would a passenger on the maiden voyage of the Titanic, looking for a more comfortable seat. No, my path on this Treadmill to Hell was to continue.

Mrs. Tomblin's cold negativism served only to further confuse children whose fragile psyches already had been dealt a punishing blow by being torn from a loving family. One should never confuse the lack of proper care with absence of love and mistreatment, as relates to home life prior to entering the orphanage. Parents were allowed to visit their children only one Sunday each month. My mother never missed a visit, and each Sunday afternoon the campus was filled with parents, siblings and relatives visiting the children of all ages.

Nearly every one of the literally thousands of children who came to live in Oxford Orphanage did so as a direct result of some traumatic circumstance in his or her early childhood. Entering this strange and foreboding environment was but another traumatic event, and to be greeted with caring and kindness would have gone a long way in lessening the hurt of the transition. It was nothing short of a travesty for these wee orphans to be met by the likes of Mrs. Edith Tomblin.

Emotionally, it was hard to recover from that traumatic first night in the orphanage hospital. Lying fetally curled up under the brown Army blanket, sobbing quietly for fear The Bitch would hear my cries and return to finish me off, I sensed my anemic body being drained of all its energy, my broken spirit suffering far worse than my swollen face and bleeding nose.

I felt a profound, never-before experienced sense of isolation, of uncertainty, of being forsaken by my family, of being so small and vulnerable. I had been tossed unceremoniously into a vast sea of despair, and no lifeguard was throwing me a Mae West.

My sense of utter hopelessness knew no reason, no ebb and flow, no apogee and perigee; it was more like a brackish, stagnant pond, and I feared that any light at the end of this cavernous maw of hell would in all likelihood be the glare of yet another oncoming nightmare.

Even today, with seemingly all the years of intervening healing, I shudder when I recall the almost indescribable feeling of floating in this Bunyanesque Slough of Despair. But it was real indeed, and it impressed forever its indelible stamp on my fragile seven-year-old psyche.

I felt at that very moment in my life a numbing emptiness, a hole, a cavernous pit in an until-then happy life. Oh, if my daddy were still there, and could ride up to this awful place on his big red Indian machine, reach down and scoop me up in his strong arm, sling me onto the seat behind him, and whisk me away to the security and comfort of 208 East Bright Street. But this was not to be. Not then. Not ever. I was on my own. Forever.

I endured a fitful night of strange, never-before experienced dreams, and awoke with an apprehension born of the previous day's (and night's) experience, to the unwelcome peal of a bell that seemed to be ringing from just outside my window. After an interminable period, the ringing of the bell ceased abruptly. This was my introduction to the ubiquitous Bell, that was to monitor my waking life's activities for the next decade.

Thus began my two-week imprisonment in Hicks Memorial Hospital, in which my initial sense of despair and hopelessness segued into what I can only believe now was depression. It was as though someone had turned on a spigot, draining from me all my feelings. At night, lying huddled under my warm Army blanket in the vacant first floor boys' ward, afraid to chance again my Midnight Escape from Captivity, strange voices and surrealistic scenes began to insinuate themselves into my nightmares.

I found myself in a totally different world, one of animosity, hate and petulance, engendered by what I did not know and could not (though I tried) comprehend. My pre-orphanage habitude was gone forever. It was going to be a long goddamn trip. "Real soon" was to become "forever." And I missed my daddy more and more as each day passed.

During my two weeks in the Wicked White Bitch's Lockup, at night my previous life failed to mesh with the present traumatic events. My daddy's laugh, mama's gentle voice, my brothers, Eoline, happy times, granddaddy's cabin at Swansboro, my daddy's big red Indian motorcycle, mama's hot biscuits and gravy, buttermilk, Saturday afternoon cowboy matinees, funny books, the ice wagon, the gunshots, my daddy's funeral, Doc's trial, mama's tear-filled eyes at the trial, flashed repeatedly before my young mind as I left behind my first life forever.

My fragile being during these two weeks endured a whirlwind of fear and apprehension, my predicament hauntingly surreal, my despair deep and foreboding. Isolated and unloved, inwardly I wanted to reach out to anyone who would be a friend, utter a kind word, show he or she cared. A light, however dim, shines brightly in a dungeon.

Well, we now know how I got into this mess. But before continuing this (mis)adventure, what is this place that Old Bitch Tomblin called an "orphanage," and how did it come about?

CHAPTER 3

The College that Became an Orphanage

By 1860 Granville County, located between the Virginia state line and Raleigh, boasted a large and prosperous tobacco crop, and was one of only five counties in North Carolina with as many as 10,000 slaves. There also existed at that time a sizable community of free blacks in the county, and the county was well known as the site of several academies of learning. The best known institution of higher learning in Granville County on the eve of the Civil War was St. John's College.

However, let us digress momentarily, for a few centuries, and we'll pick up our story later at the year 1860. The story of St. John's College, however, began much earlier . . .

Freemasonry encompasses the teachings and practices of the Fraternal Order of Free and Accepted Masons. The Order was spread by the historical advance of the British Empire. Freemasonry had its origins in the guilds of stonemasons and cathedral builders of the Middle Ages. As cathedral building declined, some lodges began to allow honorary members in order to sustain their membership. This practice gave rise to Freemasonry, and in 1717 the first Grand Lodge was founded in England.

Although not a Christian institution per se, Freemasonry contains many religious elements, including morality and charity. Application for admission into the brotherhood requires a belief in the existence of a

Supreme Being, and in the immorality of the soul. In the United States, its membership, comprised mainly of white Protestants, stands at more than two and a half million.

Masonic ideals of liberty, equality and fraternity early on found their way into American life. Masons have figured prominently in the history of our nation. George Washington and thirteen other presidents of the United States, eighteen vice-presidents and thirty-five Justices of the United States Supreme Court have been Masons. George Washington took his first presidential oath of office on a Bible borrowed from a Masonic lodge in New York, and the oath was administered by Chancellor Robert R. Livingston, another Mason and, at that time, Grand Master of Masons. Other prominent Masons have included Henry Ford, Douglas MacArthur, Lafayette, Paul Revere, Mozart, Beethoven, John Glenn, John Hancock, John Paul Jones, Rudyard Kipling, Simon Bolivar, Norman Vincent Peale and Will Rogers.

The long history of the contributions of the Masons of North Carolina to the cause of education and care of the youth of the state would fill several volumes. The one Masonic institution that by far represents the greatest outlay of money and effort had its beginnings in the meeting of the Grand Lodge in 1838, at which time a resolution was passed looking toward the establishment of a charity school under the care of the Grand Lodge.

Planning continued on the project for the next decade, and in 1850 the Grand Lodge decided the school was to be located at Oxford. At that time there were only 65 lodges in the state. St. John's College was chosen as the name for the new institution, and in 1853, the Masons purchased a 109-acre tract of land near the corporate limits of Oxford, at a price of $4,480.00. On June 24, 1855, the anniversary of the birth of St. John the Baptist, several thousand persons witnessed the laying of the cornerstone of St. John's College.

Exactly a century later, as a fifteen-year-old high school Freshman, I stood with several hundred orphans and Masons to witness the opening of that cornerstone as another was laid atop the original.

The imposing college building was an architect's dream, consisting of fifty-three dormitories in four stories and a basement within its original 122 feet by 60 feet walls. A spacious chapel, forty feet by sixty feet, with a gallery around it, seated twelve hundred persons. In addition to the dormitories, the imposing Victorian structure housed four recitation rooms, two society rooms, and four large suites for professors, each with its own fireplace. The college opened its doors to students on July 13, 1858. Its first life, however, was to be short indeed, occasioned by the infernal meddling in the lives of Southerners by those damn Yankees.

By 1860 the small but growing town of Oxford found itself in the heart of the North Carolina tobacco-producing belt, that stretched northward into the Piedmont of Virginia, and more than fifty percent of Granville County's population was slaves. When the Civil War began, 1500 able-bodied young men were formed into a fighting force known as the "Granville Grays," and the unit distinguished itself in many battles during the war. St. John's College closed its doors for lack of students, suspending operations along with many Southern schools.

Following the South's inglorious defeat, and despite President Andrew Johnson's appeals to the nation, the Radical Republicans were supported in the elections of 1866. In early 1867, over President Johnson's veto, they put into effect their plan of Reconstruction, the post-Civil War process of reorganizing the Southern states that had seceded, and re-establishing them in the Union.

The South was divided into military districts, each under the control of a Union Major General. The new state governments were organized, with the former governing class deprived of the vote.

"Carpetbagger" was a term of contempt applied to the agents and office holders forced upon the South during Reconstruction, who were interested primarily in the graft they could collect. During this period of Reconstruction, that lasted from 1867 to 1877, Oxford Orphanage was founded.

The South as a whole, including North Carolina, was pitifully poor throughout the Reconstruction era, and a series of disastrously bad crops in the late 1860's, followed by the general agricultural depression of the 1870's, greatly hurt the predominantly agricultural state.

Unlike other Southern states, North Carolina was most reluctant to sever all ties with the Union, seeking compromise until the last moment, and did not secede from the Union until May 20, 1861. Once committed to its ideals, however, North Carolina supplied more men and materiel to the Confederate cause than any other state. The state also suffered the largest number of young men killed and wounded than any other Confederate state during the War of Northern Aggression. In addition, the state suffered the ignominy of defeat and the years of instability and corruption that characterized the postwar Reconstruction period throughout the South.

The Civil War ended in 1865. In the decade that followed, several events took place that, three quarters of a century later, would have a profound effect on my life. In the South between 1860 and 1865, twenty-five percent of the white males of military age were killed. This tremendous loss of life was particularly devastating to North Carolina; having supplied more fighting men to the Confederate cause of freedom, the number of losses was staggering.

The natural consequences of such devastating loss of life were the creation of thousands of orphans in the state, and a dearth of young men of college age and the financial means to attend college. The reality of the consequences of such utter depredation brought on by the Civil War came to bear directly on a question central to our story-what was to become of St. John's College?

From the end of hostilities in 1865, until 1871, the college was operated by several educators, though none was successful, and that year a caretaker moved into the college building until further disposition of the property could be made.

At a meeting of the Grand Lodge in 1872, the salient question was, what to do with St. John's College and its property? John H. Mills, a locally prominent educator, presented a resolution that resolved that "The St. John's College be made into an asylum for the protection, training and education of indigent orphan children."

This was indeed a radical idea. Nothing of such magnitude had ever been proposed in the state. Quite literally, the Masons of North Carolina were being asked to reach deep into their pockets already rendered bare by the ravages of first war and then Reconstruction (1867-1877), to test severely their ideals of charity and fraternity in providing food, clothing, shelter and an education to what could amount to thousands of orphaned boys and girls. A quite formidable task today; an almost unheard of undertaking in 1872.

The vote when taken resulted in a tie. The incoming Grand Master, John Nichols, was called upon to break the tie, and he did not hesitate in casting his precious vote in favor of me and literally thousands of orphans over the past one hundred and thirty years. For many years thereafter, the portraits of John H. Mills and John Nichols adorned the walls of the chapel in the Main Building, a fitting tribute to these giants of benevolent insight. The transformed St. John's College was renamed the Oxford Orphan Asylum, and John H. Mills was elected its first Superintendent.

In February 1873 the first children admitted to the orphanage were Robert L. and Nancy Parrish and Isabella Robertson of Granville County, who arrived in an old battered wagon. Mr. Mills lifted the first child from the wagon, raised him high in the air, then hugged the boy. Thus began the sheltering care, training and education of many thousands; at the end of the first year alone, 109 children were under the loving care of the Masons of North Carolina. The mission of Oxford Orphanage is embodied in the original resolution, that reads in part:

> "The orphan children in the said asylum shall be fed and clothed,
> and shall receive such preparatory training and education as will
> prepare them for useful occupations and for the usual business
> transactions of life."

The plan provided that "the larger girls assist in the ordinary housework, and in the making and mending of clothes, and the larger boys assist in the preparation of fuel, care of livestock and the cultivation of the soil."

On January 6, 1875 the first issue of *The Children's Friend* was published. This weekly newspaper was the forerunner of *The Orphans' Friend and Masonic Journal*, that was published monthly for many decades, including the ten years I lived at the orphanage.

The section of the newspaper entitled "Report on the Orphan Asylum," made to "The Most Worshipful Grand Lodge of North

Carolina," reported that the receipts of the orphanage, from December 1, 1873 to December 1, 1874, were $10,783.94, that disbursements during that time were $10,701.57, leaving on hand $82.37. The editor of the newspaper acknowledged that assistance to the welfare of the orphanage had also come from Masons in Virginia, Maryland, Pennsylvania, New York, Michigan, Tennessee, South Carolina, Texas and California. The editor reported also that the old garden had been enlarged to four acres, a new one of eleven acres had been enclosed, and that "two good mules have been bought, and a stable built for them."

The newspaper reported that since the opening of the orphanage in 1873, 240 orphans had been admitted. It noted that:

> "Our rule has been to discharge them at fourteen, or sooner, if they complete a good English education, and promise to be useful in a farm, store, shop, factory or family."

An article in the very first issue of *The Children's Friend*, that, for the record, was published at the orphanage, appeared to be portentous of my life at the orphanage three quarters of a century later. The article, entitled "Prizes vs. Punishment," noted that there are perhaps no children "who can not be incited to greater diligence by commendation and hope of reward. Continual harshness and fault-finding hardens children, and confirms them in evil habits; but a word of praise will often rouse their dormant energies, increase their self-respect . . . You may punish them for indolence, increase their task, but all to no purpose. But offer the most trivial prize and the effect will astonish you."

From its ambitious beginnings in 1873 until the turn of the century, the Masons of North Carolina expanded their fledgling project at a rapid pace, in land, buildings and population, until Oxford Orphanage was transformed into a bustling community all its own.

In 1884, aided by a gift in memory of her son John Morehead Walker, Mrs. Letitia Morehead Walker invested a thousand dollars that was to be used to construct the Walker Memorial residence, home of the

Superintendent. The building was later expanded and converted into a hospital in 1904, and the Superintendent and his family moved into an apartment in the St. John's College building. The original Walker Building has remained occupied for nearly 120 years.

In 1884 the Masons acquired an additional 125 acres of land and another small tract, giving the orphanage about 242 acres in all. On June 24, 1886 the cornerstone was laid for the Industrial Building, that housed the laundry, mending and sewing rooms and clothing storage rooms. In May 1886 a shoe making and repairing department was added, and in 1887 a printing office was constructed.

Mr. Benjamin N. Duke, a wealthy North Carolina philanthropist, sensed that the needs of the orphanage required substantial housing, and initiated a construction effort that resulted in the erection of four cottages for boys, a central dining room and kitchen building, and four cottages for girls. The boys' cottages and the dining room-kitchen buildings were completed in 1897, and the girls' cottages were occupied in 1899.

At the turn of the century, the Twenty-Ninth Annual Report of the Oxford Orphan Asylum, dated November 30, 1901, reported the enrollment at 221 children and soon to become 250. That year a well, 256 feet, 3 inches deep, was bored at a cost of $1,212.21. It would pump water at a rate of 75 gallons per minute, at a temperature of 55 degrees Fahrenheit.

The total receipts for 1901 were $26,947.40, including a grant of $7,500.00 from the State of North Carolina, and the net cost of maintenance and education was $16,014.51. The orphanage was already operating "in the black." The yearly report of 1901 listed the name of each student and the county from which the student came. More orphans (13) came from Lenoir County (Kinston) than from any other county in the State.

From 1872 when the orphanage was established, until 1909, the number of affiliate Master Masons in the State had grown to about 19,000. The orphanage population had burgeoned to 325 children, and in those thirty-seven years, more than 2,500 children had been cared for by Oxford Orphanage.

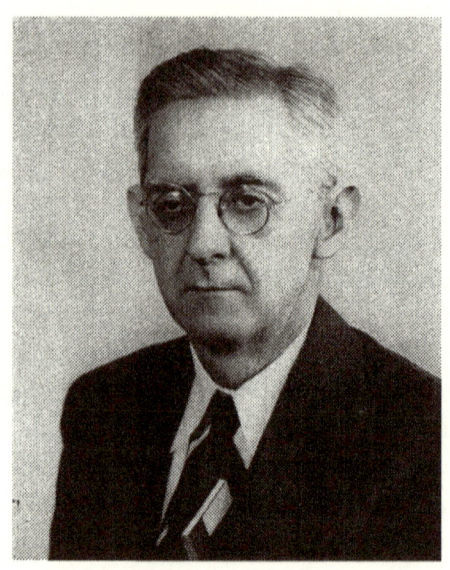

Dr. Rufus S. Jones, Oxford Orphanage Dentist.

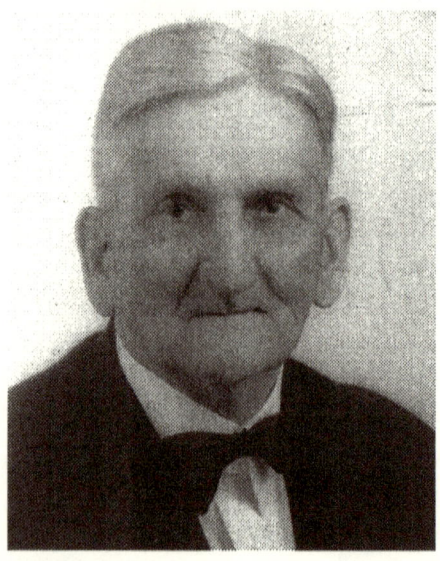

Mr. M.F. "Mos" Hill, manager of Shoe Shop, 1899-1950, and a former orphan.

In 1911 Mr. R.L. Brown was selected to be Superintendent, and the growth continued. Cottages were remodeled, and a modern fireproof school building was erected, named in honor of Past Grand Master John Nichols. A new hospital was constructed, and at the time was the only building in Granville County that boasted an elevator. The Shrine Swimming Pool was constructed, as were homes for the Treasurer and Superintendent. The Walker Building, that had since 1904 housed the hospital, later became a cottage for younger boys.

The Dunn Building, better known to generations of orphans as the "Baby Cottage," was added later and became the home of the youngest boys and girls. Another building, the Royster Building, better known as the "Annex," was later added to house young girls.

On August 1, 1928, when the Reverend Creasy K. Proctor was named Superintendent, the population of the little "city" of Oxford Orphanage stood at 393 children, with about sixty-five staff and workers. Thus at the beginning of the Great Depression the annual budget for the orphanage was approximately $175,000.00, indeed a formidable financial challenge for that era.

Founded in 1872, the Oxford Orphan Asylum was the first orphanage in North Carolina. By 1900 eight more orphanages had opened, and by the time I arrived at Oxford in February 1947, the total number of orphanages in the state had burgeoned to twenty-six.

To recap, probably your first bloody nose came at the hands of a girl smaller than yourself, on the playground in preschool. Not Little Orphan Al. And I got the strange feeling at the time that I had not been the first small seven-year-old who had had his or her face bloodied by the Nazi prison camp guard masquerading as a nurse in a sleepy Southern postwar town. A most inauspicious beginning indeed.

One thing I never wanted to become when I grew up was a dentist . . .

CHAPTER 4

The Dentist

Having been born in 1939, the knee-baby of seven children, if I ever heard the expression "regular dental checkup," it passed through my consciousness without depositing much of an impression.

Midway down the long hallway of the hospital was a room that remained closed most of the time, except for the occasional comings and goings of visibly unhappy children. I would pass by, usually rather hurriedly, and hear emanating from within the secret room intermittent whirring and grinding noises, interspersed occasionally by muffled cries and protests of small children.

By my fourth day in The Village of the Damned, Mrs. Tomblin, mayor of the Village, apparently had concluded that I was not a health risk to her and others, and I had determined my survival while in the hospital depended on avoiding her at all costs. I had been placed in isolation for the purpose of being processed in preparation for joining the general prison population and, aside from these mandatory procedures, I spent most of my time in the quiet anonymity of the playroom. And that was perfectly fine with me. I could cower in the corner when she went by, and I could, and did, cry softly as long as the White Scowling Bitch did not see me. At age seven I was already a fast study.

In early afternoon of that unforgettable fourth day, as I was standing on the cushion of the playroom couch observing through the large windows boys and girls and vehicles criss-crossing the expansive campus before me, unable yet to fathom how the driverless mule and ice (?) wagon team made it to its destination each day, my thoughts were interrupted by the soft patter of Ann's footfalls behind me.

"Let's go brush your teeth, Alton. It's time for you to see Dr. Jones." Doctor Jones? Doctor? Jones? As I tagged along after Ann to the boys' ward, I thought to myself, Brush your teeth? See Dr. Jones? How were the two events related? On my second day in captivity, Ann had given me a new toothbrush and a small red and white tin container of Colgate Tooth Powder, just like mama sold in our "convenience" store on East Bright Street.

I took my time brushing my teeth, still puzzled at what this exercise had to do with any "Dr. Jones," whom I assumed from the title to be a physician. After rinsing my mouth, I followed Ann back down the hallway in somewhat the same manner a duckling waddles after its mother. Midway down the (always) darkened hallway Ann suddenly paused, turned to her left, and the instant she opened the door to the secret room, a little girl of about ten came through the open doorway into the hall, crying softly and holding the left side of her face.

Instantly I froze in my tracks, then quickly retreated several steps, not taking my eyes off the little girl moaning in pain. Had this poor creature cried in the presence of the White-Clad Bitch, and consequently just received the "whipping of her life," as had been promised me on my first night in Hell? Worse yet, had the "whipping of her life" been administered by the mysterious "Dr. Jones?"

In a fit of panic, I bolted down the hall to the boys' ward, rushed into the bathroom, closing the door behind me, and huddled in the nook between the toilet and the wall, frightened out of my wits.

Suddenly there came a tapping, gently rapping, on the bathroom door. "Are you alright, Alton?" asked Ann, a sense of concern in her soft voice. Was she trying the old "sense of concern" ploy to trick me into opening the door? I wasn't certain of her intentions, so I tried the old standby,

"I feel sick. I don't feel good at all," hoping this lie would enable me to escape the wrath of the now presumptively elevated evil Dr. Jones, at least for the moment.

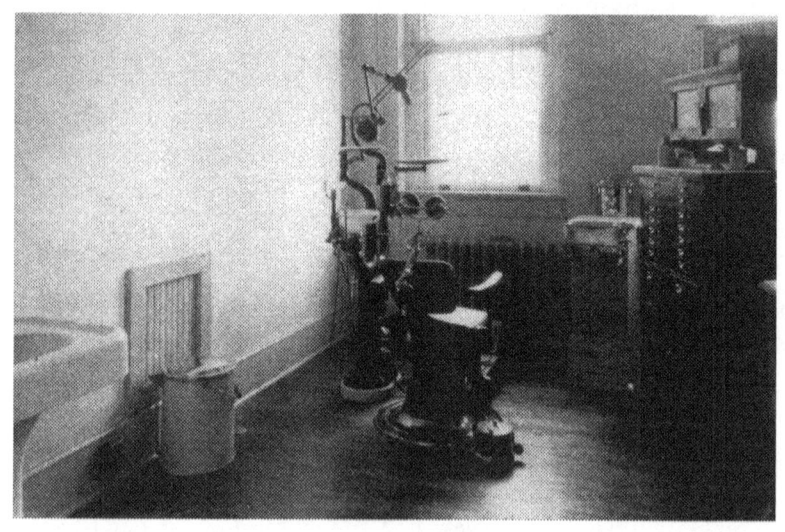

Dr. Jones' Dental Office, located on first floor of Hicks Memorial Hospital.

Apparently sensing the reason for my sudden "illness," Ann quietly assured me, "We were going for you dental checkup, Alton. Dr. Jones needs to take some x-rays and check your teeth." Yeah, you bet! By the way, I wondered, what's an "x-ray?" Could have been a bribe, like "custard."

But Little Orphan Al weren't no sucker. I wasn't about to make it easy for Ann, in case there was any skullduggery afoot.

"Why was the little girl crying anyway?" I tried to sound firm.

"Oh, Dr. Jones had to pull one of her teeth. But he's not going to pull any of your teeth, I promise."

Yeah, you bet! Promises, promises. Like, "I'll see you real soon." But Ann was my friend, and I trusted her word, so reluctantly I trailed after her, back down the hallway and into the secret room to visit the equally mysterious Dr. Jones.

What a depressing experience. Dr. Jones was a thin, slightly-built man of about fifty, with close-cropped, graying hair and sad eyes made even sadder by drooping eyelids sunken inward beneath graying, brushy eyebrows.

Climbing up onto the ancient dental chair, as instructed by Ann, the dentist apparently dispensed with the amenities of introduction and idle chitchat. Would he ask where I was from? Would I get to tell him I was from Kinston, The World's Foremost Tobacco Center, thus instantly earning his respect and accolades? 'Fraid not.

I assumed the little man was Dr. Jones, probably because of the knee-length white coat he was wearing, and maybe because besides Ann and the apprehensive "new" boy, he was the only other person crowded into the small square-shaped room. He was humming a meaningless tune when Ann and I entered the darkened room, and was humming the same discordant ditty when we departed almost an hour later.

During that frightening interval, Dr. Jones had taken the mysterious "x-rays" (reminded me of my Flash Gordon funny books) of my teeth and jaw, given me two shots in my upper right gum with a really godawful long needle, pulled one of my upper right premolars, and poked, probed and scraped my entire set of 374 teeth and gums.

I departed Dr. Jones' torture chamber much the same as the little girl before me, moaning softly and holding the swollen right side of my face with my hand, too much in pain to feel any sense of relief at being finally set free.

The only words spoken by Dr. Jones during my hour of pain, other than "Open," "Open wide," and "Open wider," were his instructions to keep my teeth closed tightly on the gauze packing placed over the empty socket, left after he had unceremoniously separated me from that upper right premolar.

I felt a little woozy from the trauma of the experience, so Ann walked me to the playroom, leaving me there to recuperate, admonishing me not to talk or laugh (laugh?), else the gauze packing might work loose, which would require a second visit to Dr. Jones' House of Pain.

Not daring open my mouth, I quickly nodded a "Don't worry about me." However, as I sat quietly in the depressing semi-darkness of the "playroom" the effects of the anesthesia soon started to wear off, and suddenly my jaw began to throb with pain. My fear of being taken back to see the sadistic dentist guy should I complain of my intense pain, by far overshadowed my discomfiture, so I kept my teeth clinched over the blood-soaked gauze compress, closing my eyes tightly in an attempt to deflect the presence of pain. Eventually I fell asleep, huddled in a darkened corner of the playroom.

After a time I was awakened by Ann's gentle voice, and I looked up to see her standing before me, holding a porcelain food tray on which sat a large white ceramic bowl.

"I know you must be in pain," she said, smiling down at me. "I've got just the thing to take the hurt away." (You want to really take the hurt away-try giving me a one-way bus ticket back to Kinston.) Placing the tray on the floor in front of me, Ann sat beside me in the semi-darkness. Taking a large white napkin off the tray, she held it up to my mouth.

"Just spit out the gauze packing," she instructed. "I've got you some frozen custard." Best stuff I've ever tasted, that frozen vanilla custard. Took away the hurt almost instantly. But I'd rather have had the bus ticket.

My assailant du jour was Dr. Rufus S. Jones of Warrenton, North Carolina, the orphanage's part-time and only dentist. During the year I arrived at Oxford, 1947, Dr. Jones examined each older student at least twice, and each younger child three times. He filled 267 teeth that year. During 1947 Dr. Jones singled out twelve children for possible orthodontic treatment, and these students were referred out to Dr. Fred G. Hale.

Before we assume that 267 teeth filled in a population of 311 children to be a great number, we must take note of the state of dental health in the United States at the time. During World War II, the primary reason that military inductees were turned down for possible military service was dental cavities.

The discovery that the addition of sodium fluoride to fluoride-deficient municipal water supplies could reduce the incidence of teeth cavities by as much as sixty-five percent was not made until the early 1940's. And it was not until 1945 that the first fluoridated water supply was initiated, in Grand Rapids, Michigan.

Given the pace of advancement of medicine, including dentistry, during and after the War, Dr. Jones was quick to pick up on this new cavity-fighting discovery. In 1948, the year after I came to the orphanage, Dr. Jones initiated a preventive dentistry program using sodium fluoride. As of December 31, 1948 about 200 of the 317 children had received the treatment, with the remaining 117 children being treated in 1949.

Dr. Jones' dental office was small and sparsely appointed. The patient's chair faced the only window in the room, that looked onto the outside of the hospital. Bolted to the floor directly below the window, and thus only about three feet from the patient, was a large castiron radiator, about three feet wide and two feet high.

During the Winter months, we kids had to suffer three equally uncomfortable things when visiting Dr. Jones' office; the suffocating heat from the radiator, the equally suffocating foul breath of Dr. Jones, and the intimidating grinding of his antiquated, whirring drill. No orphan will ever forget the godawful whirring! And the setting was appropriate; the nondescript little dental office fit well the equally nondescript little dentist.

In 1947 a "high-speed dental drill" was a misnomer. A cloth cord on a sort of pulley arrangement powered Dr. Jones' dental drill, it moving at the rate of a snail, or approximately four and a half revolutions per minute. The drill bit did not "cut" into your tooth, rather it "gnawed" through the tooth like a rodent, and the pain persisted even though the good doctor Jones had saturated our gums with Novocaine.

By the time I entered (with great trepidation) his small office on the first floor of Hicks Memorial Hospital in February 1947, Dr. Jones' shoulders already had begun sloping inward from years of bending and reaching into thousands of cavity-filled mouths, many of whom belonged to orphans. The fact that his features were inherently small and narrow only added to his general appearance of frailty.

Dr. Jones' drooping upper eyelids lent a sadness to his appearance, and he performed his dental cleanings, fillings and pullings in a businesslike manner bordering on detachment. His languid, almost distracted manner did not lend itself to conversation, which was limited to "Open," "Open wide," "Open wider," "Close," "Spit," and "You can go now." At times these stimulating conversational pieces were filled in by timeless humming.

The singular irony that struck me on my first (traumatic) visit to Dr. Jones' office the first week of my incarceration, and of which I was reminded at least twice a year for the next decade, was that this morose-looking man had been cursed with (very) bad breath. But I liked Dr. Jones, halitosis or no, even though I seemed to always climb down from his antiquated dental chair in great pain.

When it came time in my life to choose a career, Dentistry did not even make the list of possibilities. But Dr. Jones, thin, slightly built, salt-and-pepper graying hair, round rimless spectacles, drooping eyelids and foul breath, was there to help me, and I always thanked him as I left his office, holding onto my gauze-packed jaw, tears filling my young eyes. Dr. Jones was a good man.

CHAPTER 5

The Shoe Shop

"Climb on up here, son," the aged, white-haired septuagenarian gestured with a nod of his head toward a long, well-worn wooden bench, in front of which was situated a foot-high slanted wooden stand, with the low end of the stand closest to the bench.

The room smelled strongly of leather and shoe polish. "I'll be back for you. Just wait for me here," Ann said as she left the room.

The elderly gentleman with the ash-gray complexion and deep-set eyes tapped the well-worn slanted board with an equally aged and wrinkled hand.

"What's your name, son?" he asked, as he reached down, lifted my right foot, placed it on the slanted board in front of me, and began untying the frayed brown laces of the shoes I had been wearing the day I arrived at this godforsaken place five days before.

"M'name's Alton," I mumbled in a subdued manner, noticing as he knelt forward to untie my laces that his hair was much whiter even than mine. "But everybody calls me 'Cottontop' cause my hair's so white."

The old man paused pensively, then looked me in the eye and smiled. Touching the top of his head, he said,

"Then I suppose we are both cottontops." Then he added, smiling, "I'm Mr. Hill. You look kinda sad. I used to be here in the orphanage just like you are now. That was a long time ago. So I know just how you feel

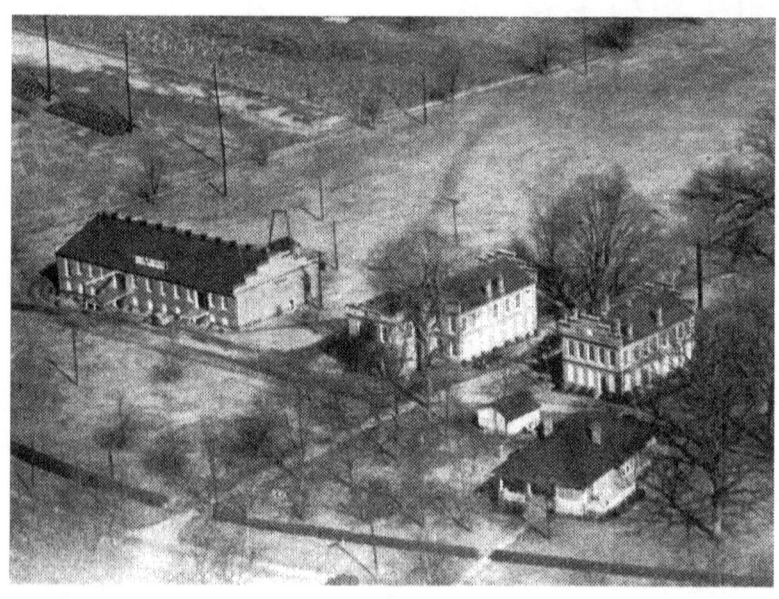

1951. Vocational Buildings. From Left: Electric Shop, Printing
Shop, Shoe Shop. The house in the foreground near the Shoe
Shop was Mr. Regan's residence. Bleachers and football field are
in upper left.

being away from home and all. But you'll meet a lot of friends here and soon you won't be so unhappy."

I was suddenly put somewhat at ease by the old gentleman's sincerity and snaggle-toothed smile.

"Now, let's measure your feet, and we'll get you a nice new pair of shoes," he said, taking my right heel in his large leathery hand and guiding my foot into a metal cup at one end of a metal clamp. Gently pressing my toes down with his wrinkled hand, he cocked his head back and aimed his bifocals for a better look at the ruler.

"I'll be right back," Mr. Hill said, as he stood and turned toward a door leading to a back room of the large, two-story well-worn red brick building.

"Hey, kid, where you from?" said a red-headed boy of about fifteen who was standing behind a wooden workbench, trying to tear a rubber heel from a well-worn brown brogan (that orphans called "brogues") that was turned upside-down on a wooden last attached to a vertical metal post. After several jerks of his pliers, punctuated by accompanying well-announced grunts of effort, the boy succeeded in removing the worn heel from the upside-down shoe.

"Kinston," I responded. Then, as an afterthought, I added with pride, "World's Foremost Tobacco Center."

"Oh, yeah," the boy said, nodding his head in certain (to me at least) recognition. Gosh, I sure was proud. Maybe if I subtly informed the Hated Bitch in White that I was from such an important town, she would treat me with the respect I surely deserved. Then again, I thought, maybe she wouldn't. After much mental debate, I decided to keep my origin a secret from her. Her loss, not mine.

Without further comment, the teenager picked up a new rubber heel, seated it carefully in place of the discarded old one, scooped up a handful of long black tacks and placed them in his mouth. I watched in awe as the boy adroitly pulled a sharp protruding tack from between his pursed lips, seated the tack, then skillfully drove the tack up to its hilt into the rubber heel with one well-aimed and determined stroke of a small metal hammer.

Simultaneously with the strike of the hammer another tack protruded from his closed lips, and I stared open-mouthed, expecting at any moment to see the boy choke on a handful of sharp tacks. After securing the new heel to the shoe, the boy spat out the remaining tacks into his hand and placed them in a large round tray of similar tacks on the workbench. Showoff.

"My name's Billy," the freckle-faced boy said smiling. "I'm from Raleigh. Ya got any brothers or sisters here?"

"My sister Eoline's here. Know where she is?" I asked expectantly.

"I don't know her by name. Tell me how old she is and I'll tell you what cottage she's in," he said helpfully.

I thought for a moment. I knew Eoline was older than I, but not by much.

"I think about nine," I answered expectantly.

"Then, she would be in the Annex. That's over yonder aways, on the other side of the campus, behind 3-G. They're not gonna let you see her, though, not til you're out of the hospital."

At last a straw of hope at which to grasp! Excitedly, I asked the boy "Can you tell her I'm here? Will you see her today?"

"Sure will. We go to dinner at twelve. So I'll find your sister. What's her name?"

"Her name's Eoline," I said. "Please tell her I'm in the hospital. I'll be in the playroom. Please?"

"I'll take care of it," the boy assured me. Then, reaching for his pliers, he deftly twisted another shoe onto the upside down last resting atop the metal post, and attacked with self-professed cockiness another well-worn rubber heel.

At that moment Mr. Hill returned through the open doorway, carrying a new pair of shiny brown ankle-high shoes. Placing the shoes on the slanted board before me, Mr. Hill inserted my right foot into one of the stiff leather shoes and began threading the aglets of a new shoelace through the eyelets of the shoe.

"Give 'em a tryout," Mr. Hill said after he had tied snugly the second shoelace. He gestured with a wave of his weathered hand toward the far wall of the room. I stood and walked slowly across the room, the new leather soles of the shoes so stiff they did not bend. I felt as though my feet were attached to two wooden boards, and after about four or five steps the toe of one shoe snagged on a crack in the aged wooden floor, and I sprawled forward quite unceremoniously onto the floor.

While I picked myself up, feeling downright embarrassed at my clumsiness, Mr. Hill laughed, revealing again his patented snaggle-toothed grin, and remarked sympathetically,

"That's all right, son. The soles will bend in a few days, and they'll last you a long time. All the kids stumble when they first start wearing shoes. And all the kids call them 'brogans,' or just 'brogues.'"

I was struck by the kindness of this old man, more likely than not because of his apparent empathy for those literally thousands of orphans with whom he shared a common bond. This aging gentleman, who always wore the same well-worn soiled apron, had been a student at Oxford Orphanage from January 12, 1886 to March 10, 1893. He served Oxford Orphanage faithfully as Manager of the Shoe Shop for more than fifty years, from September 1, 1899 until his retirement in 1950, when I was eleven years old.

At the beginning of the twentieth century, The Annual Report of the Oxford Orphanage, dated November 30, 1901, reported on page 32 that ". . . 116 more pairs of shoes have been made for the Asylum during the past year than in the preceding year," and added "Mr. M.F. Hill is still in charge of this work." And when I met "Mos" Hill forty six years later, in February 1947, this kind old gentleman was seventy years old and still going strong. Dedication.

Ten high school boys worked for Mr. Hill in the Shoe Shop, learning the cobbler's trade. Five of the boys worked in the morning while the other five were in school. After lunch the morning workers attended school in the afternoon while the other five worked in the Shoe Shop.

Except for the children in the Baby Cottage, each boy at the orphanage was issued two pairs of shoes. The leather "work" shoes were called brogans, or just brogues, and were made by the Shoe Shop boys, while the low-top leather dress shoes, that we called "Sunday" shoes, were purchased from shoe manufacturers, as were the girls' shoes. If every worker at Oxford Orphanage had had the kindness and empathy for the orphans' plight as had Mos Hill, the orphanage would indeed have been a "home." Unfortunately this was not the case.

CHAPTER 6

The Industrial Building

Wandering about the hospital, I pronounced it sparse, with minimal creature comforts. The silence alone appeared incongruously pervasive and unsettling. Even though there were no patients in the wards, Mrs. Tomblin and the high school girls assisting her spoke almost in whispers, so as not to disturb or awaken those who were not present anyway. It was, well, downright depressing and a little spooky. And it was also catching; I found myself speaking to Ann in whispers, and she to me likewise. This was a really weird place, this "orphanage." We could have been living on the set of *Rebecca*, for that matter.

Possibly Mrs. Tomblin finally tired of my crying. Perhaps I had exceeded the maximum time the administration allowed a "new" boy to remain under the protective (?) wing of the hospital staff. At the young (translate as "naïve") age of seven years I hoped that these strange and disagreeable people would exhaust their patience before I ran out of tears, and that one day "real soon" the slim, friendless bespectacled man and the neatly-dressed woman in black would materialize in the front room of the hospital to return me to the security of 208 East Bright Street and my mama. Suddenly, in my daddy's absence, mama became *my* mama.

Alas, this was not to be. One morning as I was quietly eating breakfast with the hospital staff in the kitchen, all the while making doubly sure I did not inadvertently make eye contact with the Bitch in a White Starched Hospital Uniform, the old dingbat announced,

"Ann, after breakfast, get Alton's things together and take him down to the Baby Cottage."

Of course, by that time I knew what Mrs. Tomblin meant by "Baby Cottage."

At the beginning of my second (record-setting) week at Stalag Oxford, one morning Ann collected me from my playroom-hideout and announced we were going to the "Industrial Building," whatever that was. This would be only my third excursion outside the walls of the hospital since my arrival, and though the day was cold and rainy, I was eager to get out of that dungeon.

Ann and I were bundled against a biting February wind, and because it was mid-morning, we did not encounter anyone as we walked away from the rear of the hospital. We followed a single-lane asphalt and gravel road, past a very large empty swimming pool surrounded by a concrete walkway. Adjacent to the swimming pool stood a small square wooden structure, and I asked,

"What's that little house for, Ann?"

"That's the bath house. Before you can go swimming, you have to take a bath, so you won't get the water dirty."

"Will I get to swim in the pool?" Or is that where they drown little prisoners who won't stop crying, I thought. Paranoid little twerp, I was.

"Sure you will, Alton. Everybody here gets to swim during the Summer. Since you'll be in the Baby Cottage this Summer, you get to swim in the pool first every day."

"But I don't know how to swim."

"Nobody does when he first gets here. Most 'new' kids are about your age, and most of these kids have never even seen a swimming pool."

And suddenly I had a new worry. "What's this Baby Cottage?"

"That's where you go when they let you out of the hospital. They keep you there until you're about nine years old."

Then Ann paused, laughed to herself, and continued,

"Of course, if you don't stop crying so much, they'll never let you out of the hospital."

"But I miss my mama, and I know she wants me home," I pleaded my case.

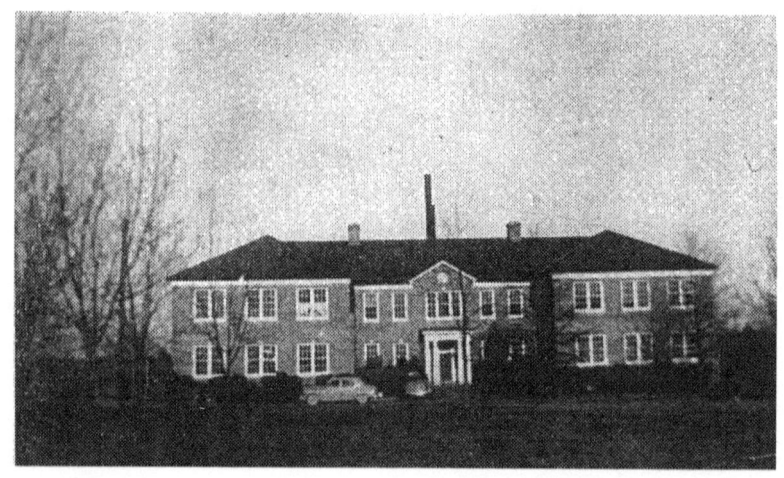

1949. The Industrial Building. Housed Laundry, mending, sewing, luggage, toy, mattress and clothes storage rooms. Basement housed athletic lockers, shower rooms and Boy Scouts Meeting Hall.

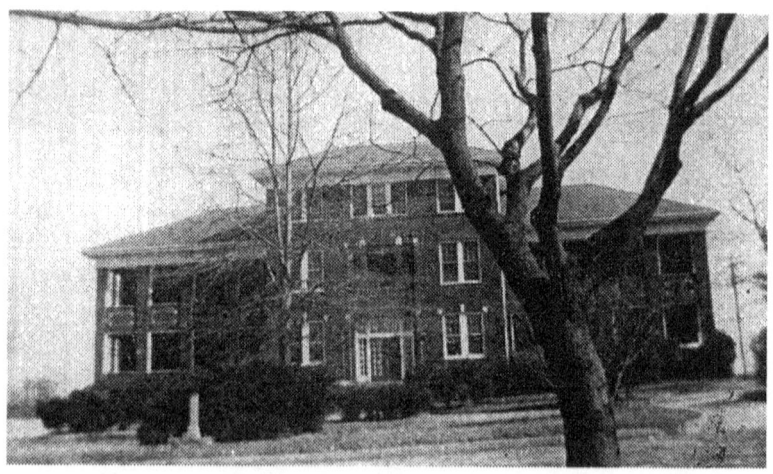

1949. Hicks Memorial Hospital

"Alton, Mrs. Tomblin and Miss Warwick can't have you crying around all the other children. So as soon as you stop crying, I believe she will let you go to the Baby Cottage."

Of the persons with whom I interacted daily, I trusted only Ann. She was so pretty, and her breasts moved inside her dress every time she took a step. Any day now I was going to ask her if she would be my sister. My brother Doc would have called her "Sweetie."

At that point, having no knowledge, or experience, with frying pans and fires, and because my only firsthand dealings had been with this "frying pan" called the "hospital," I was determined to become, or at least to appear, more agreeable to my captors, especially the dreaded "white" woman, who I firmly believed at the time, controlled my very existence on this earth. It wasn't just "concern" that concerned me; no, every time I was near the old woman, I cringed, fearing she could at any time she pleased, finish me off for good.

However, as much as I longed to be rid of the depressing hospital, I admitted to misgivings concerning the treatment to which I might be subjected once I arrived at the "Baby Cottage."

What was this "Baby Cottage?" Why was I being sent to live with "babies?" And for that matter, what was a "cottage?" Was this Baby Cottage but another transient stop along this cruel misadventure in my young life?

Control. I had no control. My welfare, yes, even my life, suddenly was in the hands of kidnappers, who surely had deceived mama (now "my" mama) into believing they would return me to my home after a day's outing, and had unashamedly reneged on that promise.

But there was a nagging thought that simply did not fit into this traumatic "orphanage" equation. Why had mama been crying the morning I left with the two strangers? Was she aware that I would not be returning home that night? And if so, was her failure to inform me of that fact intentional?

A small child's natural assumption is that his mother will always protect him, and that this maternal shield is unassailable and all-encompassing. That being the case, where was my mama? Why did this awful Mrs. Tomblin tell me I did not live with my mother anymore? As each day passed, the incongruity of these conflicting emotions deepened, and into my increasing despondency crept the seeds of a loss of faith and trust in mama.

Years later, with a great sense of embarrassment, I was to ask mama's forgiveness, for when she finally was allowed to visit me three months after my arrival at the orphanage, I refused to return her desperately affectionate embrace, but just stood limp before her, sobbing uncontrollably. Yet at that moment, how could my pubescent mind grasp the complexity of these sudden and traumatic changes in my young life?

The disturbing experience of my first few weeks away from mama was to alter and influence profoundly my psyche even into adulthood, manifesting itself as an ingrained suspicion of persons whom I would meet for the first time.

About two hundred yards along the one-lane gravel road past the swimming pool, we approached on our left an imposing two-story red brick building, whose outer walls were filled with more white-framed glass windows than I had ever seen. Entering the building through the large white front double doors, Ann led me straight ahead and up a flight of stairs. Turning left at the top of the stairs, we walked down a wide hallway, and as I looked through the open doorways on either side of the corridor, I observed young girls hunched forward at black Singer sewing machines and cutting cloth laid out on wide tables. The staccato sounds of the Singers in serious operation and the cutting of the cloth with large shears drifted into the hallway.

Near the end of the long corridor Ann guided me to the right into a large, well-lit, white-walled room where sat several young girls, busily sorting and cataloguing what appeared to be new articles of boys' clothing. Boys' boxer-style undershorts had been stacked in one neat pile, white tee shirts of various sizes in another. Multi-colored heavy plaid long-sleeved shirts occupied one end of a long wooden bench, and on the other end of the bench sat several stacks of what appeared to be brown woolen trousers that had been cut off and gathered at about knee-length. What were these strange looking pants, I wondered. Must belong to the girls. Had to.

Seated behind a small brown wooden desk at the far end of the spacious room was a petite, white-haired, pleasant-looking woman wearing a blue dress with white embroidered lace collar and sleeves. As Ann and I approached her desk, the woman looked up from her paperwork, placed her fountain pen on the desk in front of her, and smiled warmly up at me.

Immediately I liked this lady, and could sense by her smile and twinkle in her eye that she liked me. Perhaps here in Hell I had discovered my second friend?

"I'm Mrs. Hall," she introduced herself in a pleasant voice. "And what's your name?"

"M'name's Alton, but they call my 'Cottontop' at home. Some people just call me 'Cotton.'"

"Well, I'm not busy at the moment," Mrs. Hall said, pushing back her roller chair and coming from behind her desk. Taking me by the hand, she announced "Ann, I'm going to help Cotton find some clothes. We'll be right back."

I liked it that she called me by my nickname. Perhaps if things didn't work out, I could ask her if she could be my mother.

Mrs. Hall led me directly across the corridor and into an enormous room, the breadth of which was filled with row upon row of vertical wooden shelves containing neatly-stacked piles of primarily boys' clothing. Along the walls were metal racks supporting horizontal wooden poles on which hung various size and colors of boys' and girls' coats.

Starting with the coats, Mrs. Hall found the rack containing my size, and told me to try on any of the coats I liked, and after testing out several, I settled on a warm woolen brown one.

Mrs. Hall's act of kindness in giving me a choice of coats instantly elevated my spirits. This was the first time since my arrival at the orphanage that I had been given a voice in anything concerning my care, and I had the distinct impression that in allowing me a choice, Mrs. Hall was demonstrating her empathy for my predicament. Orphan kids, out of desperation for their plight, sometimes cling to a small lifesaver called "optimism" while floundering in an unfriendly grownup-controlled sea of hurt and distrust. It had to do with hope, my allotment of which was being rapidly exhausted.

Apparently sensing my appreciation, the kind silver-haired lady in blue led me to a shelf of those strange-looking aforementioned brown woolen half-trousers that appeared to be cut off at the knees. Among my first impressions of orphanage life made from my vantage point at the window of the hospital playroom, one of the more discrepant was what appeared to be knee-length short pants worn by the smaller boys but not by the bigger boys.

Taking a pair of the strange trousers from the shelf, Mrs. Hall bent forward and held the top of them to my waist.

"Go over there and try these on, Cotton. They should fit you well," she said, pointing to an area behind the coat racks. She still called me "Cotton." Good.

After trying on the trousers, I pulled the gathered bottoms of the pants down over my shins. As I walked from behind the coat rack and approached Mrs. Hall, the bottoms of the trousers crept up my calves. Unable to stifle her laughter, Mrs. Hall bent over and tugged the gathered bottoms up to just below my kneecaps. When she turned me so I could see myself in the mirror, I burst out laughing. I might as well have been an "extra" on the set of "Boys' Town," or one of the "Bowery Boys." Huntz Hall probably would be my bunkmate in the new "Baby Cottage."

Finally, after ten days of incarceration in this hellhole, someone had made me laugh! It was a wonderful feeling, as fleeting as it was. And I felt as foolish as I knew I looked. It seemed as though I were standing in two large woolen balloons, with my bare, skinny white legs connecting the puffed-out balloons with my brand spanking new brown leather brogues.

"I look so dumb, don't I?" I asked, looking up into Mrs. Hall's still smiling face. "What are these things called?"

"These are 'knee breeches,' but the kids call them 'knickers,'" she answered. "Remember that knickers go to just below the knees."

"Do *all* the boys wear knickers?" I asked, recalling that from my hospital playroom observation post this was not the case.

"No, Cotton, the 'big boys' don't wear knickers."

Big boys, I thought. Is this as opposed to "little boys?"

"What are 'big boys?' And why don't *they* have to wear knickers?"

"Well, big boys are mainly the high school boys, and they would look silly wearing knickers."

Now, just a minute, I thought. I have to look like a dunce wearing these stupid thingamagigs, but by virtue of the "big boys" being older than I, they get to escape the shame and embarrassment. The logic escaped me. I was not about to pursue this discussion, however, but I felt that if I had to look silly wearing these stupid pants, this should be reason enough not to wear them. I just couldn't wait to become a "big boy."

Next Mrs. Hall allowed me to choose four plaid woolen shirts from among several piles of warm multicolored clothing. Afterwards, without having me try them on, she selected several pairs of socks, tee shirts and boxer shorts, and placed them in a large brown paper bag.

"Now we need to get you some mittens," Mrs. Hall said cheerfully, reaching for a large box at the bottom of one of the wooden shelves. Taking out a handful of different colored woolen mittens, she placed them on the shelf before me. Without touching any of them, I pointed to a red pair.

"Good choice," she said, placing the pair of red mittens on top of the other clothes in the bag. "That should give you enough warm clothes for the rest of the Winter."

I followed Mrs. Hall across the corridor and into the large room in which was situated her desk. As we entered the room, Ann looked up from her seat and smiled with pride at my new wardrobe. One of the young girls looked up at me, snickered and whispered something to the girl seated beside her at the clothes sorting table. I knew they were talking about how farcical I looked in those godawful knickers. I felt naked standing there in the middle of the room with a bunch of females gawking at me. Worsening yet my discomposure (though I'm certain without intent), Mrs. Hall exclaimed, "Cotton, you're so pretty in your new clothes," that immediately turned my face crimson in front of the already amused young girls. Sensing my embarrassment, the girls began giggling, barely able to hold their attention on the sorting tasks before them. It was definitely time to leave this place.

Mrs. Hall bent over, placed her hand on my shoulder, and whispered in my ear, "I like you, Cotton, and I'm going to look out for you." A little more than a year later Mrs. Beulah Ward, Mrs. Hall's successor, would prove to be true to Mrs. Hall's word. And as Ann and I left the Industrial Building, the heavy brown paper bag, filled with more new clothes than I had known in my short seven years bumping against the coldest lower legs ever to wear a pair of those stupid knickers in February, I enjoyed a brief, inexplicable, euphoric sensation in having found another friend. Years later, as I reflected upon those traumatic first weeks of painful adjustment to the sudden and complete forfeiture of parental safekeeping, I came to realize just how desperately I had grasped at Ann and Mrs. Hall to fill this emotional void.

"What did Mrs. Hall whisper to you before we left, Alton?" Ann asked with a smile as we made our way back to the hospital along the tar and gravel road. "I believe she really likes you, because she sure took a long time picking out your clothes."

"Mrs. Hall let *me* pick out my *own* clothes," I answered proudly. "She told me before we left that she liked me and that she would help me. What does Mrs. Hall do anyway?"

Ann then explained that Mrs. Ora Lee Hall was the supervisor of the entire Industrial Building. Mrs. Minor, who worked for Mrs. Hall, was in charge of the orphanage laundry, that occupied half of the first floor of the massive clothing facility. The sewing and mending rooms were located on the second floor. The girls in the sewing room made dresses for all the girls in the orphanage. Mrs. Hattie Stallings supervised the girls in the mending room, while Miss Neta Edwards was in charge of the sewing room.

Every article of clothing for each boy and girl had sewn onto it the owner's name in indelible ink. This is how the children's clothes were sorted after being washed. After the soiled clothes were washed and dried in the huge metal tumblers in the laundry, the girls sorted and folded them. If upon inspection articles of clothing required mending, they were taken to the mending room, located upstairs adjacent to the sewing room.

"But why aren't these girls in school now?" I asked Ann.

"They do go to school," replied Ann. "The girls you saw work only in the morning. After lunch, they go to school all afternoon, and the girls who are in school this morning go to their jobs, mainly in the kitchen and here in the Industrial Building. There are more than three hundred kids in the orphanage, and starting in the fifth grade, the kids work half day and go to school half a day."

As we approached the hospital on our return from the Industrial Building, Ann paused suddenly.

"You know, they forgot to sew your nametags on your clothes. It's alright, though, I'll just call Mrs. Hall and she'll send the runner to get them."

"What's a 'runner?'" I asked.

"Oh, he's the errand boy who works in the Industrial Building. He carries clothes that have been mended, back and forth between the cottages and the Industrial Building. He'll pick up your clothes today, and have them back to us tomorrow."

CHAPTER 7

The Baby Cottage

I stood quietly before Ann in the center of the spacious Baby Cottage living room, feeling quite ill at ease and half-naked in a pair of ridiculous brown woolen scratchy knickers, the exposed calves of my skinny white legs still stinging from the bitter cold sweeping the campus during our trek from the hospital that bleak morning in late February 1947.

I had been assured by my sister, on her visit lasting only a few minutes, that she would contact me as soon as I was released from the hospital. But at that brief encounter, with me standing on the couch cushion in the hospital playroom, anxiously peering through a cold, sweating window at my visibly nervous sister standing shivering in the bitter cold and rain on the concrete driveway that circled Hicks Memorial Hospital, I peered mentally through her facade of assurance and sensed that she feared for the treatment I was likely to receive upon leaving the hospital.

On the occasion of that reunion, Eoline had not smiled, and her voice betrayed more of a concern for my physical safety than assurances that I would be treated well. It was not until we were teenagers that she confided to me her concern for my well-being at that time, based on her own experience of malefic and cruel treatment at the hands of a cottage counselor upon her arrival at the orphanage six months earlier.

The Rev. Creasy K. Proctor became Superintendent of Oxford Orphanage in 1928. Before that time he had served as pastor of the

Queen Street Methodist Church, only a few blocks from my home-away-from-home, the Paramount picture show. My daddy and mama, devout Episcopalians, were active members of St. Mary's Episcopal Church, situated only about eight city blocks from Rev. Proctor's Methodist church, and the two pastors knew each other quite well. Because Kinston was a relatively small town of about twenty thousand persons, in all likelihood my daddy and mama had met Rev. Proctor, and may have known him well.

My mother's sister Clyde had married a man named Vinson, and the couple had three absolutely beautiful daughters, in order of age, Grace, the eldest, then Ann and Lorena. Aunt Clyde's husband had died, and the three girls had been taken to the orphanage from Kinston. Grace Vinson, the oldest of the three sisters, had graduated from John Nichols High School in 1945, so at the time of Eoline's arrival at the orphanage in July 1946, Ann Vinson was a freshman in high school, and the youngest sister, Lorena, was an eighth-grader. The girls were very pretty, had engaging personalities, and were quite popular among their classmates.

On July 13, 1946, five months after my daddy's death in February of that year, mama had traveled with Eoline and Miss Broadwell, the case worker, to the orphanage. Just as in my experience, Eoline believed mama was taking her for an outing with one of mama's friends. Once inside the orphanage hospital, however, mama left my unsuspecting nine-year-old sister alone in the foyer, telling her only that she would see her "real soon."

Except for the cruelty of the dreaded Devil-in-Starched-White, Eoline's account of her processing at the hospital was similar to mine, and after a week in quarantine, the frightened and confused nine-year-old was assigned to the Annex, because she was too old to be sent to the Baby Cottage, and too young to be sent to 1-G.

Upon Eoline's arrival at the Annex, Mrs. Walling, the cottage counselor, immediately asked my sister,

"So, I hear you're related to those Vinson girls."

When the insecure child smiled expectantly and nodded in the affirmative, Mrs. Walling, without warning or comment, slapped my sister hard across her face, knocking her to the floor. Standing threateningly over my shocked, defenseless and frightened sister, the scowling bitch shrieked,

"You will answer me 'yes, ma'am," and 'no, ma'am,' or you'll get the whipping of your life, young lady. And you'd better not start crying!"

Later that first night, as the truculent matron turned out the lights in the dormitory, the frightened, disillusioned child began sobbing quietly. Mama and daddy infrequently had spanked Eoline with their open hand, or occasionally switched her with a handful of birch switches, but neither had ever been cruel or threatening to Eoline in any way. At the age of nine, Eoline had been at home and heard the sounds of gunfire the day my daddy died, had experienced the grief-stricken look on mama's face at my daddy's funeral, and had sat quietly beside our sobbing, distraught mother during Doc's trial, only a month before she was sent to the orphanage.

And now, only a few weeks later, she had been forced to endure the utter humiliation and indignity of a vituperous and unprovoked physical assault at the hands of a crass, abusive stranger. The soft voice of the young girl in the bed beside my sister came out of the darkness of the dormitory,

"You'd better not cry. If she catches you, she'll give you a whipping."

My sister fell asleep sobbing quietly into her pillow. However, the abusive Mrs. Walling was not finished with my sister. The following morning as the young girls were making their beds, the woman found fault with the manner in which Eoline folded her blanket at the foot of her bed.

Confronting my already traumatized sister in front of the other young girls, the contemptuous matron demanded,

"Didn't your mother teach you how to make your bed, young lady?"

Completely uncertain as to how she should answer the accusation, my frightened sister just stood still, bowed her head, and fixed her gaze on the floor. My sister did not see the hateful bitch's open hand as it landed hard across her face, the force of the blow knocking her to the floor. Dazed, my sister sat up slowly, holding her stinging face in her hands, sobbing uncontrollably. Grabbing the frightened young girl by her hair, the woman jerked her roughly to her feet, and in a shrill voice screamed,

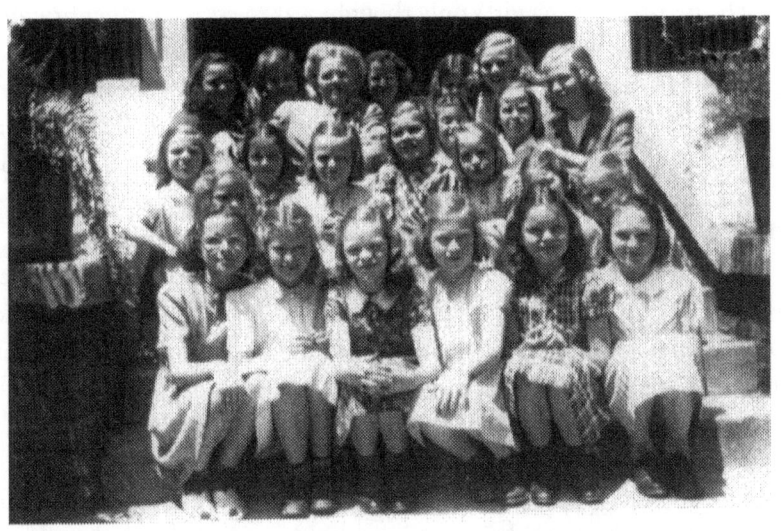

1946. The Annex (Royster Building) girls, with high school "cottage girls" and cottage counselor. The author's sister Eoline, age nine, is on first row, third from left.

"Well, since you can't seem to stop crying, it's back to the hospital with you, young lady. Now, go get your clothes."

Filled with fear and shame, the shocked young girl quickly gathered her clothes, and sat alone on the floor of the Annex vestibule as ordered.

Soon one of the older girls who worked at the hospital came to collect my sister. The two girls walked in silence to the hospital, whereupon the older girl escorted my sister to the playroom, instructing her to wait there for Mrs. Tomblin.

The petrified young girl's only thought was to escape further brutality. Moving silently to the door of the playroom, she peered both ways down the darkened main hallway. Not seeing anyone near the front door of the hospital, she crept quietly down the long hallway, staying close to the wall. Reaching the front waiting room without detection, the terrified young girl rushed to the front door, flung it open and raced wildly down the long concrete hospital steps and onto the road.

At that time of the early morning, students and staff alike were having breakfast in the large central dining hall, so Eoline found herself alone on the sprawling, unfriendly grounds. To whom could she turn for protection? Where was a safe haven?

Confused and frightened, the only building on campus familiar to the young girl was . . . the Annex. Damn! What a predicament! Because the abusive Mrs. Walling was stuffing her face in the main staff dining room, Eoline crept into the Annex and hid in one of the clothes closets. The Annex Ogre discovered Eoline later that morning, cowed and crying in the corner of the hall closet, stripped of all her dignity.

Such was the terrible secret my sister carried as she huddled in the bitter cold outside the hospital window that doleful February afternoon, fearing for my well-being, yet hopelessly unable to prevent any real or imagined harm that she feared would befall me. Adding to that continuing trauma was the fact that mama was not allowed to visit us until April 1947, nine months after Eoline arrived at the orphanage.

During the two weeks I spent in the hospital, Ann had become my island of hope in a hostile and confusing sea of apprehension. As she now knelt before me, I felt panic gripping my small body, and sensed a churning in my stomach. Suddenly, here in the front room of the Baby

Cottage, I was about to lose her protection. Perhaps sensing my vulnerability, and doubtless recalling her own unhappy experiences from years before, I noticed a redness and welling up of tears in her eyes. A lump quickly formed in my throat, and I began to take short, shallow breaths. I thought then about asking Ann if I could go back and stay with her at the hospital. She pulled me close to her, wrapped her arms around me, gave me a long, firm hug, and stood up. Tousling my mop of white hair, she whispered,

"You be a good boy, Alton, and do what they tell you to do. I'll come to see you real soon."

Now just where had I heard that before?

Without awaiting a reply, Ann turned quickly and walked out the front door, leaving me alone in the large room, clutching my brown paper bag filled with clothes, and wondering if I would ever see Ann again. Sensing movement behind me, I turned from the front door just as a slim, large-breasted blond girl of about fifteen entered the room. Approaching me with an engaging smile, she said,

"You must be Alton. Let's go to the boys' ward and I'll show you where to put your clothes."

I followed closely behind her as she turned left from the large front room, and followed a short hallway, where we turned right into a large open area with a floor made of small white ceramic tiles, with walls painted that ominous hospital off-white. I glanced to my left to observe several large white ceramic bathtubs.

I noticed as I followed the girl that her butt bobbed up and down with every step she took, so I followed her, and it, to the right into an open area walled in white with an array of square recessed wooden compartments, most of them filled with neatly-folded multi-colored shirts, knicker-type trousers, white T-shirts and boxer shorts, and woolen socks. To the right of these compartments was an open wall, with large metal coat hooks attached to a thick board nailed to the wall. Above each hook was painted a black number. The wood forming the top of each recessed space was numbered also.

"Hang your coat on number fifteen," said the young girl, pointing to the rack of hangers. I did as she instructed. She was so pretty. Visions of Miss Wellbuilt, my first grade teacher, flashed through my mind.

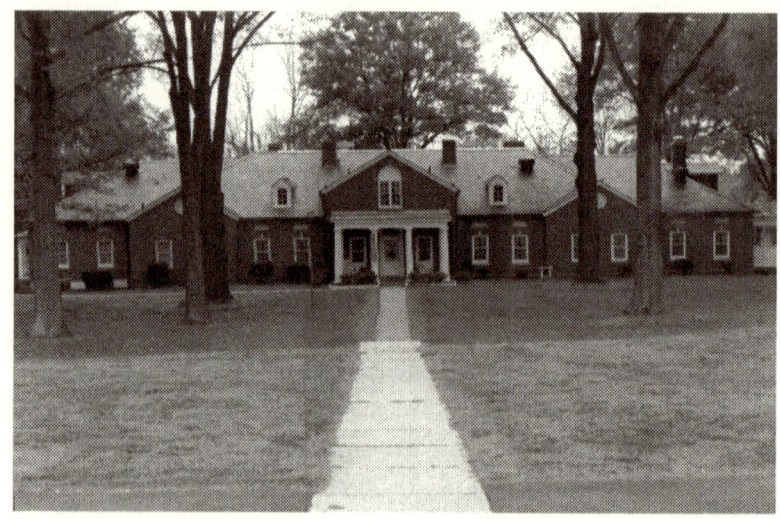

The Baby Cottage (Dunn Building). Housed boys and girls up to about eight, and had its own kitchen and dining room.

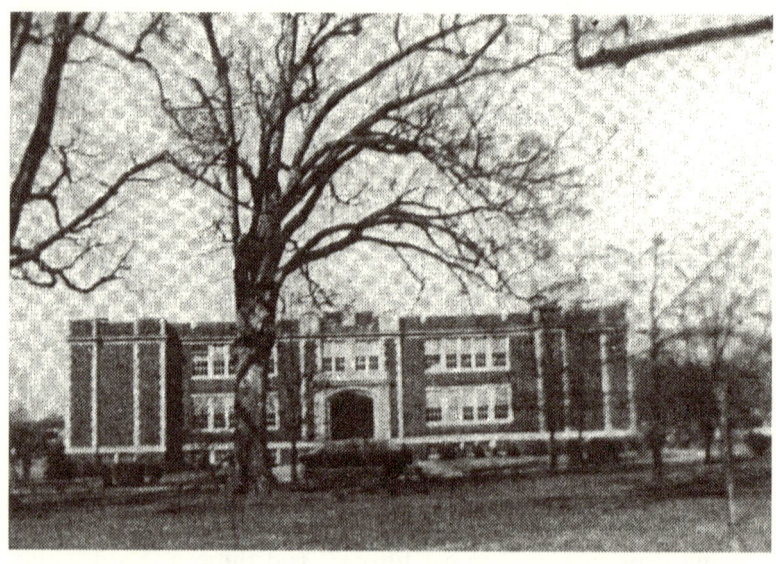

John Nichols School. Constructed in 1924, and housed grades 1-12.

Stepping to the recessed clothes storage area, Bouncing Butt pointed to the empty space above which was painted in black the number fifteen, and said,

"You're number fifteen. If Miss Warwick or one of us big girls calls you by name, or calls 'number fifteen,' you answer 'Yes, ma'am.' Do you understand?"

"Yes . . . Yes, ma'am," I stammered.

Sensing my uncertainty at her instructions, the girl lowered her voice to an almost conspiratorial whisper.

"If you do what Miss Warwick tells you to do, you won't get punished."

My perceptive mind quickly deduced the converse of this instruction, and the results therefrom. Could Miss Warwick and Mrs. Tomblin be related? I wasn't going to like this word "punished" and the ominous threat it carried. The girl's admonition was quite unsettling, and I wondered what form the "punishment" would take if I broke the rules, but dreaded her answer might heighten my fear of what my already dismal future held. Desiring no further elucidation of this distasteful word, I stood still, silently fixing my gaze in mid-space before me.

"Well," she said, apparently aware of my discomfiture. "Let's get your clothes put away."

The next few minutes were spent with the pretty girl demonstrating how she expected my clothes to be folded and arranged in my "cubbyhole," as she called the recessed compartment.

As to the aforementioned "ma'am" thingy. At the Baby Cottage, ab initio the small children were taught respect and discipline, beginning with the magic words that appear to demarcate all of life's respect and discipline, that is, "ma'am" and "sir," prefixed of course by the appropriate gender-less "yes" and "no."

Next I listened with feigned interest as the teenage girl explained that each morning "when the six o'clock bell rings at six o'clock" (sounded sorta like a redundant statement to me, even at age seven) I was to get dressed hurriedly, make my bed neatly, with square corners and all (like I made square corners on my bed at home, or something. What was a "square corner," anyway?), get a bucket of water and a washrag, and clean the baseboards in the boys' dormitory.

"All of the baseboards?" I asked with mild incredulity, that most definitely was not feigned.

"Yes, all of the baseboards, Alton. There are only two of them, one on each side of the dormitory."

"But each one is about a block long. I'll never finish them."

"Well, let's try it and we'll see."

What was this "let's" business? Even at age seven I caught on to the old "let's" ploy. And here was a teenage orphan girl trying out her juvenile psychology on a street-smart kid like myself. Just who did she think she was? I started to tell her that I lived around the corner from Dick and Jane, and then lie and tell her I had actually seen Spot run. But I let it slide for the moment. All in due time.

Abruptly from the front of the building I heard the large doors opening with a clatter, followed by the exuberant, squealing voices of young children approaching rapidly along the hallway. Poking my head out of the cubbyhole room, I stood transfixed as a swarm of about fifteen small boys tore off their multi-colored coats and hung them haphazardly on hangers on the hallway wall. Immediately the chattering swarm of tykes noisily stampeded into the bathroom, some heading for the small toilets and others for the tiny sinks along the opposite wall.

After peeing and washing their hands, and with cheeks still rosy from the cold outside, the jabbering small fry formed a makeshift line in the hallway just outside the boys' wing.

"Where are these kids going?" I asked the pretty blond teenager.

"They're lining up for dinner," she answered. "Let's wash your hands and you can eat with them."

However, by the time I had peed and washed my hands, the group of noisemakers had already departed, so I followed the girl the entire length of the hallway, by now already mesmerized by her bobbing behind, where we turned right into a large room filled with about thirty healthy-looking but now eerily still mostly seven-and-eight-year-old boys and girls, each standing quietly behind a small wooden chair, four to a table.

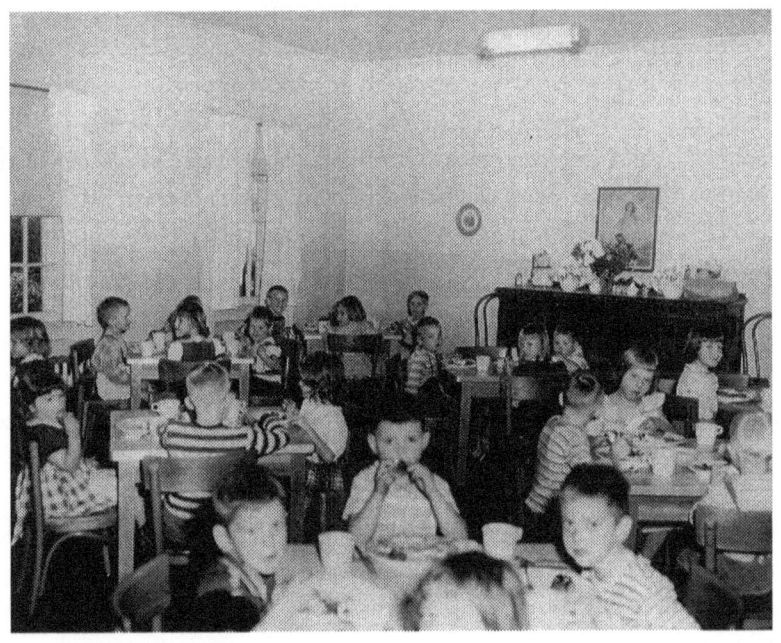

Baby Cottage Dining Room. Eight tables, each seating four children. We kids had to "clean" our plates, "or else" suffer the indignity of being "put in our place."

Spotting a vacant chair, the teenage girl led me to it and, guiding me by my shoulders, told me to "stand very still" behind the chair. Feeling quite self-conscious, I looked straight ahead into the eyes of a freckle-faced, red-headed suddenly smiling boy about my age. On either side of me stood two little girls, and as I looked from one to the other, they too smiled. I could sense myself being inspected by about thirty pairs of little eyes, and being too embarrassed to look around, I just stared at the plate that had been set before me.

The square-shaped off-white stucco-walled dining room was filled with approximately eight same-shaped brown wooden tables, each just large enough and low enough to seat four timorous, apprehensive first, second and third graders, their skinny legs dangling in space above the hardwood floor that never was touched by tiny shoes during the meal.

Oh, my god! I thought, what is this *stuff* somebody put on my plate? It was yellowish-white, squishy-looking and strong-smelling, and suddenly I didn't feel so good. I had been so homesick while at the hospital that Mrs. Tomblin (the old white-haired bitch) gladly allowed me to take my meals in the hallway playroom, so she hadn't known (or cared) whether I ate or didn't eat. Would they let me do the same here?

'Fraid not.

"Okay, children, bow your heads."

The authoritative voice of an imposing, bespectacled silver-haired matron captured my attention, and I looked in the direction of her voice. Her eyes locked onto mine for a brief instant, her stern expression causing me to break eye contact at once.

Damn! She looked an awful lot like the Aging Dimwit in Starched White I had just left at the hospital. Could they possibly be sisters? Or, worse yet, twins?

"I said, bow your head, young man," she commanded, and I quickly lowered my head.

After a silent pause, the old woman muttered something or other, and instantly thirty wooden-legged chairs scraped in unison across the hardwood floor, and we all sat down. I noticed immediately that all the kids, seemingly as one, picked up their forks and began shoveling the awful-looking, awful-smelling *stuff* into their mouths. None of them spoke a word. Just like someone had wound up thirty little eating toys and released the springs. Had I known at the time what a "robot" was, I would have thought I was in a room with thirty eating, non-speaking robots. It was amazing. I just sat there enthralled at the spectacle.

As I looked askance, and I'm certain with growing apprehension, at the preparation of hog slop splayed what-the-hell across the very large ceramic plate positioned a mere grownup's handspan from the entryway to my olfactory gland, Big Old Hateful Grandbiddy appeared to edge her bulk somewhat closer, to where the word "proximity" suddenly gained added meaning and significance. Somehow or other I equated this silent hulk with bad news. Didn't know exactly why, just a feeling I had at the moment. And she didn't disappoint me.

"You're not eating your food, young man," said the imposing presence. She then moved a little closer to my left, like she wanted to make sure I heard her.

"*Here*," she continued, with a pronounced emphasis on the word, as though to distinguish it from "there" or "anywhere else" and certainly, I thought, from 208 East Bright Street, "We eat *everything* on our plates."

Now the emphasis was on *everything*. Could there be a connection? Here? Everything? Plate? I discerned an ominous ring of finality in her voice, just a few clicks to the left of "threatening" and headed inexorably in that direction. Kids (especially small, defenseless ones, let's say, about three hundred miles away from their mothers) possess a kind of sixth sense about these things. Quickly I made the leap of the equation-Here-not home, plus Everything-no choice, plus that awful-looking and equally awful-smelling whitish-yellow gook resting about eight inches from my nose, equals I'm About to be Forced to Do Something I Really Don't Want to Do.

The very thought repulsed me. No way! Before I could reflect on the possible consequences of not being believed, I cleared my throat, looked into the expectant eyes of the little freckle-faced boy sitting seemingly equally petrified in front of me, tried to put a little wood-rasp in my voice to present a front of manliness, and blurted out the stupid comment that those little ones present that day would tease me mercilessly about for the next ten years,

"My mama told me not to eat anything I didn't like."

Silence. It wasn't working. Damn! I swallowed hard. So much for that wood-rasp in my voice. My weakly-conceived gambit was destined to fail.

I caught her out of the very corner of my eye, standing perfectly still, arms akimbo, head cocked to one side, peering down at me through the glint off her round-seg bifocal like an evil botanist looking through a microscope at a specimen of harmful bacteria. The angry edge in her voice carried a basketful of spite, a gallon of venom. She would have no part of this pissant "new" kid, this pipsqueak of a nonconformist attempting to besmirch her iron-clad authority. She would have no part of it. Nosireebob. Not this day. Not ever.

"Look at me, young man."

Dutifully, I transferred my by now thoroughly intimidated gaze from the freckle-faced boy's frightened eyes, up to those cruel light blue irises glaring a hole through my soul, and when the stocky heavy-set matron spoke, I just knew she had been comparing notes with the hated prison guard, Mrs. Edith (Mad Dog) Tomblin, when she barked,

"Your mother's not here, young man. You don't live with your mother now. You'll eat what I tell you to eat, and I'm going to stand here while you clean your plate."

Clean my plate? Does this mean what I think it means? You could have heard a pin drop on a large cotton ball in that small dining room that cold day in late February 1947. Nobody moved. Feeling like a trapped possum, I had no choice. With tears of embarrassment welling up into my eyes, with a little fear thrown in for good measure, my shaking right hand slowly picked up a fork lying to the right of my *full* plate and tentatively dipped it into the awful mass of what I was to learn later was (doubtless a double helping of) white turnips. And the cacophonous resonance of her (man's) voice had quieted instantly thirty cowering tykes.

Laboriously I ate blurry turnips and string beans, mixed with salty tears, and a cake of blurry greasy cornbread (without cracklins even) mixed with more salty tears, and stirred with more shame than any seven-year-old should ever be forced to endure, and by the time I had "cleaned" my plate as threatened, my fear and shame had become transformed into hatred, an emotion to which my puerile psyche had never before been exposed. Rage and hostility forced abruptly on a fragile seven-year-old are almost unbearable emotions to endure.

Just wait til my mama and my older brothers find out where I am, I thought, and this mean old woman will get what's coming to her. The Bully-in-a-Dress loomed threateningly and unmoving over me, til I had "cleaned" my plate, then barked triumphantly, reminding the other thirty terrified tykes of who was in charge here.

"Now, that wasn't so hard, was it, young man?"

Nervously, I tried to speak, but my now powder-dry voicebox failed me, emitting only a soft, squeaking sound, hardly a twitter.

"Well!" she boomed, "Answer me!"

"No, ma'am," came my apprehension-filled, still barely audible reply.

"Speak up, young man," she demanded loudly. She was on a roll.

I tried again. "No ma'am," I said, forcing air into my lungs, in a desperate attempt to avoid the wrath of this overweight, silver-haired threatening gargoyle.

"That's better," she said, pausing while her undisputed authority sunk in, lest tomorrow some other tyke might feel emboldened by my impudence. At this point I got this sinking feeling that my chances for survival would dwindle significantly with each new grownup I encountered.

The decision was unanimous-Miss Minnie (the old bat) Warwick was mean, and if I didn't eat *everything* on my plate, she would surely whip me. Springing to mind were the several vicious open-handed slaps across my cold face administered by the enraged Female-Devil-in-White on my first night in this godforsaken place just a few weeks earlier. I got this terrible, sinking feeling that this "orphanage" thingy wasn't going to come out in my favor. I don't know why-just a feeling I had at the moment. The Baby Cottage was fast becoming the fire to the hospital's frying pan, except that I had not jumped; rather I had been pushed unceremoniously from one torture chamber to the other. And my first day in the Baby Cottage was unraveling quicker'n rotted silk.

The Old Bat stood silently beside me, her right hand propped open-handed (ready to strike) on her hip, her weight shifted to her right side (no doubt in order to pivot when striking with the right hand), as though announcing to the other thirty scared-out-of-their-wits little ones, unquestionably who was in charge here. The tears welling up in my eyes were filled with equal portions of fear, shame and confusion.

In my mind's eye Miss Minnie Bruner Warwick and Mrs. Edith Scott Tomblin represented scowling twin vultures perched on a rotting pine tree limb, just waiting rather impatiently for Little Orphan Al to release his last breath of life. And at the rapid rate of decline occurring at that moment, this final exhalation could come at any time. I was quickly learning that the biguns around this here "orphanage" were an irascible, unforgiving bunch.

During this entire humiliating episode, the little wide-eyed boy sitting directly across the table from me gazed at me with what I sensed at the time was a mixture of pity and understanding, as if to say "I know what you are going through. I've been there myself." Old Mean and Hateful Big Bully finally dismissed us, and as I walked dejectedly and shamefully back to the little boys' ward, the boy came alongside me in the hallway and whispered advisedly, "You'd better do what she tells you, or you'll get a whupping. She's mean."

For a seven-year-old, he sure was a keen observer of criminal psychopathology. Perhaps from experience?

Miss Minnie Bruner Warwick was born in Union County, North Carolina on July 4, 1889. She was employed as the cottage mother in the Baby Cottage (the Dunn Building) from 1940 until she retired in 1950 at age sixty-one. She died near Laurinburg, North Carolina in 1961, at age seventy-one.

Miss Warwick was fifty-seven years old (seventeen years older than mama) when I entered the Baby Cottage in February 1947. I figured that during her ten-year Reign of Terror, Miss Warwick struck fear into the tiny hearts of nearly three hundred small children. The cottage "mother" was really the cottage "grandmother," a love-less spinster who never should have been the caregiver to such small, fragile, frightened children, most of whom had just arrived at the orphanage from broken homes.

Moving from Mrs. Tomblin's hospital to Miss Warwick's Baby Cottage was but another episode in my assimilation into orphanage life. My survival at Oxford depended on continuing to play my refrain of supplication, and to quickly learn and embrace wholeheartedly the concept of "place"-how to discover mine and never forget it.

Following my encounter with Miss Warwick on that fateful first day in the Baby Cottage dining room, I immediately called to mind Mad Dog Tomblin. A thought suddenly struck me. Miss Warwick's hair was the same offensive, weird, harsh tone of light blue-white as was Mad Dog's. Could they possibly be sisters? I wondered.

And I found Miss Warwick's caustic tone of voice to be almost identical to that of Mrs. Tomblin, as though they had taken voice lessons from the same tortured crow. Sure seemed like sisters to me.

The clincher, however, was the fact that Miss Warwick struck as much fear in my tiny soul as did M.D. Tomblin. No doubt about it-the two old bats were Lucifer's older sisters-had to be.

I assumed that my first horrible day at the Baby Cottage had mercifully come to an end. But there was more to come. It all had to do with hygiene, Oxford Orphanage style . . .

The Brown Smudge

At supper that first night, Miss Warwick hovered like a starved vulture near my table, just itching to make an example of this insolent, presumptuous new upstart. Harrumph! Supper that night resembled pureed leftover dinner, an attempt at making vomit quiche gone awry. But I ate it anyway. Fear. Self-preservation. Certainly not hunger or desire.

After supper, all of us kids were herded into the large study just off the front room, and Miss Warwick read us a story from a book of Bible stories.

Sitting there among thirty strange, silent kids, I noticed they all had rosy cheeks, none of them appeared to be happy, and all of them were eerily quiet. The mere presence of Miss Warwick seemed to engender an immediate silence bordering on fear. Except for the little freckle-faced boy, who told me his name was Van, none had endeavored to get to know me. I felt strangely alone and lonely. A far cry from the boisterous, outgoing second graders at home in Kinston, World's Foremost Tobacco Center.

Pretty soon the cottage girl came to gather us up and get ready for bed. When we were all inside the bathroom she announced abruptly,

"Okay, you kids line up."

I watched with curiosity as dutifully the small boys took off their clothes, stacked them in tiny piles on the floor, then, to my wonderment, turned their undershorts inside out, and formed a line in front of the slim, dark-haired teenage girl.

Completely befuddled, I followed the example of the other little boys, ending up last in line, holding my turned-inside-out shorts in front of my little button of a pee-pee in embarrassment.

Suddenly from the head of the line I heard a sharp slap of wood against skin, followed by a surprised yelp, two similar slaps, only harder this time, yelps becoming howls (a howl is longer than a yelp, both being responses of young defenseless children to brutality), then this trauma repeated.

"You'd better start cleaning yourself," the teenage girl screamed, "or you'll get the same thing next time!"

Clean yourself? Ohmigod! Quickly I glanced down at my own turned-inside-out undershorts, and there *they* were, a few (well, maybe more than a few) streaks of brown smudge, staring menacingly back at me. Instantly my heart raced, and beads of cold sweat formed on my upper lip. I was petrified with fear, and the line was dwindling rapidly before me.

Panic suddenly gripped my defenseless body. Maybe if I rubbed hard enough, the brown streaks would disappear. Rubbing the cloth together furiously for a few seconds should do it, I thought (hoped, really). Looking down, my frantic rubbing together of the brown streaks had produced, to my chagrin, one really big, really ugly brown *smudge*! The awful *smudge* looked a hundred times worse than the streaks! Streaks indicated perhaps I had not wiped myself well. A big, ugly brown *smudge* announced I had not wiped myself at all.

Glancing up quickly, I saw the two frightened tykes in front of me push their undershorts up to the girl, who didn't appear to be in a very good mood. She waved the two boys away as one would flick a finger at an annoying housefly.

Maybe I could tell the teenage girl that my mama told me I didn't have to wipe myself if I didn't want to. On second thought, don't even try that one. I girded myself for the worst, and haltingly took a giant baby step toward her. She was seated on a low chair, leaning forward, that put us at about eye level. In her right hand she (quite firmly) held a brown wooden hair brush, with a pattern of small holes bored clean through, and she was kinda waving it back and forth like maybe she not only knew how to use it, but that in addition, she had had a lot of practice doing so. And I don't mean practice brushing her hair, either. I got the distinct impression she enjoyed this part of her day, a chance to vent her anger at others upon the likes of me. Probably not a popular girl.

I was holding my undershorts with both hands, trembling. Looking down, the girl she-bitch saw the *large brown smudge*, did a sort of Oliver Hardy double-take, took a second look, and said in a hateful, demanding tone,

"Give me your hand!"

I (quite reluctantly) released my left hand from my smudged shorts, and held it out tentatively, which is a way of saying that I didn't really want to hold out my hand at all. Tentatively and reluctantly are twins.

Immediately grasping my (slightly) extended fingers with her left hand, she squeezed, pulled my hand toward her, and gave me three very rapid, very hard, very painful slaps across my palm with the back of the hole-filled hair brush.

Reflexively, I jerked my trapped left hand toward me, while at the same time moving my right hand over our locked left hands in a defensive, protective measure. Only thing was, my right hand still held onto my *brown-smudged* undershorts. I noticed brown smudge on her left hand. Mine.

Enraged, the girl flung away my right hand holding the shorts, whirled me around and struck me several times on my naked legs and butt with the hair brush. Screaming in pain and fright, I tried to dance out of her reach, but her grip was too tight, and I couldn't break free.

Finally she released my twisted hand and I fell to the tile floor, sobbing uncontrollably. Apparently realizing she had lost control, when I looked up expecting another blow, the she-bitch was gone.

For a few moments I sat motionless, naked and scared, on the cold February tiled bathroom floor. The stupid teenage girl had left, out of anger or fear of punishment by Miss Warwick, I did not know. And I really was too traumatized to care. The brutal encounter had drained away what little spirit I had remaining following my dining room bump-into with the cottage mother. The old bitch.

Sitting naked on the tiled bathroom floor in front of fifteen small boys, all total strangers, I was suddenly struck with a consuming hatred for the stupid teenage abuser and the equally stupid old cottage mother, both doubtless on loan from a circus sideshow House of Horrors. Visions of The Mummy and The Werewolf alternately flashed through my confused mind. This was not supposed to be happening to me. Where was Mama Pearl? Where was my daddy? Why were my parents allowing this abuse? Did nobody love me? How long would this nightmare continue? What would tomorrow bring?

My confused young mind had great difficulty accepting these traumatic events as real. Was this really happening to me? Or, would I awaken shortly to discover this to have been a garish nightmare? Lying there naked, sobbing and frightened on the cold ceramic tile floor, I came face-to-face with the terrible realization that this day's events would never become just a tiny blip on that larger screen called "life." No, this was a seminal occurrence in what was to become a ten-year odyssey into a search for my identity.

Each of the traumatic experiences that I was to endure for the ensuing decade would be like tumblers of a large lock falling into place, until at the end of this time the final tumbler would click, the lock would open, and I would be the person I was to become. But an abundance of tumblers lay ahead.

Later, lying alone and lonely in my bunk, I reflected on the fact that with seemingly little effort, I had segued myself from one life-threatening dilemma to another, from Mrs. Tomblin's frying pan into Miss Warwick's fire, and from there straight into the vindictive clutches of an orphan girl little older than my sister. It was too much for my confused and disoriented mind to fathom.

During the two weeks I had spent in the orphanage, an indefinable sense of fear of bodily harm coursed through my fragile body like a bolt of hot lightning. At the same time, however, indignation and a child's resentment began to smolder just beneath my veneer of fear.

But now I was too frightened to be humiliated, not knowing enough cuss words to express my outrage and the insult I felt. And again I wondered, had the cottage girl gone to fetch Miss Warwick? And would the malefic matron return to give me a further thrashing? I had usurped her ironclad authority at dinner, so I feared for the worst.

Slowly I got up from the bathroom floor, and without taking a bath, put on my pajamas and went to sit on my assigned bunk, next to last on the row to the left. When the other little boys came to bed, I found that the freckle-faced boy occupied the bunk next to mine. The baleful look on his face evidenced his empathy for my anguish. Neither of us spoke.

After the lights were turned out, I lay on my back under the brown Army blanket, the dormitory warmed from the bitter February cold by steam radiators spaced at intervals along both walls. Had I been a bad person? Had I done something to deserve the wrath of this godoxious teenage girl, who surely was an orphan just like I?

When I was home watching cowboy movie stars at the Saturday afternoon picture shows, I wanted to become a cowboy when I grew up. I figured I could learn 1) to shoot the gun out of the hand of any cattle rustler from thirty yards on the first shot, 2) to say "dadburnit" while simultaneously slapping my thigh, and 3) to appear noticeably embarrassed when being thanked for saving the farm of a heavy-shirted blond wearing tight-fitting jeans.

Later I wanted to become a private eye when I grew up. I could cock my Fedora back on my head a la Humphrey Bogart and my daddy, talk with an all-knowing authoritative drawl like Gary Cooper and James Stewart, or better still speak with a clipped irritability a la James Cagney.

After two weeks in the orphanage all that childish (but serious; the two are not mutually exclusive, you know) ambition came to a screeching halt. Suddenly I just wanted to survive so I *could* grow up. Several sharp open-handed slaps across my face by Mrs. (Big Old Bully) Tomblin on my first night away from mama, a beating with a hair brush by a teenage girl sadist, and a threat to do me a whole lot of physical hurt and then some, by Mrs. Tomblin's clone, Miss Minnie Bruner Warwick, had abruptly changed my life's long-term goal of fame and adventure, into an extremely short-term one of simply survival. This "orphanage" thingy really wasn't working out so well.

Without conscious intent I was taking stock of my situation. Apparently nonassent would not be tolerated in the Baby Cottage, and were Miss Warwick and the cold-hearted teenage girl making an example of me before the other kids? Finally, I fell asleep, thinking of mama and my daddy, wondering why mama had sent me to this awful place, this "orphanage." I had fallen through a most un-Carroll-like Looking Glass, tumbling, or it seemed to me, bumbling, into an anfractuous, mysteriously animus-saturated childhood.

CHAPTER 8

My First Day at School

Quite lamentably, my traumatic and unbesought assimilation into this constantly downward-spiraling morass called an "orphanage" was proceeding much too well on schedule. To my dismay, two weeks after my ill-omened arrival at Hicks Memorial Hospital, I had neither seen nor heard from mama, and my child's innocent and trusting mind still clung in desperation to 1) the belief that mama did not know where I was being held incommunicado, and 2) the hope that late one evening the two-thousand pound door to my prison cell in this "Baby's Cottage" would be blown off its hinges by black dynamite, and I would be rescued in timely and 1940's Buster Crabbe serial fashion by the Caped Crusader, or the Durango Kid, or perhaps even The Masked Man who, without his mask, would look an awful lot like the picture show actor Clayton Moore. We kids preferred the mask; without this degree of mystique, poor Clayton came across as "The Lone Corrugated Metal Siding Salesman." Not a pretty image.

And if at that moment Errol Flynn and the 7th Cavalry were riding hell-bent-for-leather to effect my dramatic bailout, I sure couldn't see any of their scouts on the horizon. Now that I recall, there were so many spreading-tentacled pecan trees and taller-than-the-Maker-intended oak trees on the expansive orphanage campus, we little tykes never saw the horizon anyway.

At this (dangerously low) point in my Game of Life, *somebody* sure was slinging at me a lot of nasty sidearm sinking curve balls, and I wasn't even foul-tipping any of 'em.

And the question of my imminent release had not been resolved to my satisfaction during my brief visit with my older sister three days after my arrival at the hospital.

I had been bullied and then slapped head-against-cold-red-brick-silly by the awful old bat Tomblin, threatened with more of the same by the mean old grandghoul Warwick, forced to eat food I absolutely detested (and the old biddy made me eat *all* of it), and had suffered the sudden traumatic pain and belittlement of having the palm of my open hand slapped (damn) hard several times with a wooden hairbrush drilled with holes, while standing naked in front of fifteen strange boys and a teenage girl, she appearing to enjoy the power she was commissioned and quite eager to exert over scared-out-of-their-wits tykes who, by the sheer (bad) luck of the draw, found themselves in the same untenable predicament as she.

Perhaps everybody was not out to "get me," but the brutal reality of the circumstances had caused me to be just a wee bit paranoid at that moment in my young life. Certainly somebody had tossed a giant monkey wrench into the thin glass gears of my fragile psyche.

For seven wonderful years I had been blessed with the love and protection of my mama and my daddy. Now, abruptly and stridently, this parental shield had been ripped away, leaving a timid, fragile seven-year-old exposed to the whim and caprice of strange and unbridled grownups and, even more disconcerting, under the direct control of the vagaries of a pre-menstrual orphan girl.

What defense mechanisms would my being employ to cope with this sudden assault on my mind and body? Whether or not I sensed the emotions sufficient enough to label them as such at that moment in my unworldly innocence, I am certain that genuine fear of bodily harm and distrust of grownups topped my list of newly-discovered phobias. That list was about to expand . . . exponentially, it seemed.

My first day in the Baby Cottage ended much the same as did my first day in the hospital two weeks earlier. I cried myself to sleep, wondering where mama was, and certain she knowingly would not have allowed me to be dragged to this hateful, depressing place called an "orphanage." My puerile, self-centered, unsophisticated faculties would not allow me to comprehend that at the very moment, in a darkened frame house three hundred miles to the south of Hicks Memorial Hospital, mama no doubt lay awake, crying her broken heart out, her husband tragically lost forever, facing the unbearable reality that my sister and I would never again live with her. The loving family as God had intended, would never again exist.

Early the next morning, while it was still dark outside, I was jolted to consciousness by the unwelcome and discordant pealing of a bell, that I localized as being situated about three feet outside my window, while simultaneously being shaken gently by a small hand on my shoulder.

Turning toward the source of the shaking, and squinting my eyes from the caustic glare of the sudden brightness of the large incandescent bulbs in the ceiling, I looked directly into the eyes of the little freckle-faced boy who occupied the adjacent bunk.

"You'd better get up now, 'fore *she* gets back. If yu stay in bed, she'll *hit* yu. C'mon, I'll hep yu make yur bed, then yu kin hep me."

As I had the previous night already accumulated my year's personal quota of "hits," I quickly jumped out of bed, my warm feet contacting the freezing February hardwood floor, whereupon I observed fifteen youngsters about my age, in varying stages of (hurriedly) making their beds, changing into their clothes and putting on shoes; each of them showing the urgency and calamity of a six-alarm fire drill. It came to me then that apparently I wasn't the only seven-year-old into this "hit-avoidance" mode.

"Yu get on dat side," said the red-headed kid excitedly, pointing to the other side of my bunk, which was the next to last away from the bathroom. As I moved quickly to the opposite side of my bunk, the boy grabbed the top sheet at the head of the bunk, instructing me "Jus' do whut I do."

Quickly I followed my pint-sized instructor's lead, pulling first the top sheet taut, then the dark brown woolen surplus Army blanket, then folding the top of both the sheet and blanket back toward the foot of the bed about a foot. Lastly he fluffed the ends of my pillow between his little hands, then lay the pillow neatly at the head of my bunk, patting the top of it with expertise, then smoothing out the pillow case with his hands. Like he had done it a thousand times before.

"Now let's do my bed," he ordered. "An' whut's yur duty?"

"All the baseboards in here," I responded helplessly, waving my hand around the dormitory. Perhaps from his own first-day experience, the boy seemed to understand the despondency in my voice, so he encouraged,

"C'mon, I'll help yu." I followed him as he almost ran the length of the center aisle of the dormitory to the bathroom, where he quickly poured some warm water into a shallow metal basin, then yanked a well-worn cotton rag from a small bin apparently used as storage for cleaning cloths.

Starting at one corner of the dormitory, he dropped to his knees, dipped the cleaning cloth into the water, wrung out some water, and began moving the damp cloth along only the top ledge of the wooden baseboard, purposely not touching the wide baseboard face.

Puzzled at the boy's actions, and resolved at all costs to avoid the wrath of the dark-haired bitch cottage girl's wooden-hairbrush-with-holes, I asked "Don't we got to do the whole baseboard?"

Pausing momentarily, the seven-year-old "veteran" looked at me like I was a fool or something, quickly sensed my inexperience in such matters, and, lowering his voice to a conspiratorial whisper, confided,

"It'll take yu all day t'wash this *whole* baseboard, and when *she* checks, she'll jus' run 'er finger 'long th' top," demonstrating the cottage girl's imagined inspection by a cursory swipe of his index finger along the top ledge of the baseboard.

"She's lookin' fer *dust*," he whispered. "She's only gonna check the *top*." And then he stopped, crinkled up his face, and smiled as though he held the keys to All the Knowledge of the Universe. And to me, he did.

Thus I had found my first true friend at the orphanage, and I realized in order to survive this Devil's Island, I would have to stick to him like glue. Which I did. Contrary to what I had been taught by my parents, I quickly realized that if I wanted to avoid a whipping, honesty sometimes would have to be sacrificed for expediency. The advice my young friend had offered me concerning cleaning the baseboard was a good example.

Upon being awakened each morning by the "six o'clock bell," as it was called by students and staff alike, we had about thirty minutes in which to quickly make our beds, get dressed, "do" our "duties," wash our hands and face, and be standing at the foot of our bed waiting for the cottage girl to inspect our duties and our beds.

Any tardiness, or deficiency in the quality of performance of our duties or in the satisfactory making of our beds (square corners were a "must") would be met with swift and certain physical punishment, coupled with a liberal dose of mental trauma thrown in for "effect." I was to discover in the coming years just how much the cottage counselors and work supervisors relied on this "effect" thingy.

Anyway, back to my first day in John Nichols School. My new friend had helped me make my bed and do my duty of cleaning the baseboard. A few minutes later the cottage girl inspected our work, and when she stopped between two of the bunks, bent down and ran her fingers along only the *top* of the baseboard, I was elated! Van Edwards was a young genius!

Presently the very loud bell rang again, and the boys formed a line of twos in the hallway outside the boys' ward, facing the living room, and we marched the length of the hallway, turning right into the dining room for breakfast, an event I intentionally and quite successfully turned into a "non-event" by eating *everything* on my (very large) plate, all the while fixing my gaze permanently at a point about forty-five degrees below horizontal, not opening my mouth except to shovel in whatever it was that passed for breakfast in this horrible place.

After breakfast, I followed in the wake of my new pint-sized comrades, mimicking their actions, putting on my heavy woolen coat, mittens and toboggan, and forming a two-abreast line in the lobby.

All bundled up against the biting Winter wind, that certainly seemed much harsher than the weather in Kinston, a few hundred miles to the south of Oxford, I marched two-abreast with my friend Van and the other Baby Cottage tykes, up the sloped concrete walkway from the cottage. We passed between the rear of the imposing, colossal Main

Building and the front of the equally impressive Dining Hall, down the road in front of the smaller two-story Business Office building.

When we passed the hospital on our right, I reflexively quickened my pace, while simultaneously glancing out of the corner of my eye, cautiously sneaking a peak, expecting at any moment the White Witch to come flying down the concrete steps of the hospital and give me a few open-handed slaps across my face.

My pride and my hand were still smarting from the previous day's traumatic set-to with Minnie (Mad Dog) Warwick and that stupid idiot-ass dumb-bitch cottage girl. Hope my brown "smudge" she got on her hand gave her a terminal case of infantile paralysis. Thanks to that brainless bimbo, now I would be compelled to rub my skinny butt raw with toilet paper every time I did No. 2, and my fast-learning, sharp as a new Gillette double-edged mind already had ratcheted up to hyperspeed trying to figure out ways to get around having my hand spanked again.

We were herded left at the hospital, and soon were noisily entering the first floor of John Nichols School, that imposing rectangular red brick structure that from that day forward, always reminded me of a medieval fortress I had seen often in Prince Valiant funny papers.

Doors popped open along the wide corridors, and older kids poured excitedly into the warm, brightly-lit classrooms, shedding mittens, woolen coats of many colors, and toboggans, the bedlam of voices spilling out into the hallway. I danced quickly out of the way as a rustle of kids scurried for the various classrooms.

Finally Van and I approached our second grade classroom, and fearing I was about to encounter my third tyrannical grownup in two weeks, I reluctantly entered the room. A slim, bespectacled woman in her early forties met us just inside the door. Miss Myrtle Leigh Peacock.

"And who do we have here?" she said, smiling down at me.

Despite my new teacher's seemingly genuine smile, I suddenly experienced a surge of insecurity in this, another strange and unfamiliar setting. Suddenly the newness and unwelcome foreignness were overwhelming. As far as I was concerned, I could be in a different world.

Suddenly I missed mama more than ever. I just stood unmoving before my new teacher, my gaze fixed on the floor, wanting and needing so desperately to cry out for mama, yet fearing this initially pleasant grownup would threaten me as had Mrs. Tomblin and Miss Warwick.

Sensing the shame and apprehension she had doubtless observed in hundreds of vulnerable children before that cold Winter morning, Miss Peacock leaned forward, placed her hands gently on my frail shoulders, and said in a soft, comforting voice,

"Alton, you are going to be fine here. Nobody is going to bother you as long as you are in my class."

You really mean it, lady? Can I stay here forever? I pleaded all this under my breath. Little did I know at that moment, but during the next decade I would do an awful lot of pleading, yelling, screaming and cursing (we called it "cussing") under my breath, in the presence of hated and abusive grownups and same-dispositioned older boys.

Miss Peacock guided me by my shoulders to an empty desk near a window. Suddenly I noticed that the entire wall to our left consisted of five very tall windows, such that the whole wall facing the baseball field and hospital was really one large window.

"Sit here," my teacher motioned with her hand at the desk. "I'll get you some books and a pencil." My new teacher selected three well-worn textbooks from a bookshelf at the rear of the classroom, then took two No. 2 yellow pencils from her desk drawer and brought them to me.

Accepting the books and pencils, I said softly "Thank you," then quickly added the mandatory "ma'am." She smiled, as if to let me know she understood that somebody had already straightened me out on this cast-in-stone "ma'am" rule, a conversational requirement of polite behavior that was the cornerstone of discipline at Oxford Orphanage.

Then from a table at the back of the room Miss Peacock took a blue denim bag measuring about a foot square when flattened on a table, with two double-thickness straps attached. Placing the folded bag on my desk, the teacher explained that this bag was to be used to carry my school books, and that every child in the school had one just like it.

I liked Miss Peacock from that first day in second grade. This tall (wasn't every grownup), slim, pleasant middle-aged lady with reddish-gray hair always had a ready smile for me, as though she possessed an insight into my myriad of misgivings and fears.

During the next few weeks Miss Peacock went out of her way (or though it seemed to me) to gently draw me out of my case-hardened shell of insecurity and apprehension, and at recess each day encouraged me to interact with the other children. Another battle well-fought but lost.

This poor lady had a tough row to hoe, however. I never found learning especially difficult, even in the second grade, and I spent a good part of my time daydreaming of my previous happy life, deep in the doldrums. But Myrtle Leigh Peacock, thoughtful and caring, did her best for me.

It took my third grownup to turn the trick, but at last a tiny hole had been drilled through my wall of depression, enabling a desperately needed ray of hope to break through, if but fleetingly. Miss Peacock's kindness provided a modicum of comfort, but I realized that each day after school let out at 3:15 p.m., I had to return to the depressing and fearful confines of Old Bag Warwick's House of Threats, Abuse and Very Tasteless Food.

At times a commanding presence of alcohol and other chemicals pervaded the hallways of John Nichols School. The origin of these peculiar and acute odors was a contraption called a "mimeograph" machine, that was located in the first floor supply room.

The mimeograph, or stencil duplicator, is a "duplicating machine" that uses a specially-coated stencil. A typewriter "cuts" the letters into the coating on the stencil, and this stencil is then attached to a cylinder, or "drum."

As the drum is rotated by hand, "writing fluid," that today we would call "ink," flows through the letters cut in the stencil, to enable the operator to produce copies. Real "stone-age" technology, by modern standards, in somewhat the same category, historically-speaking, as a Linotype machine, a Frieden calculator and a slide rule, all of which in my youth and in college, I used and at which I became proficient. And in their time, these machines and instruments were all considered quite efficient and well served the purposes for which they were intended.

Mimeograph copies were usually smudged and of poor reading quality. When the mimeograph was being operated, the strong chemical fumes permeated the hallways and wafted into the classrooms, often producing a mild intoxication, giving us kids a cheap ninety-proof "high." I never was able to connect the cause and effect of the sensations, but I seemed to be a little less homesick, and noticed that my classmates suddenly smiled a lot when the mimeograph machine was being operated. After all, the fumes were alcohol-based, and the mildly hallucinogenic effect rivaled that of the caffeine-laden, carbonation-filled Dr. Pepper soft drink in the late 1940's.

The word "plastics" was foreign to the vocabulary of most youngsters (as well as adults) when I entered the orphanage in February 1947. Probably the first "plastic" in widespread use was not known of as a plastic at all. "Bakelite" is a trademark for various synthetic resins and plastics, especially ones made from formaldehyde and phenol.

L.H. Baekeland (1863-1944), a Belgian-born U.S. chemist, received the patent for Bakelite. The heavy, durable (but often quite brittle) Bakelite was used in the manufacturing of telephones and various electrical insulation products. The ubiquitous heavy telephone handsets that for decades were used to discipline small children and smash large cockroaches, were made of the durable Bakelite.

A few materials in common household use were thought by some to be "plastics," but actually were composed of ingeniously put-together natural substances. "Cellophane," in everyday use as a moisture-proof wrapping for foods, etc., was not a synthetic material; rather, it was made originally from regenerated plant cellulose.

At the time of my arrival at the orphanage in February 1947, the bulk of furniture and appliances produced in the United States was manufactured from glass, wood, metal and natural cloth fibers. Our clothing was made mainly of cotton and wool. Two other substances resembling our modern-day "plastics" were Formica and linoleum.

Formica is a durable sheet made of a synthetic resin. It was fairly brittle, but was heat-resistant and chemical-resistant. By the end of World War II Formica was in widespread use as a covering for table tops and counters, in homes and restaurants.

Linoleum was made in sheets by pressing heated linseed oil, resin, powdered cork and pigments onto a canvas backing. It was used mainly as a floor covering. None of the materials comprising linoleum was synthetic, and for that era in the United States, linoleum, Formica and Bakelite were considered major improvements in the quality of life of Americans. Vinyl plastics, polymers and copolymers of vinyl derivatives, made from ethylene, either were in their infancy or nonexistent in the 1940's.

CHAPTER 9

The "How Are You. Fine I Hope" Letter

Shortly after I had arrived at the Baby Cottage, after supper one evening, Miss Warwick gathered us little snot-faced tykes together and sat us down each with a sheet of notebook paper and pencil. Immediately twenty-five little hands grasped twenty-five No. 2 yellows, scrunching tiny shoulders as if beginning a distasteful task demanding the utmost physical and mental concentration, and commenced scribbling away, hardly if ever glancing up from their important "assignment."

Now what did I miss out on, I wondered. Expecting certain admonishment from the mean old blue-haired ogress, I was not to be disappointed. Here comes Gargantua, gliding across the floor with all the grace of a three-hundred pound Nazi concentration camp guard as though we were two powerful magnets in mating season. Would she believe me if I told her, with all the conviction I could muster, that my mama told me not to write anything I didn't want to write? No, better not even attempt it. Certainly didn't work with the "eating" thingy.

Towering above me, arms already akimbo in that Oxford Orphanage patented offensive stance of chastisement, she ordered,

"Well, Alton, start writing your letter."

"My letter?" I looked up quizzically, not all the way up, though, because I feared making eye contact with the mean old biddy would be taken as an overt act of rebellion, defiance and nonconformity (all of these) of which I wanted no part. Nosireebob! My gaze got no higher than her waist level, and I waited for her rebuke-filled response.

"Each month you have to write a letter to your mother, to let her know how well you are getting along." (How *well* I'm getting along?)

"After you finish your letter, I'll put the letter in an envelope and mail it to your mother."

"Yes, ma'am," I responded, suddenly quite eager to pick up my very own No. 2 yellow and, scrunching my frail shoulders over my paper a la twenty-five other frightened children. This was my chance, and it fell right into my lap. Thank you, God!

So I carefully wrote:

> mama, I hate this place. One lady slapped me hard. The lady here is mean. They will not let me see Eoline. I have to eat everything on my plate. Come take me home. Now.

I didn't even sign the letter, for two reasons. First of all, I didn't know I was supposed to sign a letter. I was only seven, and had not written a whole helluva lot of letters in my short lifetime. Second, mama would know it was me from my wonderful penmanship. I was certain of this fact.

Because it was a personal letter from me to mama, I folded it twice, and with confidence placed the pencil and my precious letter on the small table before me. Observing that I had finished my letter, Miss Warwick approached the table, reached down, picked up the letter, unfolded it, read it, and then I heard above me the crunching of a sheet of cheap notebook paper, that sounded a lot like the cheap notebook paper on which I had just written my "I Hate This Place and Want to Go Home" letter.

Fool! Stupid seven-year-old dumbass kid!

"Young man," the stern lecture began, "We don't write this kind of letter in the orphanage. Now you pick up your pencil and write what I say."

The irritated old biddy placed before me a clean sheet of equally cheap Montag notebook paper. I picked up my No. 2 yellow and waited.

"Dear Mother."

I wrote "Dear Mother."

"How are you?"

I wrote "How are you?"

"Fine I hope."

I wrote "Fine I hope."

"Do you have a pet?"

I wrote "Do you have a pet?"

Looking down at my paper, Miss Warwick said, in a stern tone tinged with a threat of impending bodily harm,

"No, don't write that. I asked you if you had a pet at home." She was beginning to look a wee bit exasperated. Just a little bit. Another crunching of Montag's finest bond. Another clean sheet.

Presently we were down to the "pet" thingy again. In an obvious attempt to conserve notebook paper, Miss Warwick reached down and snatched the No. 2 yellow from my grasp.

"Now, do you have a pet at home?"

"Yes, ma'am. I have a cat."

"What is the cat's name?"

"Name? I just call it my cat. It don't have no name."

"Is it a boy cat or a girl cat?"

"How can you tell?" (Better still, does it really matter? I wondered.)

No answer.

"Okay. Write 'How is my cat?'"

I wrote "How is my cat?"

And on, and on, and on. Soon I had completed my very first ever letter home to mama, letting her know how well I was doing and how happy I was. As far as mama knew, her son Alton was "fine."

This was my first of what we later on referred to as the monthly "How are you. Fine I hope" letters. The letters were addressed to a parent if living, or if the child were a true orphan (no living mother or father), to a brother, sister or other relative of record. Rarely having anything of interest to write about (it's not like I had a "field trip" every day), if we had been taken to see a rare picture show at the Orpheum picture show in downtown Oxford, we were ordered to write that we had seen a picture show recently, and that we had "liked" the picture.

Apparently mama cherished our letters, for upon her death in February 1962 at age 55, Eoline collected mama's writings, that included all the letters from Eoline and me over the years.

Looking through these letters, every single one began "How are you? Fine I hope." And I always asked "How is my cat?"

CHAPTER 10

The Picture Show

One warm Spring Saturday afternoon, the two teenage cottage girls (the pretty blond one with the bouncing behind and the hand-spanking, brown-smudge-checking mean one) rounded up all us little ones, and off we marched two abreast across the campus toward the Main Gate, for what was to be my first excursion off the orphanage grounds since the beginning of my open-ended prison sentence three months earlier.

Because informing six- and seven-year-old snot-faced orphans of what was about to occur that affected their lives ranked about a twenty-nine on the Importance Scale of one-to-ten (one being the most important), as usual we had not the slightest notion of our destination. Passing through the front gate, we took a "column left" and were guided along College Street toward what, I was soon to discover, was the center of town. Six blocks later, as we turned left where College Street dead-ended at Hillsboro Street, and marched to the center of the next block, the familiar smell of hot buttered popcorn wafted up the sidewalk and enveloped us before we even got to the large sign atop the marquee that announced to my sheer delight a new-found friend, the "Orpheum."

The "picture show," as we called movie houses in that era, was located directly across the street from the historic red brick Granville County courthouse. Built in 1943 by E.G. Crews, the Orpheum was the small town's only picture show. One of the many simple pleasures I had longed for from my wartime pre-incarceration life was going to Saturday afternoon picture shows, consisting mainly of B-westerns (Bob Steele, Hopalong Cassidy, Lash LaRue, Red Ryder and Little Beaver, etc.), and following the exciting weekly episodes of "serials" at the old Paramount on Queen Street in Kinston, my hometown and the town that I was certain remained forever The World's Foremost Tobacco Center. And I never let any of the kids at the Baby Cottage forget that fact, either.

Good! I thought, as we formed an eager, pint-sized queue in front of the large red double doors to the right of the box office. Just like back home at the Paramount, the cottage girls surely will treat us to (the large size) boxes of hot buttered popcorn (they used real butter in those days), and even larger (a "both-hands-to-hold-onto") Pepsi Cola. We'll get to watch Sunset Carson, magnificent as usual in his white hat, mounted astride his Golden Palomino, rope and fight and (bloodlessly) shoot the guns out of the hands of a passel of scrungy-looking varmints in black hats, riding scrawny paints reserved as transport in the Old West for dingy desperados and the ubiquitous rascally redskins.

The dapper, reserved gentleman in the English tweed hat and dark suit took roll by touching each of us little ones on the top of the head as we filed into the Orpheum, but much to my chagrin (and disappointment and heartbreak), we were not halted in the lobby for treats, but instead were herded quickly past the glass-encased, popcorn-spewing round metal cooking stand and directly into the pitch-dark picture show, thirty little boys and girls pushing and stepping on each other's heels as the cottage girls seated us by the Braille method.

I sat through that entire damned picture show like Pavlov's dog, eyes darting expectantly over my shoulder at the lobby, palms sweating, waiting in pained anticipation for delicious, tasty, salty, hot-buttered popcorn that never arrived, listening to the envied townspeople around us crunching the fresh crispy popcorn and slurping shamelessly the equally great-tasting ice-cold Pepsi Colas, the sound of empty popcorn boxes and soft drink cups hitting the floor all around me. Just another in an increasingly long list of things to remind me of the Devil-in-Starched-White, "You don't live with your mother anymore, young man!"

However, on that particular Saturday afternoon in the spring of 1947, I was not to see Sunset or Hopalong, or Lash and Fuzzy, or Gene and Tony. Instead, for ninety minutes, mesmerized to the point of not breathing, I sat quietly in the small picture show, engulfed in the nostalgic aroma of hot-buttered popcorn wafting in from the lobby, captivated by the tear-jerking account of a young boy's love for an orphaned yearling fawn. Set against the poverty of a farm family in the post-Civil War era, *The Yearling* was the story of the unqualified love of a child for a helpless animal, the coming of age of a boy little older than I, and it brought thirty orphan Baby Cottage kids to tears and drained our emotions.

We youngsters stumbled along with tear-filled eyes all the way back to the orphanage that Saturday afternoon, and even today I debate in my mind whether I was crying because of the highly emotional picture show, or from the sheer agony of being in such close proximity to hot-buttered popcorn and not being allowed to eat it. Probably a little of both.

CHAPTER 11

I Nearly Drown and
See My First Naked Girl

In June 1947, I finished second grade, numbering among my few friends Van Edwards and Miss Myrtle Peacock, and lamenting the fact that I would not have this sensitive and caring lady as my teacher in third grade in the Fall.

Prior to entering Oxford Orphanage in February 1947, my experience as a swimmer had been limited to wading in the sand fiddler-infested ocean on the coast at Swansboro. Therefore, I tingled with expectation when I was fitted with "swim trunks" and informed that we would be going swimming every afternoon during the Summer.

Each child swam for one hour each day, except for the days when the pool was being drained and cleaned. The first swim hour in the early afternoon was reserved for the thirty or so Baby Cottage boys and girls, which meant simply that we little ones got to pee in the pool first.

Prior to going in the pool, we were required to shower in the small square yellow wooden "shower house" located adjacent to the pool. After scrubbing our bodies with the ultimate body cleansers, Octagon soap and abrasive short-bristled brushes and rinsing off, we had to line up for inspection by Mr. Regan, who supervised the swimming pool.

Orphan kids become smarter than their "keepers" because by their very station in life, they seek ways around rules, and we had oodles of rules at Oxford. We kids discovered quickly what literally hundreds of orphans had found out before our time, this being that Mr. Regan checked only two places on our bodies, the crook of one arm, where it bends at the elbow, and the outside of one foot on the soft spot just above the heel. What with all that scrubbing, by Summer's end we Baby Cottage tykes had left about twenty pounds of epidermis in the shower house.

Mr. Regan would rub both these checkpoints hard with his thumb, back and forth a few times. If he rubbed off dirt, he would harshly tell us to go back and bathe again. Didn't take us pint-sized wizards very long to figure out that if we scrubbed just these two spots well, we were home free.

On the first day of swimming, I bathed with the other kids, passed he crook-of-the-arm and ankle tests with flying colors, then the door to the shower house opened, and I anxiously followed the other squealing Baby Cottage kids and jumped feet-first into the deep water a few feet away.

And immediately sank like a rock. I didn't know how to swim. I panicked, but had the presence of mind to push myself as hard as I could off the bottom of the pool. When I broke the surface, I yelled "HELP!" as loud as I could, then quickly slid below the surface again.

Immediately, I felt a strong arm around me, pulling me to the surface. My savior, Miss Louise Pender. Assuring herself that I had not swallowed too much water, Miss Pender said, "I guess you don't know how to swim, young man."

Miss Pender continued, "Let's get you over to the 'baby' pool, and pretty soon you'll be swimming in the 'big' pool."

So for the next week, Miss Pender taught me how to swim. She showed me first how to "dog paddle," which, if you closely observe a dog swimming, you know where the term originated. "Treading water" plus forward propulsion with hands and arms equals "dog paddling." It really works quite well.

Next, Miss Pender, in my particular case the Patron Saint of Patience, taught me how to float on my back while kicking my feet. After some time, I finally got the hang of it, and she allowed me to graduate to the "big" pool, but kept me out of the deep (nine foot) end for another week or so.

In order to allow us tykes to have enough energy to swim, after lunch each day we were required to lie down on blankets in the Baby Cottage basement, and close our eyes for an hour. This period of rest was supervised by one of the cottage girls. If she caught a child with his or her eyes open, that child was ordered to stand on one foot until the child had "learned his lesson."

After leaving the swimming pool at two o'clock every afternoon, we small kids idled away the rest of the afternoon on the playground. One late afternoon was like another, but one day I had to retrieve my toy I had hidden beneath my bunk, and my life took on a different meaning . . .

The time was late June 1947, the beginning of my first Summer in the orphanage. Still, I was quite a timid child two months into my eighth year, having just completed second grade.

She was the first naked girl I had ever seen. I still remember her, and always will.

The day was a hot one. We had just returned from our one o'clock to two o'clock swim session, and we Baby Cottage girls and boys had gone into our respective bathrooms to shed our wet swim trunks. Once dressed, our daily Summer routine called for the boys and girls to meet on the small playground near the Baby Cottage, to climb the "monkey bars," ride on the "ocean wave," balance one another on the "see-saws," swing on the swings, and while performing these daily diversions, to pick our snots, giggle at the sounds of tiny farts, and engage in sundry obnoxious, meaningless and socially repugnant behavior so common among us seven- and eight-year-olds.

However, on this particular day, I had hidden a small toy under my bed while changing into my swim trunks, prior to swimming, and after dressing I had gone to retrieve my toy from its hiding place. As I returned the length of the boys' dormitory (my bed was next to last from the door), I heard water running in the boys' bathroom.

Odd, I thought. Who could this be in the bathtub in mid-afternoon? With childish curiosity, I walked quietly into the bathroom, and peeked around the tiled partition into the tub, that carried the sound of running water.

And there she stood, full-frontal, a glorious image stamped indelibly in my most impressionable young mind forever, all soapy, as though she were squeezing a freshly-lathered tortie kitten between her perfectly-shaped thighs.

Reflexively, though without cry or comment, she covered her soapy "kitten" with her right hand, while simultaneously drawing her left forearm across her full breasts, and as she half-turned away, I saw in all its beauty and glory what had been bobbing up and down beneath her thin skirt when she walked. At that moment, at the tender age of eight, I became forever and ever a dedicated "ass" man.

For a frozen moment, my entire world consisted of this absolutely beautiful naked body, truly a work of art, stamped indelibly and forever into my memory. Sensuous, no. At age eight, my puerile mind had not yet expanded to this level, and would not do so for several years. But even at such a young age, I was able to appreciate the beauty of what I beheld. Seductive only in the sense that I could not take my eyes off her.

She had well-soaped her body, that accentuated her rounded hips and large, firm breasts, and her nipples protruded like two bright red cherries through a sea of soapsuds. At first glance, I thought the mass of soapy blond hair between her well-curved legs was a washcloth, but when she made no move to take her hand away, and the "washrag" did not fall into the tub, I quickly assumed whatever it was, it was attached to her body. The deductive powers of an eight-year-old boy are at times nothing short of amazing.

The pretty blond girl's eyes met mine, and she smiled. Then I smiled because she had smiled at me.

"Are you supposed to be in here, Alton?" she asked.

Not being fully aware of what she had said because I was rapidly computing the reasonableness of the situation, in my confusion I repeated her question, confusing "me" with "her" in the process.

"Are you supposed to be in here?" I asked innocently.

Apparently realizing my difficulty with accepting the unusual turn of events, the pretty girl laughed, and when she did, her breasts, with their cherry red centers, bobbed up and down.

"I don't think either of us should be in here," she said, then added "But our hot water is not working in our bathroom upstairs, and I thought everyone had gone out to play."

I continued to stare at the soapy blond mass between her legs.

"What's that?" I asked, pointing at it.

"Oh, that," she said, looking down. "That's my secret," she said, giggling. "Now, you run along outside and play, and don't tell anybody about my secret, okay?"

"Okay," I responded, backing slowly out of the bathroom, my eyes locked onto hers. I was proud to have a secret with the teenage cottage girl. I had liked her a lot. I liked her even more now, though I didn't know exactly why. Several years later, this reason would hit me like a ton of bricks, right in the groin.

In the Baby Cottage, spare time wreaked havoc on my psyche. As long as we kids were busily going about our daily activities, I did not think about home and my family as much. But at bedtime, having pulled the toilet paper padding from between my butt cheeks and flushed it down the toilet, passed "inspection" by the super-bitch cottage girl, and was in bed, I never once fell asleep without passing my "before" life on my mental picture show screen, and I fell asleep many, many times with tear-filled eyes.

And during spans of idle time, I noticed little boys and girls on the playground, some gazing off toward the horizon, deep in thought, wondering what kind of life awaited them on the other side of those eyes-high hedges that made up the periphery of their compressed world, calmly rooting for boogers while practicing farting and waiting their turn on the "ocean wave." And while we're on that subject . . .

A "fart" is defined as "an audible expulsion of intestinal gas." Farting is something disgusting little seven- and eight-year-old Baby Cottage girls did-a lot! By the time they moved up to the Royster Building (that we called the "Annex"), these same smelly little wind-breakers were taught that farting is a gross and socially unacceptable act, so, fast-learning little she-devils that they are, they quickly resorted to "pooting."

However, you'll not find "poot" in the dictionary. Perhaps it is one of those "nonce" words (words that are invented, or just used in a particular situation) that doubtlessly spring up in a closed society of more than three hundred orphan children.

These same little she-animals learn then, that by squeezing their butt-cheeks together just right, they can, following a lot of practice, eventually learn to turn a socially indecorous fart into a silent one, that we kids called a "poot." A poot, then, may be further defined as a "silent fart," or "a fart that's lost its voice." And, fast learners that they are, these little munchkins quickly hone this disgusting practice to a fine art form.

A similar transformation did not seem to come about with us nine- and ten-year-old Walker Building boys because, being unprincipled little troglodytes that we were, such refinements in social etiquette were not expected of us. To review then, small boys and girls are little more than animals that have learned to walk upright, and (occasionally, if reminded constantly) wash their front paws before eating. Gender-wise, they are distinguishable only by whether they fart or poot.

Case in point: When my nine-year-old sister was in the Royster Building (Annex), home of about thirty or so, nine- and ten-year-old girls, the girls sat four to a table during the nightly two-hour study hall, during which time no talking of any kind was allowed.

One school night the cottage mother, Mrs. Walling, who sat on a chair in study hall in order to enforce the "quiet" rule, was stationed near the table around which were seated my sister Eoline and three other young girls. Suddenly, my sister smelled something really awful that she described to me as a six-day old dead goat, and as if on the same cue, the cottage mother's eyes darted up from the book she was reading and, according to my sister, audibly sniffed at the air like a coon-sniffing hunting dog on the opening day of hunting season.

Unable to immediately pinpoint the source of the breathtaking stench, the cottage mother ordered the four frightened young girls into the bathroom.

"Who did *that*?" she demanded angrily, looking from one girl to the other expectantly.

"Not me, ma'am."

"Not me, ma'am."

"Me neither, ma'am."

"Me neither, ma'am."

"All of you take off your panties immediately!" demanded the enraged matron, reeling from the olfactory shock.

In turn, each of the intimidated young girls removed her panties and held them up to the infuriated woman. In turn, she pushed her nose into the panties and breathed deeply.

Nothing.

Nothing.

Nothing.

Nothing.

Eoline said to me later she supposed the cottage mother was hoping to locate a "hanging poot."

Suddenly, my sister said, before she could even flinch, the huge cottage mother's open hand caught her on the left side of her face, knocking her to the floor. The other three girls received a similar slap across the face and the four girls began to cry.

"Now, I know *one* of you girls did *that*," she shrieked, "and if I find out who it was, you're going to get the whipping of your life. Now put your panties back on and get back to study hall."

Eoline said that none of the girls ever owned up to it. However, she said, they all knew who it was, because the poor girl pooted-a lot.

I believe the point in life wherein a small child begins his or her protracted, arduous road to maturity, enlightenment and social awareness is reached when the witless youngun discovers, much to his or her dismay and disappointment, that farting in a public place, with or without an olfactory warning, is looked upon by grownups as an indecorous and thus proscribed act.

CHAPTER 12

End of the First Year-1947

As of Christmas 1947, V-E Day was two and a half years into the history books, and the baby boom strummed along unabated as ex-servicemen and their wives continued to make up for half a decade of war and separation. Universities were jam-packed with veterans taking advantage of the G. I. Bill, and affordable tract housing was well on its way to providing desperately needed shelter for growing families.

Christmas Eve found me especially sad; this was the first Christmas I had spent without my family. Parents were not allowed to visit their children at Christmas, and I had seen mama only a few times during my ten months' incarceration. I had learned to eat most of the food on my plate; really awful-looking mushy and foul-tasting garbage I stuffed in my pockets or my mouth at the end of the meal, then hurried to the boys' bathroom, where I could spit it out or throw it in the toilet and flush it when nobody was looking.

Petrified at even the thought of the sadistic dark-haired cottage girl beating my stretched palm with her wooden hair brush upon discovering a harmless "brown smudge" on my undershorts, I walked around a good part of the time with a wad of toilet paper tucked between my butt cheeks. As I was fast learning, fear is the mother of many inventions.

My repertoire of cuss words was still limited to "damn" and "hell," without yet the prefixes "god" and "go to," and I had to be extra careful when using these-the stupid little Baby Cottage girls relished in "telling" if they heard us boys cussing. Stupid little pint-sized bitches. Their reward for "telling" should have been a quick drowning, their last utterance a gurgle.

My mental list of "friends" at the end of 1947 included Van Edwards, Newton Wilder, Lawrence Strum, Alvin Gibbs, Bill Herrington, Miss Ora Lee Hall, Miss Myrtle Peacock, Ann from the hospital, Miss Pender for teaching me how to swim, the blond cottage girl with the bouncing butt for being so understanding and for showing me her "kitten."

My list of "enemies" was formidable and growing. Miss Warwick and Mrs. Tomblin, both having the status in my mind of sadistic concentration camp male guards, headed the list, followed closely by Mr. Regan for nearly allowing me to drown. The dark-haired, "brown smudge" detecting, palm-paddling cottage girl occupied a special place on the list, along with a few nameless snot-faced little Baby Cottage girls who wouldn't allow me to openly express my displeasure with my lot in life without "telling."

And at such a young age, I had already learned to hold a grudge, with the same iron grip as I would hold onto a new Indian Head nickel; an emotion I never knew even existed during my first seven years of life.

Even at the not-so-tender age of eight, I refused to either forgive or forget intentional and mean-spirited physical and mental abuse. Having been blessed with loving parents and a stable home life for seven years, I was outraged and insulted by the unbridled verbal abuse and threats of physical harm under which we tender-aged and highly impressionable Baby Cottage children lived.

The absence of love and praise, and the lack of encouragement during our time spent in the Baby Cottage and Walker Building, say, between the ages of seven and eleven, undoubtedly led to a poor self-image among many of these children. Others, including myself, met this affront to our dignity by stuffing food we disliked into our pockets and mouths, and flushing it down the toilet, completing just enough of our morning "duties" to get by, and devising methods like our butt-cheeked toilet paper sandwich to flaunt our audacity and the certain punishment that followed if caught.

Children who live in orphanages are referred to collectively as "orphans." Nothing wrong with this-as a group it is a convenient means of classification. Technically speaking, however, the universal dictionary definition of an "orphan" is "a child whose parents (plural) are dead." This definition was used also by Oxford Orphanage administrators.

As of January 1, 1947 there were 308 children residing at Oxford Orphanage. A year later, on December 31, 1947, the student population was 311, consisting of 150 boys and 161 girls.

Of this year-ending total of 311 children, 32 were true "orphans" (both parents deceased), 65 whose mother only was deceased, 176 whose father only was deceased, and 38 had both parents still living. Thus in 1947, the classification of true "orphans" comprised the lowest percentage of the children at Oxford Orphanage; to put it another way, the majority of orphans living at Oxford Orphanage was technically not really "orphans." In fact, there were more students who had both parents living (38) than who had both parents deceased (32). Of the 311 children, nineteen percent were children of Masonic parentage.

In 1947, nineteen students were taken from the orphanage by relatives, one child was expelled and five children ran away and did not return, giving a total of twenty-five children who left the orphanage who did not graduate. Of the twenty-three who did graduate (fourteen boys and nine girls), fourteen entered college or nursing school, two enlisted in the U.S. Navy and seven found employment. Statistics show that more children "left" the orphanage (25) than graduated (23).

During 1947, of the 311 children at the orphanage, all except thirty gained weight, the average gain being 5.6 pounds. The William J. Hicks Memorial Hospital, that operated under the direct supervision of Mrs. Edith S. Tomblin, a Practical Nurse, and under the general direction of Rives W. Taylor, M.D., cared for an average of eight patients per day in 1947.

On April 9, 1924, the first red brick was laid in the foundation to John Nichols School. The cornerstone of the new two-story brick structure, complete with a full basement, was laid on St. John's Day, June 24, 1924. The building was erected at a cost of $85,000.00.

The new school was named in honor of Past Grand Master John Nichols. The fireproof, state-of-the-art building was completed in 1925, and was occupied in September of that year.

From its very beginning, the school was accredited by the State Board of Education and by the Southern Association of Colleges and Secondary Schools. Prior to 1931, John Nichols School operated as a private school, with all expenses of the school, including teachers' salaries, financed by Oxford Orphanage.

The ground floor of the impressive all-brick structure housed grades one through six, in ascending order from right to left as one entered the front doors. If someone had placed cannons at the parapets along its ramparts, we could have had our very own medieval castle. Prince Valiant would have felt at home in John Nichols School.

The second floor contained grades seven through twelve. At the end of the full basement facing the boys' cottages was situated the music room, and the opposite end, toward the hospital, was home to the school library. The music room and library were accessed by sets of stairs and also by stairwells leading up to the ground level at each end of the building. When I arrived in February 1947, Miss Laura Hammond was the school librarian. She was replaced on June 1, 1948 by Mrs. E. E. Fuller.

In 1931, John Nichols School became a part of the North Carolina state school system, occupying a unique situation within that system as a "state supported public school." Although most of the teachers were paid by the State of North Carolina, the state did not pay entirely the expenses of operating the school; neither did Oxford Orphanage lose entire control of the school or in the management of its affairs. Mr. E. T. Regan became the school's fourth principal in 1943, and became the Assistant Superintendent of Oxford Orphanage on November 25, 1946.

Grades one through four began class at 8:30 a.m., and got out at 3:15 p.m. Beginning with the fifth grade, all grades were divided into "A" and "B" sections, alternating each grade. Section A, comprised of grades five, seven, nine, and eleven, attended school from one to five, and did vocational work in the mornings. Section B, comprised of grades six, eight, ten, and twelve, attended school from eight to noon, and did vocational work in the afternoons.

Thus, from grades five through twelve, for example, if a boy were in the eighth grade, he never went to school with children in the grade below him (seventh) or the grade above him (ninth). This same situation applied to vocational work. This accounts for the alumni being able to recall some of their friends more than others.

In addition to the 311 orphanage children, there were an additional 136 "town" children from Oxford and the surrounding area, bringing to 447 the total number of children attending John Nichols School in 1947. The state of North Carolina paid the salaries of fourteen teachers at John Nichols School. The school library contained 6,267 books. The varsity football team, composed of thirty-four boys, was undefeated in conference play and won the conference championship. The new Daniel Memorial football field, complete with bleachers and lighting financed by the Oxford Orphanage Alumni Association, was presented that year.

Mrs. Ligon taught high school Latin in 1947. This wise and gentle lady was to become an inspiration to me in the coming years. Mrs. Ligon's husband, Luther Ausborne Ligon, born March 30, 1894, died on January 20, 1946. Mr. Ligon had served as Baker-Storekeeper at the orphanage in 1916 and 1917, and later between 1925 and his death in 1946.

The orphanage provided more than enough religious instruction to go around. Mr. Gray directed a Vespers worship service each Sunday evening that we kids referred to as "Bible babble" because Mr. Gray talked well over our heads most of the time.

Children at the Baby Cottage did not attend church. All children above the Baby Cottage attended the church of their parents' religious affiliation. Baptists must breed like flies. There sure were lots of them in the orphanage. The grammar grade children attended Sunday school on campus, then marched to church in Oxford, grouped according to religious denomination. High school boys attended Sunday school and church of their choice in town.

During 1947, the orphanage part-time and only dentist, Dr. Rufus S. Jones, filled 267 teeth, and examined each child at least twice during the year, while cleaning each child's teeth at least once.

Thomas Hugh Cameron, born April 4, 1889, started working at the orphanage in 1936 as the dairy manager. He died of a cerebral hemorrhage on August 31, 1947. D. P. "Soapy" Peake again assumed the supervision of the entire farm and dairy operations. Three months later, on December 1, 1947, Edwin G. Kerr joined the orphanage staff as Dairyman.

The Orphanage Shoe Department was still operated in 1947 by M. F. Hill, who as a small orphanage boy remembered when the Shoe Shop, as he called it, had been constructed in 1887. In 1947, Mr. Hill had been in charge of the Shoe Shop for 48 years. In 1947, nine boys worked in the Shoe Shop. In addition to making and repairing all the work shoes worn by the 311 children, Mr. Hill was responsible for keeping in repair all of the harnesses of the ten mules on the farm, the athletic shoes, pants, helmets, baseball gloves and even the baseballs.

In 1947, the administration noted that the Walker Building, that housed twenty-four small boys, ". . . is the only serious fire hazard on the campus in which any personnel is in danger."

In 1947, in addition to about forty boys who worked on the farm, five colored men were employed to handle the farm machinery, haul coal and saw wood. Livestock consisted of ten mules, forty-six milk cows, twelve heifers, ten calves and two herd bulls. The farm workers killed and dressed 68 hogs to supply meat and lard for the orphanage. The Mule Barn housing the ten mules burned to the ground on December 27, 1947; fortunately no animals were lost. A new Mule Barn was constructed almost immediately.

In 1947, the state of North Carolina contributed $37,500.00 to the general upkeep of the orphanage.

Such was the state of affairs at Oxford Orphanage in 1947, the first year of my imprisonment.

In late 1947, that pesky varmint that refused to go away, polio, again reared its ugly head, and before I made the journey across campus to the Walker Building in June 1948, the campus was under quarantine, and all vacations were canceled for the Summer.

For Little Orphan Al, Little Orphan Annie's spit at and stomped on kid brother, 1947 ended on the same depressing sour note as was being played on D-Day, February 15, 1947. Only in my case, "D" stood for Death. During the nearly two weeks of downright terrifying inner mental distress I suffered upon arrival at Hicks Memorial Hospital, my fragile psyche was rudely bounced through alternating and repetitive cycles of denial, disbelief, fear, anger, and grief.

Acceptance of this tragic circumstance into which I had been so rudely thrust never became a part of my responses to what my young mind perceived as a pattern of gross injustice and raging insult.

My frightened seven-year-old mind strove to find some perspective, some reason, some order in all that had happened to me. But to no avail. Mrs. Edith Tomblin was one of those cold, heartless adults who in her own mind no doubt equated discipline with physical abuse and mental cruelty.

Psychologists and sociologists generally agree that an unjustly accused or wrongfully incarcerated individual at some point of desperation asks himself if what is happening to him really his own fault. Did he actually do something to deserve these abuses? In searching for some threshold semblance of reason to my sudden misfortune, this emotion surfaced intermittently throughout my early years at the orphanage.

Even at the artless age of seven, I had noticed immediately several differences between children in my grammar school in Kinston and my tiny comrades in the Baby Cottage. Two dissimilarities were noticeable within a few days. While at play, the Baby Cottage children tended to push and shove one another, and definitely were more aggressive on the playground. Conversely, when alone or with only one or two of their classmates or cottagemates, these same children appeared overly quiet to the point of seeming withdrawn, as though in deep thought.

So perhaps we should not equate boundless energy with state of mind. Healthy children possess limitless vitality that they exhibit outwardly, especially when in a group setting. Only when you separate a child from the pack can you really observe his or her true vein. The Baby Cottage children's behavior tended toward the extremes, that is, too boisterous when in a group setting, and too withdrawn when alone or with only one or two friends.

Aggressiveness among peers when at play and a demonstration of an inordinate degree of laughter may well be the masking of deep-seated apprehension and insecurity. And while not able vocally to express what was occurring, at age seven I wondered if each of these thirty children had not suffered the sudden emotional trauma as when my daddy was killed, resulting in the breakup of our close-knit family, and had not endured emotional and physical assaults similar to my experiences during my first two weeks in the orphanage.

I sensed I had become trapped, enmeshed in a seemingly revolving nightmare, a surreal trauma from which I feared there would be no escape. And I believe this feeling pervaded our young lives. Some children in the Baby Cottage carried with them often a look of vacuous incomprehension, and I got the feeling that this was not a "home" in any sense of the word, but a warehouse for orphaned children, the same as pallets of dried tobacco awaiting the auction in Kinston. Oxford Orphanage was indeed a place lacking in love. During my ten years at Oxford, never once do I remember the orphanage referred to as "home" by any child. We kids just called it "the orphanage." Home was for most of us a rapidly fading, distant, unreachable memory.

My early on, simple definition of a "friend" was "one who cares." In this cold and lonely place called Oxford Orphanage, friends seemed as rare as a June bug in January, and when I found a friend, I stuck to him or her like an indelible tattoo. After several months in the orphanage, I could count my friends on the fingers of a three-fingered man; in short, Ann at the hospital, Van Edwards, and the pretty blond cottage girl. And I feel certain that my list of friends was three times longer than that of many other small children in the Baby Cottage.

Sometimes, in my despondency, I felt that I was slipping into a bottomless crevasse, and had great difficulty sorting through a confusing jumble of emotions. At times I would get one of my "vacant" spells, so uncertain was I of my future. Nor was I alone in my confusion.

Physical abuse. On second thought, this is definitely an all-capper. Let's give the subject its due. PHYSICAL ABUSE. Its actuality, the threat of by the orphanage staff, teachers, and older boys, and the fear of, by the younger boys and girls, was the single most immutable fact of my life from the day I entered Oxford Orphanage in February 1947 at age seven, until my rebellion against such trauma on the steep banks of an off-campus fish pond one hot July afternoon shortly after turning thirteen.

By an innate universality, fragile children strive to hang onto life, to seek desperately a place where they can "fit in" and are loved. Along that arduous and seemingly never-ending, pitfall-filled country road whose street sign reads "Growing Up," some adults always manage to find new ways to cheapen and degrade the innocent dreams and aspirations of small children. Quite sadly, Oxford Orphanage was cursed with more than its fair share of such grownups.

It was as though I were a passenger in a car, traveling down a smooth highway on a clear, cold day, with nary a worry in the world. Then suddenly the car hit a patch of ice, my daddy's death, and I was propelled headlong into a nightmare called Oxford Orphanage. During periods of hurt, or depression, or slight, or humiliation, the sounds and smells of that fateful afternoon of February 9, 1946 stampeded with a vengeance into my memory, that day when the course of my life-no, my very life itself-was suddenly and inexorably blown apart as though sitting on a keg of ignited dynamite.

In the confusion and heartache of my youth, I spent many a day communing with the majestic oaks, the skyward-reaching pecan trees and the wondrous gray squirrels frolicking beneath those branches. This definitely was not a period of profluence in my life. Seemed as though for every baby step forward I managed, some stupid grownup knocked me two giant steps to the rear. Goddamn grownups. Crass, uneducated, emotionless bastards. T. S. Eliot had nothing on Little Orphan Al. I too spent many a night lying awake, calculating the future, trying to unweave, unwind, unravel and piece together the past and the future. Not until I reached adulthood was I able to fully understand that what I had experienced for years as a small child at Oxford was depression, along with other small children engulfed in this morass of anonymity into which we had been thrust through no fault of our own.

Self-doubt, left to its own inertia, can snowball like a runaway Colorado avalanche and quickly segue into self-doubt's offspring, a poor image of self worth. Discipline and control. How does one maintain discipline and control over more than three hundred children, ages six to eighteen, whose one tie that binds them all is the fact that each entered the orphanage at a young, impressionable age, apprehensive and dispirited, from a broken home?

Does one nurture these lost souls with love, care and understanding? Or does one simply warehouse these unfortunate children, and maintain order and discipline by coercion, threats and physical abuse? And, throughout all this travail, who supervises the supervisors? Apparently, at Oxford Orphanage during the decade 1947-1957 and beyond, nobody.

In dealing with defenseless and vulnerable children, why did some teachers and staff use caustic cannons when kind words were needed? The answer is a combination of two factors, an innate propensity to physically assault small children, and a total absence of restraints imposed on such conduct.

The group of adults authorized by the orphanage superintendent, the Reverend A. DeLeon Gray, to administer corporal punishment, by slapping, kicking or beating, was all-encompassing, and included work supervisors, teachers, cottage counselors and administrators. A high school teacher, who will remain anonymous at her request, years later confided to me that when she arrived at the orphanage, she was informed that corporal punishment (read as physical abuse) was tolerated, as long as no "marks" (objective signs of physical abuse) were evident upon visual inspection. That such ongoing and pervasive physical abuse was encouraged is shown by the fact that during my ten-year stay at Oxford, no adult was ever fired or asked to leave employment at the orphanage because of child abuse.

In my first (pre-orphanage) life, I minded my parents out of respect for the love and care they gave me. Even the one time mama put the birches to me at midnight for refusing to release *my* mongrel dog from the garage, she did not raise her voice, and after that night never again mentioned the incident.

Bill and Kenny, though, refused to let it lie. They resolved to milk it for all it was worth. Afterwards, Kinston's own version of the Katzenjammer Kids pointed out to me every stray dog they saw, offering to take the mutt home and lock it in the garage for me. Bozos. Yahoos.

However, I minded the adult staff (and the Big Boys) at the orphanage for an altogether different reason, a real and present fear of immediate and grievous bodily harm.

CHAPTER 13

Out of the Frying Pan and into the Walker Building

As of January 1, 1948 I had been languishing, demoralized and overwrought, in Minnie Warwick's boobyhatch for ten damnlong months, doubtless the unhappiest of the 311 students in the Oxford orphans' 'sylum on that date. And by year's end, December 31, 1948, I was one of nearly thirty youngsters living in that "known fire hazard," the Walker Building, the population of our little "city" having increased during the year to 317.

The twenty-four member graduating class of May 1948 consisted of fourteen boys and ten girls. Ten graduates entered college or nursing school, eleven became employed and three entered military service. During 1948, sixteen children were taken home by relatives, four ran away and never returned, and two left for "other reasons." Thus only two more children graduated (24) than left for the reasons mentioned just above (22).

As of December 31, 1948, there were 25 true orphans (both parents dead), 68 whose mother had died, 170 whose father had died, and 54 who still had both parents living. Again, there were more than twice as many children in the orphanage with both parents living (54) than who had lost both parents (25). Only twelve percent of the student body was of Masonic parentage. The greatest change among these four groups was the category with both parents living, which increased from 38 in 1947 to 54 in 1948.

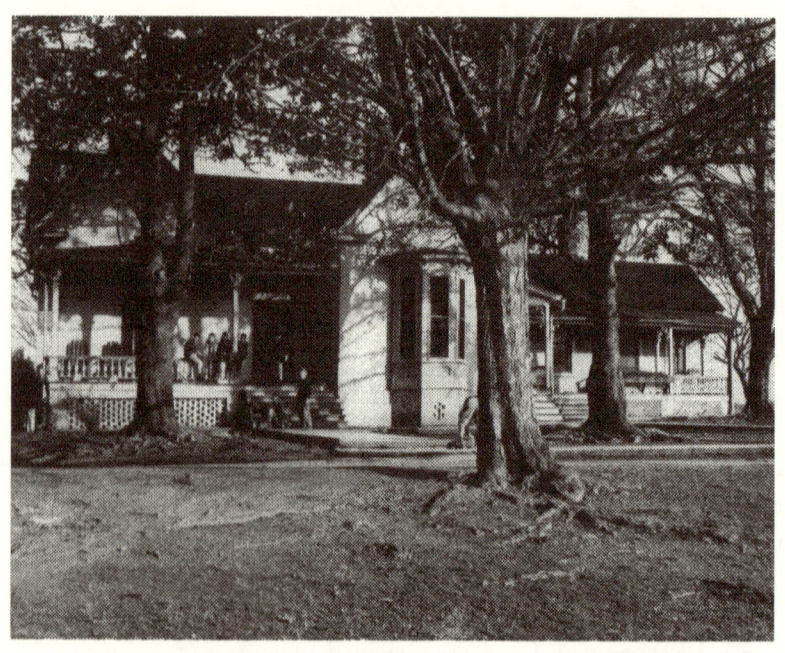

1948. Walker Building. Constructed in 1884 as superintendent's residence, converted to hospital in 1904, and later became cottage for twenty-five boys ages nine and ten.

My incarceration in the infamous Baby Cottage lasted from February 1947 until June 1948. Some survival skills learned during this sixteen-month period included:

1. To avoid the sharp sting of that stupid bimbo bitch teenage cottage girl's hair-brush-with-holes-in-it on my open taut palm, I had to keep an ample amount of toilet paper stuffed between my skinny butt cheeks. That way, I hid the telltale I'm-not-smart-enough-to-clean-myself brown stain on my undershorts. On my deathbed at age 125, I'm still going to wonder just how stupid I could have been at age seven to think that if I rubbed together three (large) streaks of brown on my undershorts, these three (large) brown stains would just by some miracle disappear!

2. If another little boy (or girl) shoves you, immediately shove back, only with more force than he (or she) uses against you. This instant reprisal admonishes your peers not to "mess" with you. My experiences showed that little boys don't push a lot. Boys know their "place." Little girls know their "place," but they want yours too. In this regard, girls believe this blessed license from the Maker to be a permanent one, lasting a lifetime.

3. If another little girl (seldom a boy) "tells" on you for breaking the rules, don't be obvious in your retaliation, lest she "tells" on you again. Wait until she hitches a ride on the ubiquitous "ocean wave," and when it gets up to about forty-five miles per hour, gently bump her off. I must have bumped Betty Jean Moore off that ocean wave a dozen times, and she probably deserved it two dozen more times. I was just being considerate. My captors had turned me into a conniving little bastard.

4. Learn to like cooked squash and okra because both are squishy and almost impossible to clean out of your pants pockets.

5. Master the art of looking the hated cottage (grand)mother or stupid cottage girl straight in the eye, and defiantly and unflinchingly uttering the words, "I didn't do it." Of course you did it, but a good bluff works well about twelve percent of the time.

Thus on a misty, steamy morning in June 1948, having just turned nine and fresh out of Miss Simpson's third grade, still detesting slimy cooked vegetables but fast developing a liking for peanut butter, molasses, pimento cheese and deviled eggs, well on my way to becoming an international terrorist, I bade farewell to that unforgettable learning experience called the Baby Cottage. In the company of by now my best friend and four other apprehensive nine-year-olds, chaperoned by the blond cottage girl with the bouncing behind, I trekked the length of the expansive campus to my new home, Miss Bertha Hobson's Walker Building, where I was to become once more the reluctant recipient of that accumulation of really bad experiences known universally as "the facts of life."

The Walker Building was home to approximately twenty-six boys between the ages of nine and eleven, or, more specifically, boys in the fourth and fifth grades. The grade and not the age was the determining factor for placement in cottages. For example, Van Edwards was a year older than I, and Frank McMillan was two years older than I; however, we three stayed together in the Walker Building. The reasoning for such placement was as follows. Children in grades one through four attended school from 8:30 a.m. till noon and again from 1:00-3:15 p.m. Any work performed by these children was restricted to menial tasks in or around the cottages, or policing the campus to pick up trash by the Walker Building boys.

The day-to-day operation of the orphanage was carried out by the boys and girls in the fifth through twelfth grades, under the supervision of the orphanage staff. Such an operation required that some children work mornings and others, afternoons. In order to accomplish this goal, the children in the sixth, eighth, tenth and twelfth grades attended school from 8:00 a.m. till noon. At 1:00 p.m. these children reported for work at their assigned departments. These children were in Section B.

Children in the fifth, seventh, ninth and eleventh grades, who made up Section A, worked in their assigned departments from 8:00 a.m. till noon, and attended school from 1:00-5:00 p.m.

North Carolina state law mandated six hours of supervised schooling each day. In order to fulfill this state education requirement, as well as

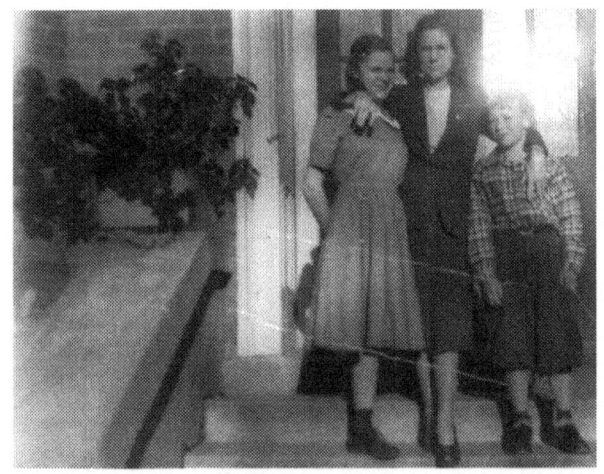

1949. Mama, Eoline and the author, age nine, on steps of Main Building. Note the stupid knickers.

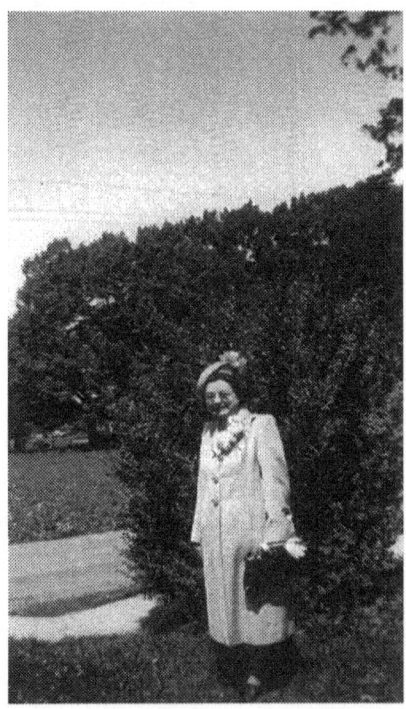

1949. Bertha Hobson, Walker Building Cottage counselor.

allowing the children to complete their homework, each boy and girl was required to sit through an absolutely quiet study hall, supervised in person by the respective cottage counselors, from 7:00-9:00 p.m., Monday through Friday.

Miss Hobson warmly greeted the nervous and apprehensive six of us in the entryway of the one-story white frame and stucco building. With a constant twinkle in her eye and engaging smile, the short, round, dark-haired lady with the rimless glasses reminded me of a dumpy elf I had seen in numerous Christmas advertisements. We six had evolved from being big fish in the small Baby Cottage pond to small fish in the big Walker Building pond, and here we huddled together anxiously in the front room, clutching brown paper bags containing our belongings, while she gave us a brief welcome speech with all the enthusiasm of an eighty-year-old beginning her fiftieth year as a tour guide at the local cemetery and mausoleum.

Of primary importance (at least to Miss Hobson) in our indoctrination into life at the Walker Building was the assignment of our "duties." No more washing baseboards for me. That was kid stuff. I had been "promoted" overnight to the responsible position of . . . Yard Raker. Miss Hobson explained to me that when the "six o'clock bell" sounded (at six o'clock, she said, like I was a fool or something), I was to get dressed hurriedly, find a fan rake in the outside tool bin, and rake half the yard on the side of the Walker Building facing the one-lane gravel and tar road that led to the main campus.

One of the other "new" boys was assigned the task of raking the remaining half of the west side of the yard. Initially, I was not overjoyed with the idea of raking a yard, or even half a yard for that matter, that is, until I learned that another of the new arrivals had been assigned the task of scrubbing the bathroom toilets each morning. The Duty God had smiled on me, or so I gloated on that muggy first morning in June 1948. Four months later, however, raking the yard definitely was not the "duty" evoking envy. Odd thing about leaves is, in the late Fall they die, and about fourteen million billion of them (each day) fall, and I was certain I could hear each of them laughing as it hit the ground.

In the Baby Cottage, the boys dormitory consisted of sixteen beds, neatly arranged in rows of eight beds each, with plenty of space between beds and a wide aisle separating the rows. However, the dormitory in the Walker Building consisted of two large rooms separated by a thick wall in the center of the room that once had been a fireplace, with the metal bunks jumbled together as though arranged with all the orderliness of a 7.7 Richter scale earthquake. Miss Hobson assigned each of us a bed, though in that maze I doubt any one of us found the correct bed when we put ourselves to sleep that first night.

After being assigned our "duties" and our beds, we followed Miss Hobson in mother duck-duckling fashion to the other side of the sprawling building, where we were assigned a number (mine was 16) and a bin in which to store our clothes. The number system was used because it was much simpler to write numbers than names on clothes bins, coat racks, etc.

The clothes bin area was situated just off a large room containing six large rectangular, timeworn wooden tables, each surrounded by six equally well-worn wooden chairs with straight backs. Along the wall was a row of numbered hooks on which we hung our coats. The clothes bins were large enough to accommodate the storage of our books, so most of the boys kept their books in these "cubbies." For study hall, which lasted from seven till nine each weekday night, Miss Hobson assigned us a specific place at the study tables.

The large open room in the center of the Walker Building was heated during Winter by means of a large pot-bellied coal stove just off the center of the room. The end of this room opposite the clothes storage area opened to the right into the bathroom and shower area, and to the left into the crowded dormitories.

Whereas in the Baby Cottage we had bathed in bathtubs, the Walker Building boys showered together in one large open shower area. A row of sinks ran along the wall closest to the shower stall, behind which was a row of open toilets and urinals. This arrangement afforded no privacy whatever, nor was there any intent by the orphanage staff to do so.

Because we had lived together for more than a year in the Baby Cottage, we six "new" boys had each other for comfort in our assimilation into our new life in the Walker Building.

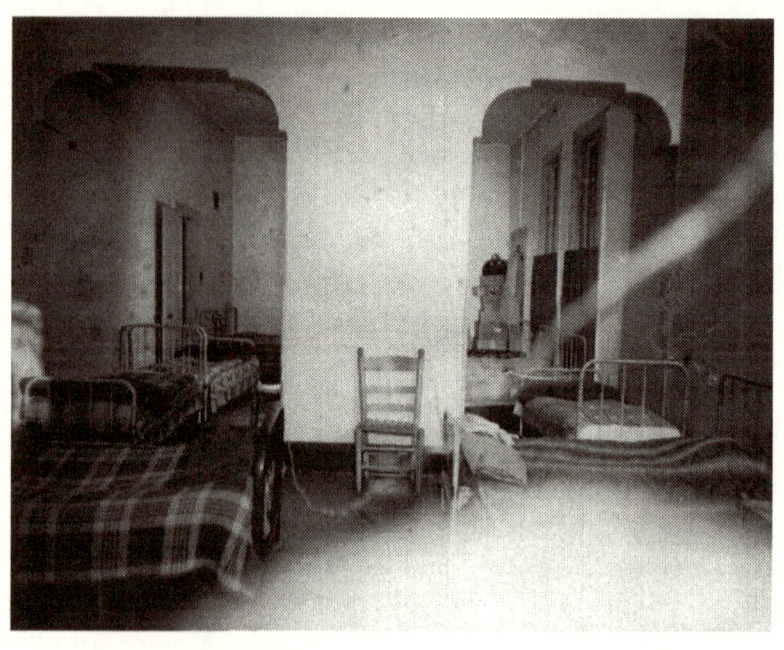

1948. Section of Walker Building dormitory. Note brown "Army" blankets and muli-colored "Indian" blankets covering the rickety, chipped metal cots. The dormitory was unheated, even in the "Dead of Winter."

Assisting Miss Hobson in our care (and discipline) were two high school boys, whom we addressed by their first names and referred to by either their first names or simply the "cottage boys." The two boys lived with us in the Walker Building, ensuring that we all hopped out of bed pronto at the sound of the six o'clock bell, made our beds and began performing our duties.

At night, the cottage boys confirmed that we showered and got into bed at the proper time. Rarely did Miss Hobson venture into our bathroom or dormitory, but was content with supervising us during study hall, and always left the door of her small apartment she occupied at the front of the Walker Building open in case we needed her assistance.

During the school year, we took our showers and prepared for bed after study hall ended at nine o'clock. However, just before bedtime year round, we would take our assigned seats in the large study hall, and sit quietly while Miss Hobson read to us from her large book of Bible stories, as I recall it was entitled *Hurlburt's Book of Bible Stories*, and sometimes she would read a few passages from *The Holy Bible*.

When Miss Hobson had read the last story in the book of Bible stories, the next night she would begin the book anew. During my two-year incarceration in the Walker Building (June 1948-June 1950) our young minds became totally saturated with stories from *The Holy Bible*, having listened to the story of Joseph and his coat of many colors, Daniel in the lions' den, the birth of baby Jesus, Noah and the flood, etc., ad infinitum and then some, so that, by the age of ten Miss Hobson had produced twenty-six God-fearing, Bible-totin', hellfire-and-damnation-spouting child evangelists that would have turned Elmer Gantry green with envy. In two years we listened to Miss Hobson read to us stories from the Bible on more than seven hundred occasions. By the time I turned ten, I could recite the books of the Bible with one hand tied behind my back, and could spout off the Twenty-third Psalm backwards, with my eyes closed. We Walker Building boys sensed we had been present with Mary that blessed night in the manger, felt as though we had tried on Joseph's coat, stood shoulder-to-shoulder with Daniel amongst all those smelly lions, and I had a sudden urge to do pee every time Miss Hobson mentioned the words "Noah," "ark," or "flood."

At the time I moved from the Baby Cottage to the Walker Building in June 1948, most of the other cottages on campus were heated by coal-fed furnaces located in the basement, that supplied heat to radiators located along the walls of the room, or heated forced air through ducts located in the floors. Of course, at that time there was no kind of central air conditioning, even up to the time I left the orphanage in February 1957. To obtain "air conditioning," we just opened all the windows on the ground floor study hall and the second floor bedroom-dormitories, and sweated through the hot Spring and Summer months.

However, the Walker Building had no basement, and no second story. There were two main dormitories, connected by a wide passageway, so it was really one very large room that slept up to thirty of us preteens.

Oxford is located only fifteen miles from the Virginia state line. While in the orphanage, because of Oxford's map location, each year the area experienced several deep snowfalls, and many a Winter night the temperature outside the Walker Building dipped well below freezing.

And because there was no heat of any kind at night, we youngsters figured that at night the temperature in the dormitory was about a full one and a half degrees warmer than the outside below-freezing conditions. But what the hell, we were just nine- and ten-year-old kids, and because we didn't know from nothing about anything, we naturally assumed that all the cottages were not heated in the Wintertime. And we assumed also that during those freezing temperatures, every kid on campus talked through chattering teeth.

So during the Winter of 1948, we had to pile as many Army blankets on top of us as possible as insulation. It was not unusual to awaken in the morning to find a thin coating of ice on the inside walls of the dormitory.

There were only two sources of heat in the Walker Building during most of the Winter of 1948. A coal-burning stove in the bathroom kept the bathroom area warm, and also heated water in the hot water heater. The other source of heat, though not at night, by golly, was a cast-iron stove in what some boys called the "playroom" but was in reality the "study hall."

The "rising bell," that we all called the "six o'clock bell," rang, as I recall, for three minutes, each morning at six o'clock. At 5:30 a.m., one of the two high school cottage boys got out of bed, started the two coal stoves, then went back to bed. Usually the bathroom and study hall were warming up when we got up a half hour later. We boys kept our clothes folded up under our covers at night. When the six o'clock bell sounded, we hopped out of bed, grabbed our clothes and shoes, and rushed out to the warmth of the study hall to crowd as close as possible to the hot coal stove, and there we put on our clothes and shoes.

The Seventy-fifth Annual Report of the Board of Directors and Superintendent of the Oxford Orphanage, states on page 21:

The Walker Building, thrice worn out, remains on campus, being used as a cottage for twenty-four small boys. It is the only serious fire hazard on the campus in which any personnel of the orphanage is in danger.

This Annual Report was dated December 31, 1947, six months prior to my arrival at Firetrap Towers in June 1948. And as I suspected at the time, I, quite literally, was being unceremoniously pushed from the Baby Cottage "frying pan" into the (potential) fire (hazard) of the Walker Building. And the wise sage who made the statement noted above had not changed his mind a year later.

Under the heading "Housing" on page 21 of the Annual Report of the Oxford Orphanage for the year ending December 31, 1948, my first of two cold Winters in the Walker Building, is reported:

> All of the cottages are in excellent condition with the exception of the Walker Building, a cottage for small boys. The Walker Building is part stucco and part frame construction, having been used in three capacities, and at the present time houses twenty-four small boys. It is a very serious fire hazard and constantly endangers the lives of these boys who occupy it and is completely inadequate for the use it fulfills.

During the refrigerated Winter of 1948, we covered our skinny nine-year-old frames with brown woolen Army blankets, folded when not in use at the foot of the cot, and a mish-mash of multi-colored so-called "Indian blankets." On many a hibernal night the last thing I glimpsed just before ducking my head beneath the covers at lights-out was my breath.

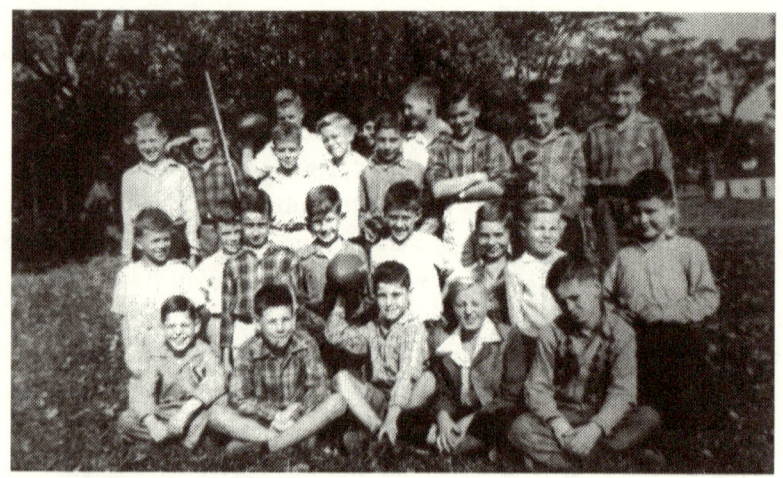

1949. Walker building misfits. The author, at age nine, is on third row, fourth from left, blonde hair, squinting. Only ten of these twenty-four boys graduated John Nichols High School. Sadly, fourteen boys either ran away and never returned, or were taken back home by relatives.

To call what we slept on "beds" would indeed be quite gracious; squeaky, rickety old cots would be a more apt description. Uniformity in billeting was most assuredly not the order of the day. But even a kid with a short memory and a lack of appreciation of aesthetics-and our little group was generously represented in both categories-could tell his cot by the unique design of his Indian blanket and the pattern of chipped paint on the frame of his metal cot.

In late Winter of 1948, a fire started in the wall that separated the two dormitories, and the fire department was called out from Oxford, while we huddled outside in the freezing night. Shortly thereafter, the orphanage had installed an oil-burning furnace in the hall between the two dormitories and an oil furnace in the study hall. My second Winter at the Walker Building, the Winter of 1949, was a whole lot warmer.

Most of us Walker Building boys never complained about the absence of heat in the building at night. That's just the way it was, and we accepted the situation. I learned at an early age not to spend a lot of time and energy complaining about things over which I had no control.

At the orphanage, once you got past the Baby Cottage, each boy owned two pairs of shoes, that for obvious reasons were called "work" shoes and "Sunday" shoes. Socks were of either cotton or wool, depending on the season. The most popular sock design during the late forties and early fifties was the black and white diamond pattern. Each article of clothing had the boy's name printed in indelible ink on white rectangular cotton tags, sewn onto the garment.

At Oxford, nobody ever accused us kids of having to wear uniforms. This total lack of uniformity in clothing was such that one kid could spot it immediately should his cottagemate "borrow" a shirt or pair of trousers.

The most comical sight on campus was a ten-year-old Walker Building boy wearing a well-worn pair of stupid hand-me-down brown corduroy or plaid woolen knickers, with just one of his ankle-length brown brogans having swallowed up one of his ill-fitting, non-elastic white cotton socks. Many of the boys sported "cowboy" belts, flashing baubles and all, that had been given as presents (or necessities) by visiting relatives. We were misfits in more ways than one.

As of the middle of the twentieth century, elasticity as it relates to woolen coatsleeves apparently had not yet found its way to Oxford, so we kids would hold onto the ends of our coatsleeves and stuff our hands into our coat pockets in an attempt to prevent Old Man Winter from crawling up into our coatsleeves. The style of clothing in vogue during my Decade of Enlightenment at Oxford could best be characterized as Southern Illfitting, and the orphanage staff did its level best to further this cosmopolitanism throughout the campus.

We boys wore tweed suits to Sunday school and church that fit each of us as though our hand-me-downs had been handed back a few years later. In a photograph taken when I was in the Walker Building in the Spring of 1950, the buttons on my tweed coat appeared to carry on a tug of war with their buttonholes. In the 1957 yearbook, *The Log*, the last year I was in the orphanage, I appeared in the same manner.

When I moved "up" from the Baby Cottage to the Walker Building in June 1948, I assumed I had left behind the obligation to pen my once a month brilliant letter to mama. And I figured that, even though I had always asked mama how my cat was getting along, for all I knew, in my poor cat's despondency at my prolonged absence, he (or she, for that matter) had tied a short rope connecting its hind leg to a twenty-pound cinder block (as we called them in those days), and jumped into the Neuse River at high tide, or had purposely walked in front of a fully-laden tobacco truck on its way to the tobacco auction in The World's Foremost Tobacco Center.

However, as soon as I got to the Walker Building, I was rudely introduced to what was called "quiet hour" that unfortunately was observed throughout the campus every Sunday from 2:00 p.m. to 3:00 p.m. We youngsters were required to sit quietly in study hall, and one Sunday each month, had to write one of those stupid aforementioned obligatory "How Are You? Fine I Hope" letters to a parent or other relative.

In late Spring, the lush greenery blanketed the wide ball fields around campus, and with it came a not too unpleasant invasion of June Beetles, which all the kids called "Junebugs," pronounced as one word, and bumblebees, those fat, hairy creatures that, although initially frightful in appearance, were really quite sociable, existing in harmony with their close neighbors, the slow-moving, metallic green Junebugs.

The annual population of Junebugs and yellow-and-black bumblebees was inadvertently decimated by the kids, especially us twenty-five to thirty Walker Building boys, whose job each morning after breakfast during the Summer months was to "police" the entire campus as a swarm, picking up any trash we found.

We youngsters were not required to wear shoes during the Summer, so all of us Walker Building boys went barefooted, and we thirty boys policed the campus daily, in the process squashing literally dozens of the minding-their-own-business Junebugs underfoot.

The cute little bumblebees, who spent most of their waking hours flitting from the dense head of one clover stalk to another, gathering nectar, also were subjected to the indiscriminate squashing by nine-year-old toes and heels.

However, over the long haul, the Bumbles fared better than the Junes. Once we had moved up from the Walker Building to 1-B, we were free to roam the outstretched farm of several hundred acres on Saturday and Sunday afternoons. These treks invariably took us through the cow pastures, on which was deposited daily an abundance and then some of fresh cow manure, amid an ample population of Junebugs. Through painstaking scientific research we kids discovered that Junebugs really did not like cow manure. We found that if you place a Junebug on top of a pile of fresh, still wet cow manure, the small creature will literally tread dung. Furthermore, if you take a stick and push the defenseless little devil under the surface of the cow cake, it will very quickly dig its way to the surface. And as in many of these childish adventures, I was the only boy who did not take part in such goings-on.

Many a bet was placed on many a hot Summer afternoon by many a bored eleven- and twelve-year-old orphan as to whose "dunked" Junebug would be the first to emerge from a hot cow cake. But, what the hell. We were just kids.

During the long Summer months and on weekends during the school year, after policing the main campus, we Walker Building boys would often while away (or "wile" away) the hours playing various games, among these being pickup sticks (using wooden popsicle sticks), mumblety-peg (that we pronounced "mumbly-peg"), dabs (a game known to the World-Beyond-the-Main-Gate as "marbles"), horseshoes (real, well-worn metal "mule" shoes), hopscotch, jack rocks, using real rocks or small green acorns, and croquet.

We youngsters had not yet "discovered" the fine art of "pocket pool," so for fun we kids slung farts at one another and picked snots a lot, in an attempt to make meaningful, productive use of our time. Thus, our idyllic Walker Building Summers of 1948 and 1949 were spent policing the main campus, swimming, playing games and indiscriminately decimating the defenseless "June" and "Bumble" population.

We youngsters played a game called "jack rocks," not "jacks." We called the game "jack rocks" because in the nearly always absence of the small metal jacks, we used instead tiny pebbles, or rocks, that could be found in abundance anywhere on the orphanage grounds. Thus, we needed only a small rubber ball to start a game of jack rocks, and it was not uncommon on a rainy Winter weekend to find several games of jack rocks being played simultaneously.

"Pickup sticks" was another game that was quite competitive, yet required no outlay of money. In that era, popsicle sticks were made only of wood, and we always saved them or our parents or relatives brought them to us, just for the purpose of the game.

For games of horseshoes, we used the worn iron horseshoes found on the farm. Many years afore, two iron rods had been driven into the ground at an agreed-upon distance, and left at that location, such that the iron rods, that we called "stobs," ended up in the center of well scooped out depressions. What we orphan kids called a "stob," others might call a "stake." However, neither a stob nor stake would be confused with a "stick." A stick was longer than a stob. If pressed for the difference, I would have to say that a stob was a piece of wood or iron no longer than two feet. A stick would be any slender piece of wood or tree branch longer than two feet.

Now, a stake would seem to be shorter than or the same length as, a stob. A stake and a stick indicate wood; a stob would be either wood or metal. And this is why we threw horseshoes at a stob.

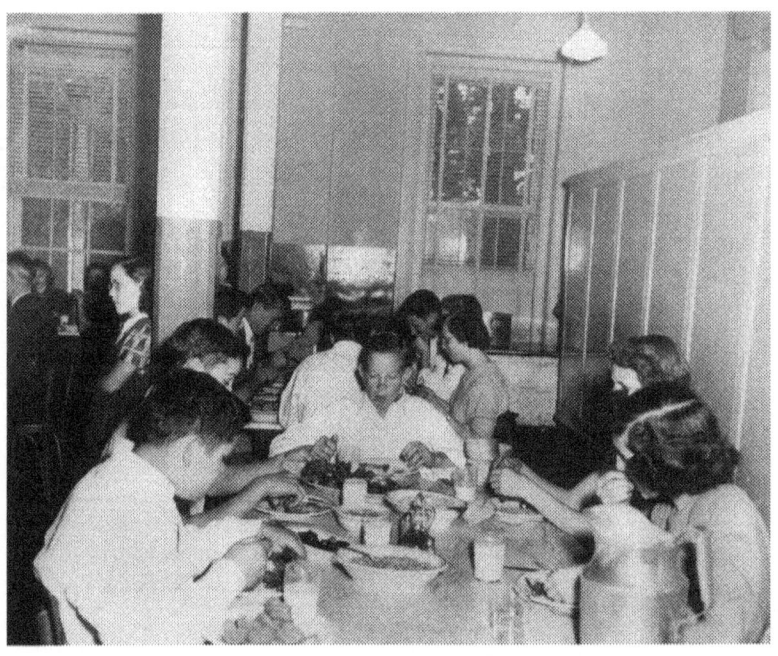

1951. Section of Main dining room. A waitress ("head girl") is standing beside a support column. Note large milk pitcher and food bowls, and stacks of sliced bread to Archie Capps' left.

Similar to the well-worn horseshoe stob depressions were hopscotch areas. Hopscotch squares and rectangles were laid out precisely and carved deeply and meticulously into the hard ground with the end of a broomstick. Even after the heavy rains one had only to retrace the well-worn outlines with a "stick," broom or not (as opposed to a "stake" or "stob," of course) to restore the hopscotch form to its original definition.

Jackknives and other sharp knives were strictly forbidden. A cottage mother's discovery of such a knife led to swift confiscation and certain punishment. I thought I would use the term cottage "mother" this once, just to let you know that I never referred to these mainly women as my cottage "mother." To me, they were only cottage "counselors." The only "mother" I ever acknowledged, even by name, lived at 208 East Bright Street in Kinston, North Carolina, the World's Foremost Tobacco Center.

However, many of us boys kept knives. My brother Bill gave me my first pocketknife, a trusty "Barlow," on a visit in the Summer of 1950, shortly after I moved up to 1-B.

During the Summer months, we kids played these games under the huge oaks situated in the field between the Walker Building and Tom Adams' house. During the cold Winter months, we used the area in front of and to the Tom Adams side of the Walker Building.

Occasionally, one of the kids would receive as a gift from his parents on visiting day (that being Sunday) a harmonica, universally known to youngsters as a "harp," and if you were lucky enough to be known as that fortunate kid's friend, eventually you might be allowed to play the kid's harp. If you were really fortunate enough to be bigger in size than the owner of the harp, "eventually" somehow segued miraculously into "immediately," or "right now," whichever came first in time. Or else.

Even as a preteen Walker Building inmate, my buddy Van Edwards exuded an abundance of confidence, and his sharp wit and smart mouth earned him a spot on the dreaded "Mr. Gray's List" on a fairly regular basis.

At the same time, however, Van presented another side to his emerging character, that of a conniving, brown-nosing little ass-kisser should the situation warrant such conduct and an opportunity arose to gain therefrom. As in the case of "Van's Harmonica."

When we were in the fifth grade, Van's job on campus the half-day we were not in school was that of Main Building "office boy," a non mentally-taxing position that required all the brainpower of a medium-sized clod of red clay. In my young friend's case, the job requirements matched perfectly the employee's qualifications. To a "T."

At about this time, Van's yearning to develop his musical talents instilled in him the desire to possess his very own harmonica, having honed this musical skill by constantly harassing any other kid who owned such a musical instrument.

And at about this exact time, the kind and gracious Miss McGinness was employed as the eighth grade teacher at John Nichols School. And as the Main Building office boy, it didn't take very long at all for enterprising little Van Edwards to become tagged by his peers as the unassuming lady's "pet."

Somehow or other, doubtless by incessantly "suggesting" such a gift, Miss McGinness, sooner than later succumbed to the constant whining of my young friend, and purchased for Van a brand spanking new "M. Hohner" harmonica, and almost overnight Van's list of "friends" appeared to grow exponentially.

However, being classified (by myself) as what one might call a "true" friend, I was allowed to use Van's harp on a fairly regular basis, and I would sneak off around the back of the cottage where nobody could hear me, and practice the patriotic *Battle Hymn of the Republic* and the perennial favorite *From the Halls of Montezuma* over, and over, and over again, very quietly, lest I be discovered by one of Van's many "false" friends.

Unspoken etiquette dictated that the young harp player, before relinquishing (always grudgingly) the harp to his friend, would first slap the harp against the palm of his hand or his thigh, to expel the spit. By the age of thirteen, nearly every boy in the orphanage could play *From the Halls of Montezuma* on the harp, and some of the kids became fairly accomplished harp players. Every boy at the orphanage tried his best to become good at something, so as to gain the respect of his peers. But alas, I quickly discovered that, just like dabs, my talents did not lie in playing the harp.

In October 1950, the contract was let for construction of the Masters Cottage, a two-story, all-brick structure, to replace that "known fire hazard," the Walker Building, at a cost of $74,789.36. The ceremony dedicating the Masters Cottage was held on October 11, 1951, a little more than a year after I had moved up to 1-B. The Walker Building was converted into apartments for orphanage staff, and as the orphanage entered the twenty-first century, was one of only two (the Baby Cottage being the other) buildings remaining in regular use of all the structures in existence when I arrived at Oxford in February 1947.

CHAPTER 14

The Watering Hole

Almost immediately upon my arrival at the Walker Building in June 1948, my keen-as-an-owl hearing was drawn to the familiar and welcome sound of jingling coins, emanating from the pockets of some of the Walker Building, 1-B and 2-B boys, and somewhat louder sounds of coins of similar denomination, doubtless due to a greater volume, coming from the pockets of the older boys in 4-B and 3-B.

My sharp-as-a-tack mind reasoned that these kids had a secret financial source of which I was not privy, and the discordant jingling and jangling bothered me to no end, simply because the familiar sounds did not emanate from the deep (and quite empty) pockets of my own pants. And this fact disturbed me greatly. It was as though my very best friend, God, had decided to remove my position from the financial food chain. Egads! This would never do!

Early the next month, Miss Hobson marched us as a group to a small two-story red brick building just off the Main Building, and told us to form a line outside the door of the Business Office, situated to the left as we entered the building. This was the office of Maurice Parham, the orphanage business manager and treasurer.

When came my turn in line, I stepped forward expectantly, and a pleasant woman, holding loosely in her fist a handful of silver mintage, pressed one of the precious coins onto the palm of my (really) outstretched hand. This was the first money anyone had given me since

Mama packed me off to this godforsaken place nearly sixteen months before, and the feel of the shiny silver coin against my sweaty palm was an eye-moistening and welcome experience. I didn't know whether to cry or pee in my pants. Monetary deprivation, to me at least, was a burden hatched in hell. An awful feeling.

Mimicking the refrain of the kids who preceded me, I parroted "Thank you, ma'am," and quickly turned on my heels and left the building, clutching tightly my first ever "allowance," a whole quarter of a U.S. dollar. This welcomed ritual was to be repeated each month until I left the orphanage nearly a decade later. Dispensing the coveted and much eagerly awaited monthly allowance was Ernestine Taylor, Mr. Parham's secretary.

Children in the Baby Cottage were sheltered from the main campus population, and in North Carolina in 1948, the little tykes probably would not have understood the concept of an "allowance" anyway. Beginning with Walker Building boys and Annex girls, each child received an allowance around the first of each month. For the Walker Building boys this was a token (to us at least) twenty-five cents, increased to fifty cents for 1-B and 2-B boys, a dollar for 4-B boys and finally two dollars for the older boys in 3-B.

The administration offices on the first floor of the ancient Main Building opened onto spacious wooden covered porches, and the boys in 2-B, 4-B and 3-B loitered here while awaiting the final bell calling everyone into the dining hall. The large side room of the Main Building, that faced the sprawling dining halls and kitchen at the rear of the building, was affectionately known as the "Candy Corner," the orphanage equivalent of a nineteenth-century Old West "watering hole."

We youngsters in the Walker Building attached a certain unspoken degree of maturity and freedom to that monthly quarter, most if not all of it being spent within the first day at the Candy Corner. The proverbial expression "shortest distance between two points" no doubt originated at Oxford Orphanage, and was the distance between Mr. Parham's office and the Candy Corner in the Main Building, or more succinctly phrased, between the hands of Ernestine Taylor and Betty Evans, the raving-beauty teenager who operated the Candy Corner most of the time.

Press a whole shiny quarter into the eager, appreciative palm of a candy-starved nine-year-old orphan boy, point him in the general direction of a place to spend that quarter of a dollar, and the two of them (boy and quarter) will part company within the half-hour. And so it was with me the first few times I was given an allowance. Save for a rainy day? What's a "rainy day?" And for that matter, what's "save" mean?

However, after the first few months the smart ones among us learned our lesson, and I began saving my money, spending only a few pennies at a time, realizing I had to make that meager twenty-five cents last a whole thirty days. Certainly was hard to do. Even harder on those months that had thirty-one days. You ever heard the old song *"What a Difference a Day Makes?"* Most certainly does if you are a candy-starved orphan kid in the Walker Building, it's July 30th, and the next day isn't August 1st.

The monthly allowance was for the most part immune from claims of "Leffuns!" except toward the last few days of the month, when some hungry chowderhead older boys in 4-B, having foolishly exhausted their allowance, tried to bully their younger, smaller, frugal schoolmates into sharing candy or chewing gum purchased with the last few pennies of their allowance.

We smaller children, knowing who these bullying beggars were, tried our best to avoid the leeches, often a difficult task because the older predators tended to linger outside the side door of the Main Building, ready to pounce on the unsuspecting as we left the Candy Corner, goodies in pocket.

One door of the square, high-ceilinged Candy Corner opened onto the rear covered porch facing the dining room and kitchen. The other, side door, opened into a vestibule that led to the spacious side porch facing 1-B. Just off the center of The Most Popular Room on Campus, Bar None, stood a large glassed-in display case, about six feet long and two feet deep. The height of the glass enclosure years before had been set at "drool" level, in order to accommodate customers of any height, from Walker Building to 3-B.

Displayed invitingly inside the glass cabinet on several shelves, were neatly-arranged paper boxes and other containers filled with assorted and attractively-wrapped penny candy, candy bars and gum, both chewing and

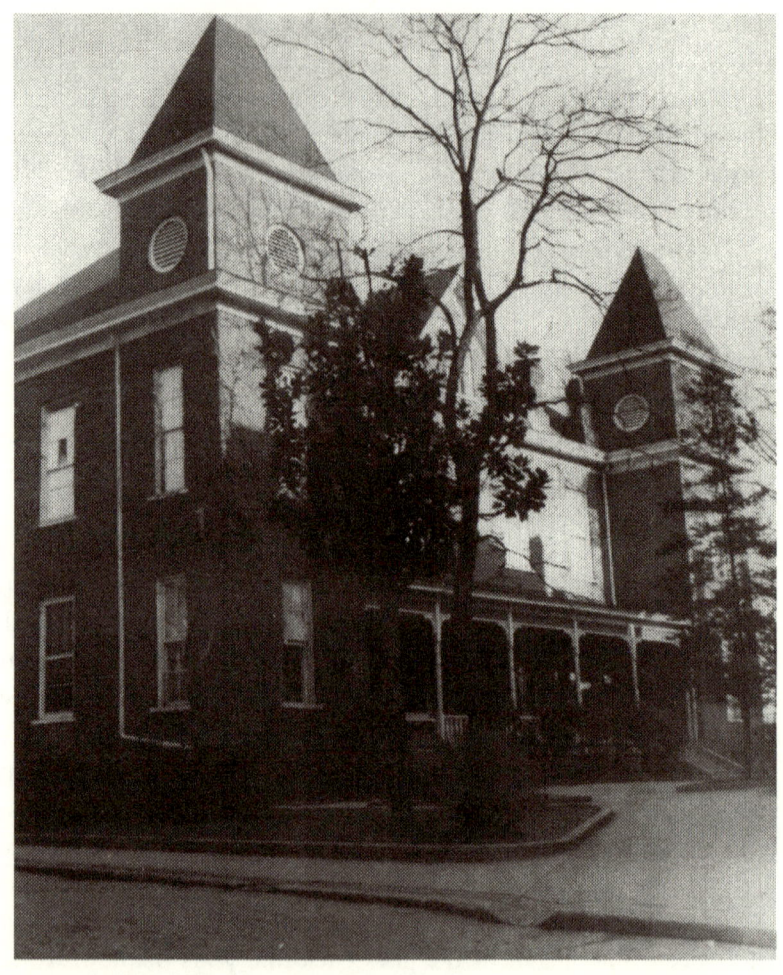

Massive dining halls and kitchen. Top floor was the Masonic meeting hall, later converted into a basketball court.

bubble. One of the older girls, usually Betty Evans, was on duty behind the "Candy Counter," as it was called, before and after dinner, and before supper.

Orphans' love affair with the Candy Corner was legendary. The monthly "Candy Cycle" began a few days before the first of the month, that is, before "Allowance Day" that, at least for more than three hundred candy-starved kids, many years before had been elevated to the revered prominence of a national holiday.

These few days preceding Allowance Day constituted the "Planning Period" of the Candy Cycle. A whole slew of kids congregated before dinner (the noon meal that those who don't know any better call "lunch") at the counter in the Candy Corner, that, as previously mentioned, was called the "Candy Counter," mouths watering, debating among themselves the relative merits of Mary Janes, Bazooka bubble gum, B-B Bats, Juicy Fruit chewing gum, Baby Ruth, Butterfinger and Payday candy bars, and an assortment of hard penny candies. Small fingers pointed here and there; firm decisions were made, only to be changed abruptly a moment later.

I loved Mary Janes, those cream-colored, individually wrapped chewy taffy candies with the peanut butter-filled centers. My other favorites were Bazooka bubble gum, Payday candy bars and of course, the ever-tasty B-B Bats.

The Candy Corner was one of those great "levelers" among children of all ages in the orphanage. One kid may be bigger, or meaner, or faster, or be able (like me) to pee farther in a January snowdrift than other boys in the orphanage, but his nickel wouldn't buy a larger candy bar or pack of Juicy Fruit chewing gum than anyone else's five-cent piece. And this was the never-ending appeal of our beloved Candy Corner.

The prominence our revered Candy Corner held in our lives is underscored by its inclusion in the Statement of Assets and Liabilities noted each year in the Annual Report of the Oxford Orphanage. Under the heading "Endowments and Special Funds" for the year ending December 31, 1947, my first year at the orphanage, is listed "Candy Corner Fund-$3,538.00." It was listed in the same column as the "Neal Trust Fund-$366,577.12."

Money was set aside for our Candy Corner Fund each of the ten years I was at the orphanage, the last being for the year ending December 31, 1957, in the amount of $4,096.93. We kids that year were just as proud of our Candy Corner as the orphanage was of the $617,066.77 Neal Trust Fund.

The Candy Corner was an orphanage institution, never founded to earn a profit for anyone, but perhaps unintentionally shed a ray of light and hope for more than three hundred young travelers on their way to grownupland.

My sister Eoline, two years my senior and the Salutatorian of her 1955 graduating class (Clare Regan, lovely daughter of the Prince of Darkness' rabid dog, was the class Valedictorian that year) recalls one year saving her allowance for months in order to purchase a special hair brush she had seen at the Five-and-Dime in Oxford. She recalls that not being able to spend her meager allowance at the Candy Corner for all those months in order to save for her hairbrush was an agonizing experience, and taught her just how much she must sacrifice at times in order to achieve her goals.

I told my sister that, if I had been in the same situation, that hairbrush would have gathered dust on the shelf in the Five-and-Dime. And, being somewhat curious, I asked her casually, how did she get by all those months without candy. Don't you remember, she said, that toward the first of each month I would ask you if you had any "spare" candy? Stupid me. Stupid, dumb-headed younger brother. Sucker.

A comment concerning the ever-present "spongers" who seemed to spring from the side and rear porches of the Main Building in the waning days of each month. Certainly in any cross-section of small children there are those who set upon their peers for free handouts of food. Some call these intruders "freeloaders." We kids used the denigrating term "spongers."

A boy who seemed never to have candy of his own, yet always kept his lips slightly parted in order to form almost instantly the "le" in the magic word "leffuns" at the slightest crinkling sound of a B-B Bat candy wrapper or an elbow bent with the forearm and hand moving in the general direction of his "friend's" mouth, rapidly earned the moniker "sponger," and the other kids learned quickly to avoid him like his middle initial was "P," as in "polio."

CHAPTER 15

Mr. Gray's List

Upon returning to the Walker Building from the noon meal (that we called "dinner") one cold Saturday in late October 1948, Miss Hobson called the twenty-six of us into the study hall. After we quieted down, she announced,

"When I call your name, I want you to go out into the hallway and sit against the wall."

She began to read from a list she had written on a stenographer's lined note pad.

"Coley Lee."

We knew immediately this was not a "good" list. Freckle-faced, left-handed, loud-mouthed Coley Lee was always getting into hot water with Miss Hobson. Likeable as Coley Lee was, we all had come to believe the poor kid had been cursed, born either under an evil star, or still yet, on a night devoid of stars.

"Terry."

Almost as dangerous as Coley Lee. At least Terry was not left-handed. Tow-headed and gregarious, one could believe, however, that Terry well *could* be on a list with Coley Lee.

"Newton."

Friendly, mild-mannered Newton. Kept out of trouble and got along with everyone. Certainly not in the same league with Coley Lee. Or Terry. Fleetingly, one could sense doubts arising from our group as to the purpose of this list. Perhaps it was not a "good" list, but maybe it wasn't a really "bad" one either. Room for hope.

"Frank."

Our collective psychological pendulum abruptly began swinging the opposite way. Bad news. Any list that included Coley Lee and Frank was on its face highly suspect. This kid would not take your word for anything. You had to prove everything to him. What could be more vexing than a paranoid nine-year-old orphan? Frank thought that everybody over the age of ten was out to do him harm. As I was soon to learn, however, a double dose of paranoia was often an orphan boy's best defense. It at least put a kid on his guard.

Finally, looking up from her notepad, Miss Hobson looked straight into my blinking eyes and said,

"Alton."

Damn! Jeeeeesuuuuus Kuuuuuriiiiiiiieeeeest! My palms began to sweat. Moisture quickly beaded on my upper lip, cooled by rapid evaporation. My entire body felt suddenly hot, then cold, then hot again, and I had a sensation of lightheadedness, of floating in the air. I didn't move. The other kids still seated in the study hall turned and stared at me. Nobody made even a sound.

Suddenly, I realized the meaning of the list, and I knew it was not a "good" list. I also knew why my name had been called. I was in a lot of trouble. I knew what was about to happen to me. Omigod!

A few nights before, a group of us had been taking our nightly showers. It is an unwritten rule that children cannot take showers on a cold October night unless the water is hot enough to peel the skin of a wild boar. That's only natural, and in this regard orphan kids are no different from other children.

Anyway, all at once two boys flushed their toilets in unison, immediately drawing off the cold water, and scalding the kids in the shower, including Terry and me.

"Fuck!" yelled Terry. "Tell us before you flush that toilet, dammit!"

"Sorry," answered the two errant flushers in unison.

I didn't know what "fuck" meant, nor could I recall hearing the word during my months in the Baby Cottage. Had I so known, most assuredly I would have worn out the word; excuses for its use blossomed exponentially with each day passed at Oxford.

Apparently, it was a word of displeasure because the two flushers apologized when Terry yelled at them. Consciously, I gave it no thought. However, my mind must have deemed the new word significant, and incorporated it into my subconscious vocabulary, figuring that although I did not fully appreciate the word, I might find it useful at a later date and under the proper circumstances.

There was really no heat in the two large dormitories, so to keep warm we piled as many of the warm woolen Army blankets on top of us, just shy of being crushed or smothered by the weight, and enough to provide adequate insulation during the bitterly cold Winter nights.

When the six o'clock bell sounded each morning during the Winter, we hopped quickly out of bed, snatched up our brogues and clothes, and gathered around the large black pot-bellied coal stove in the center room of the Walker Building, in order to change from our pajamas into our clothes.

The morning following Terry forcing this new word into my subconscious, I bounded from my warm bed to the warmth of the pot-bellied stove, hurriedly put on my cold clothes, then reached into my brogues for my socks. No socks. And the left brogue was as empty as was the right. Feeling that immediate sense of uncontrolled frustration possessed by all small boys in similar circumstances, and drawing on my newfound though subconscious expression no doubt meant for use on this very occasion, I blurted out,

"Fuck." And immediately I skedaddled off to the cold dormitory to retrieve my errant feet covers.

Racing back to the pot-bellied stove, I found Miss Hobson standing in the center of the room, arms akimbo, surrounded by twenty-five very, very quiet little boys, sitting as though flash frozen in the moment, becoming an instant audience to the rapidly unfolding drama.

"What was that word you just used, young man?" Miss Hobson demanded.

"When?" I queried expectantly, innocently unaware of the meaning of the cottage counselor's question.

"Before you left the room, young man."

"Oh," I responded. "You must mean 'fuck.'"

I could almost hear the quietness in the room get quieter.

"And just where did you learn that word?" she asked, her voice rising sharply.

"I heard Terry say it last night when we were taking a shower."

"Oh, he did, did he?" Miss Hobson's voice seeming to rise an octave with each word, her face reddening to a soft mushy Alabama Tide crimson.

"We'll see about that, young man." And she turned sharply and stalked off in a snit.

The three "young mans" uttered almost in the same breath. Absolutely unheard of in the annals of child abuse at Oxford Orphanage. This was tantamount to receiving a death sentence. Three!

"I said 'Alton Provost,'" repeated Miss Hobson, jolting me out of my stupor of sheer terror.

"You go into the hall with the others." I distinctly sensed a tone of vengeance in the cottage mother's voice. And she followed me into the hall. Coley Lee, Newton, Frank, and Terry got to their feet as we approached. Addressing us five nine- and ten-year-olds, the silly-assed old fogie announced,

"You boys go on up to the business office and see Mr. Gray. He wants to talk to you."

So, frightened out of our wits, the five of us headed out across the baseball field, not saying a word, past the hospital, where we stopped in front of the business office, a small two-story red brick building located adjacent to the large kitchen and main dining building.

Coley Lee was the only one of us boys singled out by Miss Hobson for this latter-day Bataan Death March, who questioned being selected for this dubious honor. The other four of us were so shocked and frightened at hearing our names called aloud in front of the other kids that we were afraid to question the reason for having been selected. Or rather, accused.

Certainly the calling of my name had been a big mistake, some sort of easily explained clerical or administrative error, and momentarily Miss Hobson would smile at me and say, "Oh, Alton, there's been a mistake. Let me just cross your name off this silly old list."

Didn't happen. Wish it had. No such luck. At least my fears were confirmed-Miss Hobson was a mean old biddy, and she held a grudge. My name appearing on that stupid old list was enough to convince me of that fact.

It became obvious to the four of us why Coley Lee had been asked to join this little jaunt into Hell. He was a cocky, ballsy, mouthy kid who possessed so much nervous energy that he expended it by biting his fingernails and sassing Miss Hobson. Coley Lee was one of those kids who had great difficulty locating the ever-elusive "be," always where he shouldn't and never where he should. Be, that is.

Anyway, before we enter the business office, allow me to tell you a little about this "Mr. Gray" and how it came to pass that he was the one Miss Hobson had said was going to "talk" to us five miscreants. "Talk," my eye. Just whom did she think she was kidding? We five kids may have been stupid, but we weren't no fools. Well, maybe Coley Lee was.

Alan DeLeon Gray

Alan DeLeon Gray was born in Brighton, Alabama, on August 1, 1908. He was three years younger than my daddy and a year older than my mama. Mr. Gray graduated from the Divinity School at Duke University in 1941, when I was two years old. Thus, when I arrived at the orphanage on February 15, 1947, Mr. Gray was only thirty-eight years old.

My sister and I had been accepted for admission into Oxford Orphanage while the Rev. Creasy K. Proctor was still Superintendent. So Mr. Gray was only forty years old when I made my first (of many) appearances on the dreaded "Mr. Gray's Lists" in the Fall of 1948, at the age of nine.

The Rev. Creasy K. Proctor, who had been pastor of the Queen Street Methodist Church, about eight city blocks from my home on East Bright Street, had served as Superintendent of Oxford Orphanage since 1928. On June 15, 1946, four months after my daddy's death, Rev. Proctor suffered a heart attack while working in his office and died the same day. Thus, when my sister first arrived the following month, in July 1946, the orphanage did not have a Superintendent.

On November 25, 1946 the orphanage Board of Directors met in Raleigh, and the Rev. A. DeLeon Gray, as the old bastard was known to those outside the confines of the orphanage, who at the time was serving in his second year as pastor of the Methodist Church in Snow Hill, North Carolina, was selected to succeed the late Creasy Proctor as Superintendent of Oxford Orphanage.

In fact, Mr. Gray's appointment as Superintendent came a mere two months before I was dragged in chains to Oxford Orphanage as a frightened seven-year-old, on February 15, 1947.

Mr. Gray's office was on the first floor of the business office, and as we approached quietly and with great trepidation, we found his office door open and him seated in a high-backed brown leather chair on the far side of a large mahogany desk cluttered with papers.

"You boys come on in," he intoned in the classic Southern preacher didactic monotone, "and stand over there," waving his hand toward the wall opposite his desk.

This was my first encounter with this flamingly pedantic, somber Southern Methodist preacher, and as he peered sullenly and accusingly across his large desk at us five pint-sized arch-criminals, I was at once disconcerted by his stern, downright unfriendly appearance, underscored by cold and distant eyes peering at us from behind the old Sirmont eyeglass frame ever so popular in that era.

Mr. Gray's face was thin and elongated, his skin olive-colored, and I thought with certainty that if one were to give his family tree a good old-fashioned light pecan-tree shaking, out would likely tumble a goodly number of Cherokee Indians. Picturing in my mind's eye this half-breed Indian mauler of young defenseless children, suddenly appearing on The Lord's Day replete in ecclesiastical vestments was beyond comprehension.

Most assuredly, Mr. Gray was not a likeable person, and I sensed, standing frightened before him that Saturday afternoon, that my relationship with him was not going to work out very well. And I was beginning to get a sixth sense about such things.

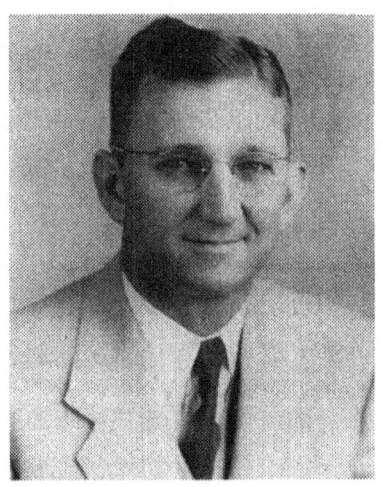

1949. Mr. E.T. Regan, Assistant Superintendent of Oxford Orphanage.

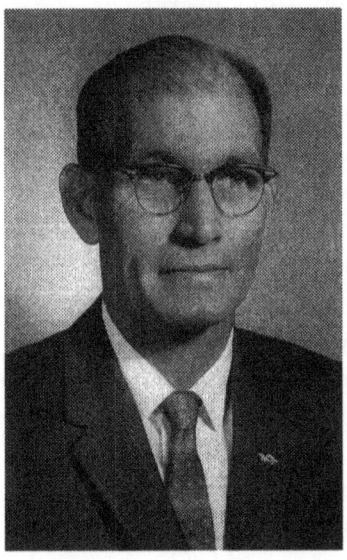

1949. Reverend A. DeLeon Gray, Superintendent of Oxford Orphanage.

Mr. Gray's demeanor could best be described as aloof and condescending, and he exuded an air of unfriendliness bordering on hardness; a pseudo-patrician indeed. His priggish air of self-importance spoke loudly of vanity, and his haughty manner certainly did not engender a great deal of trust in us Walker Building misfits. I felt a sense of foreboding that this would not be my last visit to his office. My fears proved to be justified the following Saturday, but first to continue with my initial visit to Mr. Gray's one-man Star Chamber.

Sitting back pontifically in his high-backed brown leather chair, as if holding court over some unruly riffraff in his kingdom (which was about the gist of it) and before addressing us further, Mr. Gray slowly (and I believe certainly for "effect") pulled open a drawer on the left side of his large desk, and extracted a piece of wood approximately twelve inches long, four inches wide and about a half inch thick. One end of the piece of wood had been carved in the shape of a handle.

Slowly and deliberately (that "effect" thingy again) he placed the board on the blotting pad in front of him, as though preparing to bargain with us for possession of this Instrument of Terror and Loose Bowel Initiator. Facing him across his wide desk, we five pint-sized reprobates suddenly knew damn well the swift and certain fate that awaited us. "Talk," hell; this weren't gonna be no "talk."

In an action designed no doubt to intimidate (didn't take much), Mr. Gray grimaced and folded his hands on the desk in front of him. For a long moment (he was really into this "effect" idea) he did not speak, but looked from one frightened child to the next in line, making eye contact with each of us.

When he finally spoke, his voice matched his appearance and demeanor to a "T." Standing before him, fidgeting and nervously shifting my (very little) weight from one spindly, trembling leg to the other, I suddenly got this uncontrollable urge to do pee-a lot of pee. Should I ask Mr. Gray if I could go to the bathroom?

For a fleeting moment I considered begging his forgiveness, but nothing in his mannerism tended to suggest that he would entertain such adolescent frivolity. Or, worded more succinctly, Mr. Gray appeared to be greatly put out, and I didn't want to be the one to cause his pot to boil over.

At the sight of his fearsome Board of Small Ass Realignment, the leather soles of five pairs of worn brown brogues commenced an audible and nervous shifting on the hardwood floor.

"Stop that moving around!"

This stern rebuke put an immediate end to the Hardwood Floor Getaway Shuffle, and to ensure that any escalation of our danger would not be of my doing, I stopped moving, stopped breathing and held onto (mentally, that is) my micturation valve.

But hold on here just a minute. Hadn't Miss Hobson said that Mr. Gray wanted to "talk" to us? He probably intended only to scare us. Yes, that was it. He would now say something like "If you boys ever have to come in here again, this (and he would hold up the wooden beating instrument adults attempt to lessen in severity by calling it a paddle) is what you are going to get." And he would then dismiss us with a stern lecture, and all would be right with the world. After all, Mr. Gray was a preacher, a man of God. Right?

But alas, this was not to be. Mr. Gray's religious credentials belied a downright sadistic nature. Must be his dormant redskin ancestry surfacing.

Again, without taking his gaze off us five frightened wretches, he extended his arms in front of him, then swept them back laterally like a swimmer demonstrating a dry breast stroke, at the same time commanding in a stern voice raised about two and a half octaves from when we first entered his office,

"Okay, you boys spread yourselves along that wall, and turn and face the other way." Shocked and scared out of our wits, our anal sphincters suddenly contracting to the point of pain, we hurriedly did as instructed.

"Now you boys bend over and grab your ankles."

And when in our confusion we did not respond immediately, he repeated his command, his voice again rising.

"I said for you boys to bend over and grab your ankles."

Hurriedly following Mr. Gray's imperative, and no doubt resembling a pint-sized ballet troupe, in unison we bent at the waist, and as soon as I grabbed my ankles, I felt the tightness of my woolen knickers across my skinny ass. Because I had been the first to enter Mr. Gray's office, I ended up the farthest from the door. Staring at the hardwood floor about a foot below my face, I could hear my heart thumping rapidly as I anticipated the awful blow, and suddenly I could feel a dampness in my armpits. I don't even remember the sound of Mr. Gray's shoes approaching along the hardwood floor. The sound that shattered the terrifying silence was a sharp, loud "Splat!" of the board across Coley Lee's skinny butt, followed almost instantly by Coley Lee's "Yoooow!" There followed in rapid succession three more "Splats!" accompanied by as many sharp screams of pain and terror, and I closed my eyes tightly, expecting the worst.

And then I felt it, the sharp sting of the large board across my fragile backside, followed instantly by a strange, never before experienced burning sensation. I felt as though my knickers were on fire.

But I didn't yell. I don't know why, but no sound would come from my throat. Tears streamed from my eyes, making tiny raindrop splashes on the hardwood floor, and I was shaking from fright. It was as though my voice box was paralyzed. I tried but could not utter a sound. A large, rock-hard lump formed in my throat.

"Stay down!" came the harsh voice from the "preacher" behind us. "I didn't say you could get up!" Man of God, my eye. Goddamn butcher.

Four more times each of us suffered the sting of Mr. Gray's blows, each painful strike certainly seeming more severe than the preceding one. My tears had come together to form a small puddle on the floor below me. My butt seemed as large as an inflamed pillow, and I was still trembling with fright, the lump still lodged in my throat.

"Okay, you can stand up and turn around."

As I glanced to my left upon rising, I noticed through my still blurred vision four more tiny pools of tears staining the hardwood floor. Or were they pools of pee?

The five of us stood, shaking and sobbing before Mr. Gray, our eyes fixed on the floor in front of us, ashamed to be caught crying in front of each other, yet relieved the trauma had ended.

We five nine-year-old boys had not been "reprimanded," or "paddled," or "punished." No, we five young unfortunates had suffered a cruel beating, the severity of which exceeded ten-fold the degree required to alert us to the fact that our conduct (real in the case of the other four, imagined in my case) the cause of which merited this Saturday afternoon "talk" had been socially unacceptable.

Far worse than the pain of the (large) board could ever be, was the awful humiliation we endured, because each of us was acutely aware we had received an unwarranted beating at the hand of a cruel and uncaring sadist. At the same time, however, we nine-year-olds were orphans, and had just suffered physical abuse at the hands of Mr. Gray, who was *the* Superintendent of Oxford Orphanage. To whom could we report such abuse? That, of course, was then a strictly rhetorical question.

None of us uttered a word as we left Mr. Gray's office and walked quickly down the concrete steps of the business office, fearing that at any moment the Superintendent might determine we had not had enough of his physical assault, or that he needed more practice, and invite us back for more of the same.

We were about halfway across the wide ball field on our way back to the Walker Building, when suddenly one of my four cohorts blurted out,

"Fuck! Fuck! Fuck! Fuck!" and began laughing aloud.

Spontaneously, we all joined his chant, laughing and giggling, no doubt to release the nervous tension and to allow our anal sphincters to return to normal tonicity. I did not have the slightest idea of the meaning of the word before that time, but apparently it was a "bad" word, and this was our childish way of snubbing our noses in the face of authority.

Was the purpose of Mr. Gray's cruelty to punish us for some real or perceived transgressions as reported by Miss Hobson? Or was the beating administered to deter us from committing said real or imagined gross breaches of institutional conformity? If such mistreatment was designed to act as a trammel on our youthful rebellious nature, in that sense it certainly failed. The five of us felt our punishment to be grossly abusive and certainly unwarranted, and in order to make my feelings known to the cause of our troubles, i.e. Miss Hobson, I refused to rake the leaves on my side of the Walker Building yard the following week, as was my daily "duty."

Forcing nine-year-olds to bend over and grab their ankles, then proceeding to beat these frightened youngsters with a board was on its face cruel and inhumane punishment, and Mr. Gray should be forever damned for his cavalier, insensitive treatment of small children and for the arrogantly unforgivable abuse of the trust placed in him by the Masons of North Carolina.

I was there in real time, suffering on more than a few occasions his physical abuse, and I know that of which I write as fact. Passage of time does not right egregious wrongs, nor does it mask outrageous and abusive conduct.

We Walker Building boys did not convey to our parents or other relatives the physical abuse we suffered routinely at the hands of Mr. Gray, although quite often we debated the issue among ourselves out of earshot of Miss Hobson.

Alas, however, we nine-year-olds were quite literally intimidated against informing our relatives of our mistreatment by Mr. Gray. We had been taught by example the harsh reprisals that followed on the heels of what we referred to as "telling," or "snitching."

And early on Miss Hobson had discovered that she did not have to discipline us; that on a whim she merely could call out a boy's name on Saturday afternoon, and that unfortunate child was sent to Mr. Gray to receive a thrashing. On our second "visit" to Mr. Gray's office in two weeks, Henry Lee had openly questioned Miss Hobson as to why his name was on the dreaded "list," and Miss Hobson ignored him.

When we entered Mr. Gray's office, the superintendent noted that Henry Lee and I had been sent to his office the previous week. When Henry Lee attempted to ask Mr. Gray the reason he was being punished, Mr. Gray interrupted the boy. However, Miss Hobson was not required to give a reason for having Mr. Gray assault us, and likely Mr. Gray never asked Miss Hobson the reason for our being sent to him for punishment.

I found that children react to wrongs committed against them (be these wrongs real or imagined) in several different ways. My response to the Superintendent's gross and unwarranted physical abuse was a mixture of hatred, anger and utter defiance, emotions that were fast becoming incorporated into my youth and early adult psyche. Although our feelings remained unspoken among us, simmering below the surface of our conversations for fear our words would find their way back to Miss Hobson,

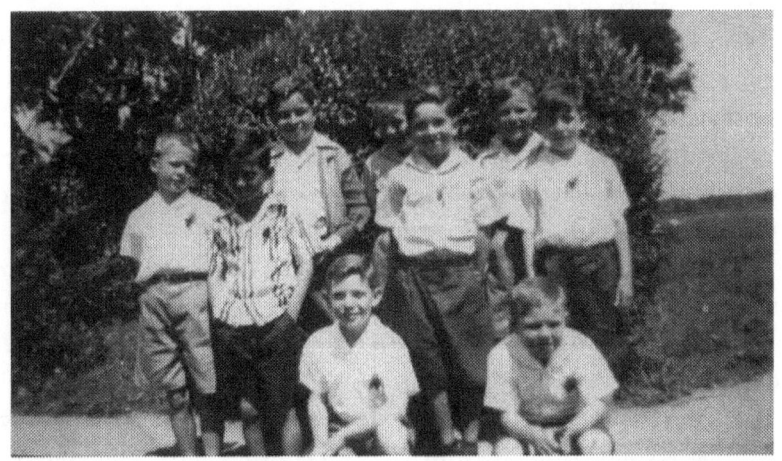

1949. Some Walker Building nine-year olds. The author is at far left, trying to act like he doesn't belong with this bunch of hooligans. First row (kneeling): Phillip Edwards, Coley Lee Hackett. Second row: Alton Provost, Bill Herrington, Jimmy Frederick, Robert Pace. Third row: W.T. Bass, Alvin Gibbs, Newton Wilder.

we Walker Building boys shared an utter contempt for Mr. Gray because of his unchecked and indiscriminate physical abuse of young children.

Thus, it was no surprise that after assembling us in the study hall after dinner the following Saturday, Miss Hobson began her, what we were soon wont to call, "Mr. Gray's List," with Henry Lee, followed by Alton, and three other unfortunates du jour, forming what would be the nexus of Mr. Gray's wrath. Despite Henry Lee's repeated whines to Miss Hobson, "What did I do wrong?" soon we were waiting outside Mr. Gray's office door again.

The Big Boys, i.e., those boys of high school age at the time Mr. Gray assumed his duties as Superintendent in December 1946, never were made to suffer the sharp sting of his board across their backsides; thus, to that group of students Mr. Gray appeared to be a capable administrator. Unaffected persons tend to view another in terms of their personal relationship to that person.

Because we were sent to Mr. Gray's office to receive an unmerited thrashing, our puerile minds quite naturally assumed that *any* boys seen in the Superintendent's office on Saturday afternoon were summoned to receive like mistreatment.

Trudging laboriously up the concrete steps and into the business office that second Saturday, with Henry Lee whimpering and sniveling all the way from the Walker Building, we approached Mr. Gray's office to find the door closed and Mr. Gray's voice intoning, "Well, maybe you can do even better next week."

Presently, the door to Mr. Gray's office opened and out filed six high school boys, who at first glance did not appear to have been the recipients of just-administered physical abuse. But again, we collectively surmised that boys that big would not cry when whipped. As each boy left the office, he looked back and said, "Thank you, Mr. Gray."

Once the Big Boys were out and gone, Mr. Gray's stern voice commanded from behind his large desk, "Okay, you boys come on in!" We (quite reluctantly) filed into his office, and in true Pavlovian style, spread out along the near wall facing his desk. Odd that the desire to cooperate and thus curry favor with one's enemy when imprisoned is so quickly learned at such an early age. Amazing. We kids weren't too proud to grovel, if it would help.

Old Man Gray looked across the room at me, and it seemed as if he were peering into my thoughts. Gaugin might well shade the old bastard pedantic, heartless and brutal, while simultaneously that same famous color-dauber would pigmentize defenseless little Alton as cowering, hurt and petrified with fear of his certain, imminent and absolute extinction.

"You were here last week, weren't you, boy?" He kinda spat out the "boy" part at the end of the question, like he had a bad taste in his mouth.

"Yes, sir." I uttered the words softly, again not wanting to antagonize my sadistic captor.

"And so were you," he said, his piercing gaze fixed down the line in the general direction of Henry Lee.

"Yes, sir but-"

"No 'buts,' boy. You wouldn't be here without a good reason."

"Okay, you boys turn around and face the wall," he commanded impatiently, his voice rising, and we heard wood sliding over wood as the left-side desk drawer opened, and his chair rolled back from his desk.

Again this time, I did not cry out when struck; this time from defiance. And I refused to cry. Damn him, I simply was not going to give him any satisfaction. And one or two of the other boys refused to cry out in pain. Again, as the week before, five hard, stinging thwacks across each of our backsides, and again my pants literally seemed to be on fire.

"Now, stand up and turn around!" he ordered. Then, giving us a stern lecture concerning obedience and responsibility, he said,

"Now, you boys go on back to your cottage, and I'd better never see any of you in here again!" He didn't add "or else" but the assumption was that we would suffer grievous bodily harm if again we were unfortunate enough to make another "Mr. Gray's List."

Now, upon entering Mr. Gray's office earlier, Henry Lee had ended up at the far end of the wall, and would be the last to leave. Apparently in a stupid, childish, desperate attempt to ingratiate himself with the Superintendent, a la the just-departed Big Boys, as he left the room Henry Lee looked back into the room and, forcing a smile through his tears, said,

"Thank you, Mr. Gray."

Taken aback and incensed by what he perceived to be a derisive, baldly impertinent comment, the Superintendent bellowed,

"Come right back in here, boy. What did you just say to me?"

Utterly confused, Henry Lee just stood, looking at the Superintendent's welling up anger, completely speechless. No answer Henry Lee could muster would ever soothe Mr. Gray's perceived insult, and the poor lad knew it. So he just stood there crying.

The other four of us (the smart four) stood motionless in the hallway, fearing that at any moment Henry Lee's big mouth would get our butts scorched again. However, we were spared Henry Lee's fate. Perhaps there was a God after all.

Opening his office door wider than required to admit the small boy, Mr. Gray bellowed,

"You get back in here, boy, and bend over and grab your ankles!"

The door closed behind the by now terrified child, and we heard five resounding blows, the pitiable lad yelping in pain after each one found its mark.

From outside the closed office door, we heard the unremitting sobbing of a humiliated and terrified child, who had just suffered a vicious beating at the hands of a cruel, callous and merciless bastard masquerading as a preacher and orphanage administrator. His repulsive, insensitive actions had crossed the line of reprimand, punishment, and discipline and had entered boldly the realm of the brutal manhandling of defenseless, innocent children entrusted to his care by the state of North Carolina and the Masons of North Carolina.

But as usual, we five ass-burned kids had the last laugh. Halfway back across the ball field that day, once well out of the old man's listening range, we picked up the chant "Thank you, Mr. Gray. Thank you, Mr. Gray," and sang it all the way back to the Walker Building. For the next several months, we would be standing around doing nothing in particular, and one of the five of us would look at another of us and smile and say, "Thank you, Mr. Gray." And we would both laugh at our misery. And this is where I learned as a young boy of nine to laugh at adversity.

Plainly put, Alan DeLeon Gray was an insensitive prick who was clearly out of his element in his position as Superintendent in charge of more than three hundred orphans. For those students who were already in high school when Mr. Gray arrived in December 1946 to assume the office of Superintendent, the aforementioned characterization might seem misplaced, or even unfair. This group of children would include those who graduated in 1947, 1948, 1949 and 1950, who for the most part were past the age at which Mr. Gray would have inflicted corporal punishment.

And why did Mr. Gray get a second crack at Henry (Stupid) Lee on that fateful Saturday mentioned just above? We found out later that the high school boys had just the night before won a close football game, and the six football players had been called to the business office by Mr. Gray to receive congratulations. Those short brown things each boy carried as he left Mr. Gray's office and passed us in the hallway, we found out, were cigars given to the boys by Mr. Gray, even though smoking of any kind was strictly forbidden.

Chapter 16

I Meet the "Big Boys"

Hatred. Even the sound of the word carries with it an offensive quality, a harshness that should not be part of the psyche of a nine-year-old fourth grade orphan. But I was forced to hate at an early age.

It was late October 1948, and Winter was coming on strong that year. That "certain slant of light on Winter afternoons" really was quite depressing and did nothing to ease my terminal case of homesickness. I was a few months into Miss Ellie Parrish's fourth grade, and I recall that the most fascinating part of the school day was history class. The "pictures" (as we called them in those days) in our history book were of the old "woodcut" designs. I might as well have been in grammar school (as we called it in those days) with Chuck Dickens, my favorite author of all time.

Apparently one of the prerequisites of becoming an orphan is that you have a "sweet tooth." Every kid I knew at Oxford loved sweets. I was certainly no exception.

That Sunday mama came to see Eoline and me. Her unannounced visit was a welcomed surprise, because mama had made the three-hour automobile trip with my older brother J.B., his wife Mary and their two small children. Eoline and I had not seen our oldest brother since 1945, when he left home to join the U.S. Merchant Marines, and I was delighted to see him.

Mama took a lot of pictures, nobody ever called them "photographs" or used the word "photos," one of which shows us all huddled together in the cold, with me clutching (with both hands) a (very) large brown paper bag filled with assorted candies and Bazooka bubble gum that J.B. had brought me.

It was a happy day for Eoline and me, and it really gave me hope that I would see more of my big brother. All went well. That is, until my relatives departed at around 4:00 p.m. There were hugs and kisses all around, promises to come again "real soon," and as on every one of mama's visits, I cried and asked her to come and take me home because I really missed my cat. When? Why, "real soon," of course.

Following this heart-wrenching ritual, I waited on the top concrete step of the Main Building until J.B.'s car passed through the Main Gate entrance and turned left toward the center of Oxford. The most depressing scene at Oxford, for all the children, was that disheartening left turn our relatives' automobiles made on a late Sunday Winter afternoon.

Then, still crying softly, and still clutching my (very large) brown paper bag of goodies, I left the Main Building, walking past the Business Office (hurriedly, lest Old Man Gray suddenly open the front door waving that goddamn large board of his at me) and was at the edge of the baseball field near the hospital on my way to the Walker Building, when suddenly out of the corner of my right eye, I noticed two teenage boys kinda sorta veer off their announced path toward the school building to where even at that young age it was obvious they had a purpose in their abrupt detour.

"Whatcha got in dat bag, kid?" The attendant smile was derisive in nature and effect, and I sensed suddenly that I might be in trouble.

"Some candy." I tried to put a little wood-rasp in my voice to show I was not afraid of the boy. Didn't work, though. Didn't really think it would. I found that a nine-year-old orphan could put enough wood-rasp in his voice to overflow a bushel basket, and it wouldn't faze these sadistic bastards. Especially if the unfortunate nine-year-old kid was crying and clutching (with both hands) a heavy-looking brown paper bag, walking from the general direction of the place where the orphan's relatives had just departed for home. Don't take no bloomin' Einstein to figure out what's in that heavy-looking brown paper bag.

"Lemme see here, boy," Bully's cohort mocked, snatching the (very) large brown paper bag of goodies from my clutching hands.

"Gimme back my bag. It's *my* candy. My big brother gave it to me." Tears welled up in my eyes, crowding out the homesick ones already there, blurring my vision. I reached for my bag of candy.

But Bully's partner easily jerked the bag from my reach, at the same time shoving his large hand into my frail chest, and I fell sprawling backwards on the ground.

"My big brother gave me that candy," I screamed, crying unashamedly with hurt and anger. I knew then that I would not get my (large) bag of candy back.

"Leffuns, kid," mockingly laughed the first bandit. And then the foreign word turned into a mocking taunt.

"Leffuns. Leffuns. Leffuns."

"Yeah," chimed his buddy, rummaging around in what was now "his" large brown paper bag full of candy, "You didn't say Venny leffuns."

And laughing, the two "highwayboys" walked away, hands deep into what had until a few seconds before, been a gift from my brother J.B.

When I arrived at the Walker Building, I was still crying, and one of the older boys asked me what had happened. I told him, then added,

"I'm gonna tell Miss Hobson."

"Better not, Al," he advised in a serious tone.

"Why not? They took my bag of candy."

"If you tell, they'll find out, and they'll beat you up when they catch you." His advice was sincere, and I took his warning to heart. Gone was the isolation and the attendant protection of the Baby Cottage; we in the Walker Building ate our meals in the large dining hall building, so getting to me would be easy for those scumbag thieves.

"Next time you get candy from your family, Al, just stuff it all inside your shorts and pockets. If those guys don't see a bag, sometimes they won't check your pockets."

"Sometimes?"

"Yeah." And, then pausing, he added, "And sometimes they do."

So, on a cold October Sunday afternoon in 1948, at the tender age of nine, I learned to hate. I had feared Mrs. Tomblin, Miss Warwick and the stupid, mean cottage girl in the Baby Cottage, but the emotion of hate was somewhat new to me and equally as confusing.

But the worst part of the situation was that I did not know of any way to retaliate, and that made the insult hurt to the quick. For the next several weeks, every time we assembled at the dining hall for meals, I sought out the two bullies, and tried to think of ways to repay them for what they had done to me. However, in my situation I could not even say anything to them, for fear they would beat me up. It was an absolute, total feeling of utter helplessness.

And, I wondered, what is this business about "leffuns?" And equally as perplexing, who in the world is this kid named "Venny?" Leffuns? Venny Leffuns? And to add insult to injury, during the "shakedown" one of the hoodlums had been picking his nose, while the other petty thief pumped his right leg like he was stomping the starter pedal of an Indian, then laughed and farted simultaneously. God, this was one really weird place.

I suddenly realized I had an awful lot to learn if I were to survive (using the word in its literal sense) this Black Hole called Oxford Orphanage. The words "Big Boy," "leffuns," "venny leffuns," "boy," and "sponger," as well as many others, were quite foreign to me; however, within a year or two these strange expressions would be stamped indelibly into my consciousness, and as much a part of my day-to-day existence as my name. Oxford Orphanage and its (at that time) nearly eighty years of odd customs, traditions, and unwritten laws would grab an artless, unsophisticated and pitiably gullible city boy from 208 East Bright Street, roughly by the nape of the neck, and within a few short years transform him into a paranoid, conniving, lying, street-smart young mercenary who could hold a grudge with the best, taste revenge as though it were dessert, and plan, plot and scheme his way out of any seemingly impossible predicament.

When I refer to "Big Boys," I capitalize the two B's not out of any great fondness but moreso from a mixture of respect (about eighty-four percent) and fear (about sixteen percent). I refuse to honor this group with "all-cappers;" these hooligans do not deserve to be referred to as

"BIG BOYS," but in certain aspects of life, a hierarchy once established becomes a part of one's existence. So it is with "Big Boys."

In reality, most of the Big Boys on campus were good to us youngsters, or ignored us altogether. Being ignored by a Big Boy was a blessing. Any insults, obscenities, slurs, scorn and other and numerous denigrating comments are reserved for that thirty percent or so of twits, bottom-feeders, low-lifes, simple-minded dolts who clearly deserve to be torn asunder by steeds mounted by the Four Horsemen of the Apocalypse, galloping at breakneck speed to each of the four winds.

I have reluctantly refrained from calling any of these goons by name because most assuredly, some of them became hitmen for the Charlotte Mafia. If one of these thugs tells you "There's more than one way to skin a cat," you can bet your last peanut butter and molasses sandwich that he's speaking from experience.

Generally speaking, age and not size determined the status of a Big Boy. This was a term used to refer, only in the third person, to another boy generally five years or more older than you. A Big Boy would be what the American mafia refers to as a "made man," meaning that you could not "mess with" such boy, and if a Big Boy told you to do something, you did it without comment, under threat of certain bodily harm. It was an unwritten rule that the status of a Big Boy of small stature (i.e., a "puny" Big Boy) was protected by his fellow Big Boys; to disobey his wishes was tantamount to inviting a beating from the other Big Boys. It all had to do with respect. And fear. And knowing your "place." And more fear. Lots of it.

"Leffuns" and the associated defensive disclaimer, "Venny Leffuns," are complicated concepts indeed, but I'll try to explain them. To give some instant perspective to these ideas, Al Capone in 1930 certainly would not have uttered "Leffuns" to a timid Chicago South Side store owner. He wouldn't have to. By the same token, this timid store owner would never claim "Venny leffuns" to Al Capone. He knew better.

To the two evil Big Boy "Capones" who confiscated Little Orphan ("timid store owner") Al's (very large) bag of candy in 1948, "leffuns" and "venny leffuns" had absolutely no meaning; that's why they mocked me with those words.

"Leffuns" is very likely a variation of the word "leavings," meaning the remainder, or residue, of food, visible to the naked eye, and in one's actual physical possession. The word "leffuns," when spoken aloud (or more often, shouted, in order to stake one's claim to the exclusion of potential nearby claims jumpers) attached a moral obligation to share anything edible, visible on the person addressed, and which was not a part of a meal that had been served in the dining room, with the following exceptions.

Technically, a soft drink fell under the moral obligation of the leffuns rule; however, because leffuns was given grudgingly, the recipient never could be certain that the reluctant giver had not slobbered purposely into the soft drink bottle. Thus, leffuns was claimed on a soft drink only if the claimant were nearly dying of thirst, or was very best friends with the other boy and could trust his friend (or hoped he could) not to slobber in his soft drink. I did not like to hear the cry "Leffuns!"

One day I was standing in front of a bathroom mirror in the basement of 2-B, practicing eating a real live Baby Ruth candy bar without moving my lips or mouth, and I thought I had it down pat, when Ersul Sowers walked behind me, took a quick glance in the mirror, and said "Leffuns on whatever it is you're eating." He had me. What I had not had a chance to practice on yet was telling a boy that I was not really eating a Baby Ruth candy bar, without moving my mouth or lips. I'd have to work on that.

And there's "Venny leffuns." The word "venny" apparently was an orphanage nonce word, i.e., one made out of whole cloth, and meant "There are no leffuns," or "I deny anyone's claim to leffuns." The word had absolutely no meaning when used alone or as part of any phrase other than "Venny leffuns."

In order to deny to another boy or boys the right to something edible (other than food served in the dining room), the boy in possession of the food was obligated to announce in a clear voice "Venny leffuns," before his hungry friend could stake his moral claim with an equally loud "Leffuns." Thus, negation of the obligation attaching to the cry "Leffuns!" was a preemptory cry of "Venny leffuns!" Once "Venny leffuns" was invoked, the boy making such cry was free of the obligation of sharing.

The ethical duty to share, i.e. "Leffuns," applied only to food, fruit, or candy given to a boy, and not to something that the boy had purchased with his own money. And this duty extended only one "generation." If one boy claimed "Leffuns" and received something from the giver, the receiver of the food was not obligated to a further claim of "Leffuns." The receiver's diligence in ambushing the boy with the food was rewarded by being allowed to keep that which he had claimed.

The defense of "Venny leffuns" could be invoked only against one's peers. Try such a stupid stunt against one of the meaner'n hell Big Boys, and just to teach you a lesson he would confiscate *all* your candy, give you a swift kick in the pants and send you packing. Similarly, an attempt to claim "Leffuns" against a Big Boy would amount to a gross insult, leading to a similar swift kick in the knickers. It is easy to understand why "new" boys, being unaware of the ingrained, cast in stone social hierarchy and punitive order, received a lot of swift kicks.

When I was growing up, the word "boy" was just as belittling and demeaning to young white boys as it was to colored folk. It fell into the same personally offensive category as did the words "young man," for what followed as either a beating, or at the very minimum a vilifying lecture. Usually both.

And at the orphanage, even the more truculent of the older boys used the slur "boy" when addressing younger kids whom they were going to beat up or take money or food.

"C'mere, boy. Wha'cha got in yer pockets?"

"C'mere, boy. Take off yer shoes. Let's see if ya got any money in 'em."

"C'mere, boy. Gimme summa dat orange. Nah, gimme all o' it."

Sorry bastards. Lowlife, good-for-nothing scumbuckets. And after June 25, 1950, "Go to Korea and don't come back alive."

We nine- and ten-year-old youngsters in the Walker Building and 1-B hated the heartless older boys with the same fervor as we did Old Man Gray. Likewise, we feared them equally. Treading softly was the order of the day in this damn place. Survival definitely was my goal.

CHAPTER 17

The Toy

On one of mama's visits in the Fall of 1948, she brought me one of those little fluorescent doohickeys that were so popular with youngsters during the late 1940's. It was circular in shape, about two inches in diameter, with an embossed likeness of an eighteenth century schooner in the center. Light green in color, it glowed in the dark. None of the other kids possessed one like it, so the small toy quickly became the diversion du jour for us Walker Building boys.

The "glow" effect was accomplished by first holding the small toy close to an incandescent light bulb for a few seconds. Then, turning out all the lights in the room, the absorbed radiation would cause the toy to "glow" in the dark for several minutes. At bedtime, after Miss Hobson turned out the lights, I would pull my ubiquitous Army blanket over my head, and in the total darkness the ship appeared to glow a more vivid green.

I had possessed the toy for about two weeks, when one night one of my buddies noticed that I was hiding under my covers. Before you could say "jackrocks," four of us were huddled beneath my blanket, passing the toy back and forth.

At about that time Miss Hobson was going through the dormitory, checking for "lights out," when she was drawn to the animated chatter coming from beneath my blanket.

"Just what are you boys doing under there?" the cottage mother demanded, with great irritation in her voice.

Careful not to allow any light under the covers, Butch Mitchell poked his head from beneath the blanket, and answered excitedly,

"Alton's got this little thing that glows in the dark."

"I'll bet he does!" Miss Hobson exclaimed. "What's going on under there? You boys come out this instant!"

The four of us slowly pulled back the blanket, and (quite reluctantly) I held up the toy, that had lost its glow now that she had turned on the lights. Miss Hobson, apparently quite nettled at the disruption in the dormitory, snatched the toy from my hand.

"Now, you boys go to sleep," she said, and putting my toy in her apron pocket, left the dormitory in a snit.

A week passed before I mustered up the courage to ask Miss Hobson to return my toy, and I figured Sunday afternoon was the best opportunity. That Saturday night, some of the Big Boys came to visit Miss Hobson, and one of my friends told me he saw these older boys passing around my toy.

The next day, I apologized to Miss Hobson for having the toy in bed, and asked her to return it to me. She told me I could not have it.

"But that's *my* toy," I protested defiantly. "My mama gave me that toy, and it's *mine*."

Mind you, the small object was not just a toy. It was a gift from mama. Probably didn't cost more than a dollar. But it was a gift, it was my link to a better place; it was hope, it was personal and it meant a lot to me. When I crawled beneath the covers at night and watched my toy sailing ship fluoresce, I was holding a link to mama, to my family, to my pre-orphanage, happy life. I desperately needed to maintain this contact with my past. So when Miss Hobson confiscated my toy, she also robbed me of this essential bond. Silly-assed old fogie.

Standing before Miss Hobson, the gross inequity of what she had done, taking from me a gift from my mother, overwhelmed me, tears welled up in my eyes, and I said angrily,

"You took my toy. All I was doing was playing with it. If you don't give it back, I'm gonna tell my mama."

Bridling at my impudence, but at the same time angered and quite embarrassed by being addressed in such a disrespectful manner in front of the other children, Miss Hobson's gaze bore into mine, and she said,

"I've had about enough of your snippy attitude. We'll see what Mr. Gray says about that, young man," and turned in a huff and walked back to her room. There was that "young man" thingy again. Troubles brewing for little Al.

I never again saw my fluorescent toy. A few days later, two of the kids informed me they had seen one of the Big Boys, who frequently visited Miss Hobson, showing my toy to some other boys as we were grouped together awaiting the final supper bell. Either Miss Hobson had given the boy my toy, or the boy had stolen it from her, which, to my bruised feelings, was truly a distinction without a difference.

So here I was yet again caught smack-dab between the proverbial "rock and a hard place." Not only had I lost my toy, I had incurred the wrath of Miss Hobson, for which I could expect to pay dearly.

Certain that I would receive a severe beating from Old Man Gray, the following Saturday, immediately after dinner, I hurried to the Walker Building, ran to my cubbyhole where I kept my clothes, and found that I had only two pairs of boxer shorts. I quickly took off my pants, put on the two extra pairs of boxer shorts over the pair I was wearing, then "borrowed" two pairs from my buddy Bill Herrington's cubby located next to mine, and put those on over my three pairs.

None of us Walker Building boys had hips, so our pants were always loose and falling down anyway, so if "Old Man Gray" (we nine-year-olds' "expletives deleted" vocabulary was not sophisticated enough to have a vulgar name for him) did not possess a keen ear, perhaps the sound of his board making sharp contact with a pair of trousers and five pairs of boxer shorts would not sound too differently from the same board hitting a pair of trousers and one pair of shorts. And as I expected to receive a sound thrashing because of the back-talk I had given Miss Hobson (the hateful old biddy), any amount of padding would be a godsend.

So, when Miss Hobson assembled us in the study hall at 1:00 p.m. I was seated already, my butt feeling like a fluffed-up pillow with all that padding, not fearing so much Old Man Gray's board as his discovering my subterfuge. I realized consciously that I was taking a big chance, and had misgivings from the very first (or second, rather) pair of shorts I had put on.

Twenty-six pairs of nine-year-old eyes were locked onto me as Miss Hobson began calling names of those hapless wretches who were to assemble in the hallway outside her door. The last of the five names announced was that of the kid who had once owned a nice fluorescent toy.

The Longest Walk in the World was the two hundred yards between the Walker Building and the Business Office on an early Saturday afternoon. It was like (to us at least) taking that final walk to the electric chair, and fear was our constant and unwelcome companion every dreaded step of the way.

I entered Mr. Gray's office that afternoon with anguish in my heart, hate on my mind and extra padding in my pants. Standing solemnly before him, gazing intently at that definite spot of empty space between my eyes and my brogues, I felt the sadist's eyes were on me, and sure enough, he addressed me personally.

"I hear you've been sassing Miss Hobson, boy."

Boy? Young man? They were the same; each of these belittling and demeaning words trailing at the end of a sentence uttered by a truculent grownup almost always, at least in our confined little world, signaled either a beating, or at a bare minimum, a vilifying lecture. Usually both. No, ninety-nine and forty-four one hundredths percent of the time both.

Having learned painfully by now that any attempt at explaining or defending my conduct would be met with an insulting rebuke, I just kept my head bowed and my mouth shut. If nothing else, orphan kids are fast learners.

Anyway, because I did not answer Mr. Gray's "non-question" statement of accusation, he let it slide, and instead slid open the top left drawer of his large desk and extracted his dead-serious board. Sure was big.

"I see that you boys have been here before," continued our tormentor.

"So line up along that wall (waving with a dramatic flourish his right hand like he was Moses parting the Red Sea waters or something), turn around, bend over and grab your ankles."

I had made sure I was the first of us five recidivists to enter the office, so I was the last in line, and I ended up facing the far wall, nearly in the corner of the room.

If the old bastard possessed keen hearing, and discovered my duplicity, I was doomed for sure. He would beat me to death right then and there. My promising career as an arch-criminal/international terrorist would come to a premature, hideous and bloody end in the darkened far corner of A. DeLeon Gray's private office, and I would never see 208 East Bright Street again. An ignominious end to such a promising young life.

The superintendent/preacher/prison guard/fascist quickly started down the line of the five pint-sized prisoners, and I distinctly heard each contact of his board.

A resounding "SPLAT" followed by

A resounding "SPLAT" followed by

A resounding "SPLAT" followed by

A resounding "SPLAT" followed by

A muffled, anemic "thump."

I held my breath, expecting the worst. However, without comment, Mr. Gray started Round Two at the other end of the line. On each of his five passes, I heard four distinctly sharp "SPLATS" followed by a (welcomed) muffled "thump." "Thumps" are better'n "SPLATS" any day under God's bright sun.

And with each blow, I timed my terrified yelp of "pain" with the moment of contact of his board across my five-shorts padding. I hardly felt a thing.

Returning to his side of the desk, Mr. Gray ordered us to stand up and turn around, and I whimpered and sniffled in unison with my four battered comrades. Following his usual (falling on deaf ears) admonition concerning the dire consequences we would suffer if ever sent to his office again, The Great High (Phony) Priest dismissed us, and four scorched (and one barely touched) butts waddled on back to the Walker

Building. Fooled you, you stupid, arrogant prick. A small victory is still a victory, and still goes in the "W" column on the sports page.

Butt Cheeks in the Snow

Much to the dismay of twenty-odd Walker Building preteen misfits, Mr. Gray's List proved to be neither seasonal nor fair-weather dependent.

One especially bleak and freezing Saturday afternoon in late January 1949, following the previous night's knee-deep (to us Walker Building preteens, anyway) snowfall, Van Edwards and four fellow mini-hooligans were informed by Miss Hobson that they had "made" Mr. Gray's List, as the vindictive, squat, elf-like cottage mother called it, but that in reality should have been called the "Hateful Old Biddy Hobson's List."

Anyway, different Saturday, same physical abuse. *C'est la vie.* Following the requisite threats, admonishments and intimidation that constituted the "foreplay" for this weekly exercise in child abuse and, having informed the frightened quintet of the dire circumstances that surely would befall the pint-sized recidivists should their names ever again appear on "The List" after that date, the terse order emanated from behind the massive mahogany desk to "spread out along that wall, turn around, bend over and grab your ankles," and the stinging brutality ensued, after which the nickel's worth of intimidated boys filed quietly out of the Torture Chamber and scurried quickly out the front door of the Business Office, heading across the foot-deep white powder-blanketed baseball field toward the Walker Building, some two hundred yards distance.

During the four of five fairly heavy snowfalls that swept across the northern third of God's Country each Winter, we kids enjoyed making the well-known "angels in the snow."

Anyway, on this particular snowy Saturday afternoon, about fifty yards into the ballfield (and thus about the same distance out of earshot of the Business Office and you-know-who), without preamble or comment, one of the ass-burned kids stopped abruptly, unbuckled his belt, dropped his woolen knickers and boxer shorts onto the knee-deep snowdrift, promptly planted his skinny bare ass in the freezing snow, and began chanting "Asses in the snow. Asses in the snow," all the while laughing aloud.

Orphan boys being by their very nature copycats, immediately there were four more nine-year-olds, scratchy woolen knickers and boxers jerked down around their snow-encased ankles, making tiny butt cheek impressions in the snow, then moving to their right or left to form additional like depressions, freezing their shriveled testicles and laughing uncontrollably at their predicament, as they chanted in unison, "Asses in the snow. Asses in the snow."

I grew up with some very strange boys who, though oftentimes not endowed with a surplusage of reasonableness, discretion and logic, made up for these shortcomings with an abundance of defiance and audacity. At Oxford, being a little crazy at times enabled us orphan boys to maintain our sanity.

CHAPTER 18

The Errand Boy

In the Fall of 1949, shortly after I entered Baby Elephant's fifth grade, I mustered up the courage one day to go to the Industrial Building to have a word with Miss Beulah Ward, who had succeeded Miss Ora Lee Hall as supervisor of the massive clothing facility.

My ostensible complaint centered around being forced to wear again that Winter those really ugly, stupid, itchy woolen knickers that seemed so popular during the thirties and forties. Utilizing my by that time finely-honed Holmes-like powers of observation and deduction, I had concluded that sane and reasonable persons throughout the free world had decided not to wear the silly baggy trousers ever again but, rather than just toss them out, had dispatched entire railway boxcars full of the ill-fitting knickers to Oxford Orphanage, along with specific instructions that these articles of undesired clothing be delivered forthwith by means of oversized transfer trucks to the Walker Building. Or so it seemed to us Walker Building boys.

I felt like some kind of circus side show freak wearing the baggy woolen pants that ended abruptly just below the knees, leaving my skinny bare legs freezing in the Winter. With a pair of high-topped brown leather brogues on my feet, my spindly legs resembled two toothpicks stuck in brown thimbles. I looked so, well, how do I express it . . . so much like, well . . . an orphan. I know the young girls laughed at us Walker Building boys because of the knickers, which certainly did nothing for my self image, already in tags and tatters. And if I had to wear the stupid knickers, why didn't the Big Boys have to wear them?

So much for official reasons. My underlying complaint was as follows. It centers around the most basic of all instincts-survival. Most of us fifth graders in the Walker Building had been assigned that Fall to the farm work detail, where we picked beans, shucked corn and hoed fields, after which we hoed fields, picked beans and shucked corn. Farm life at Oxford Orphanage was one monotonous, continuous loop. Inmates at prison farms didn't work as hard.

Anyway, when it rained and we had to seek shelter under the shed, or the Snug House, some goddamn heartless, sadistic scumbag Big Boys forced us youngsters to fight one another. If we refused to hit our friends, the Big Boys would beat us up.

I knew I had to escape from this singularly traumatic dilemma. Besides that, I might be forced to fight Terry "Blockhead" Johnson, or worse still, Newton "Mad Dog" Wilder, and I wanted desperately to live to see 1950. At age nine, I was already well into this "survival-at-all-costs" thingy. Anyway, I had looked into the mirror and found that I liked my face just the way it was. Re-arrangement is for furniture.

So when I went to see Miss Beulah Ward-she was so pretty and blond, and reminded me of the actress Virginia Mayo-I quickly poured out my tale of woe about the Big Boys (sick bastards) making us Walker Building boys fight each other. She asked me about the circumstances that caused me to be sent to the orphanage. As I related to this kind lady my story, all the unhappy memories flooded back, and I stood beside her desk and began to cry. Miss Ward pulled me to her, put her arms around my shoulders, and whispered "I'm going to make it right for you, Alton. Don't you worry." And (Saint) Beulah Ward was true to her word. Three days later, Miss Hobson told me to report to Miss Ward, and for the school year Dalma Evans and I became this kind lady's errand boys.

Miss Ward was slim, pretty, blond, dressed immaculately always, usually in high heels, wearing a dark suit that accentuated her fair skin and blond hair, worn it seems on alternate days in bouffant and pompadour styles. Each day I looked forward to being near her, and she seemed the only person who could allow me respite from what I feared was terminal grief at being trapped in this hellhole called Oxford Orphanage. Before long, Miss Ward was picking up Dalma and me on Saturday afternoons in her automobile, and the three of us would enjoy a Saturday matinee at the Orpheum picture show, together with a box of (real) buttered popcorn and a caffeine and carbonation-filled soft drink. And lots of ice.

For the most part, my job as errand boy for Miss Ward entailed picking up and delivering clothes requiring mending, to the cottages, hospital and kitchen. Before long, I knew each of the cottage mothers well, and when I had to make deliveries to the hospital, steered well clear of Mrs. Edith (Mad Dog I) Tomblin. Ditto for old Minnie (Mad Dog II) Warwick in the Baby Cottage. I was learning.

In my spare time (which was most of the time), Miss Beulah (My Very Best Friend in the Whole Wide World, Bar None, having surpassed my friend Dave at the Standard Drug Store and then God, who took care of my best Christmas ever) Ward, allowed me the run of the massive clothing facility, and I quickly came to know the different departments and supervisors quite well. I became fascinated with the old pedal-operated Singer sewing machine, so Miss Edwards taught me how to sew. Before long, I became a pretty good seamstress (or is it "seamster") and was mending torn articles of clothing, darning socks, and sewing name tags on shirts, pants and underwear. Mrs. Stallings and I got along famously.

In 1947, the standard black Singer sewing machine was the workhorse of the day, utilizing the broad rotating foot pedal for power. Miss Edwards taught me how to secure the appropriate needle in the needle guide, the thread in the thread guide, and to move the slide plate presser foot back in order to insert and secure the bobbin, the spool that holds the thread used to sew the garment.

Thus, the trick to learning to sew on the old Singer involved a certain degree of coordination of the foot pedal to get the rhythm required to keep the machine going. It just took practice, then a little more practice, and finally enough practice to become an expert. I caught on to the operation of the Singer pretty fast and could probably do the job better than the girls assigned the task. And it was something to busy myself with when I wasn't getting into things and making a nuisance of myself with Miss Ward. A big part of it was just the challenge. And I especially liked Miss Neta Edwards because she reminded me of my first grade teacher, Miss Wellbuilt. And even though she was a grownup, she was pretty and her butt bobbed when she walked, just like the blond Baby Cottage girl's behind.

The big difference between the upstairs sewing/mending rooms and the downstairs laundry room was the fact that the young girls in the sewing/mending rooms sat down to do their work, while the laundry room girls stood to perform their tasks. Several of the teenage girls in the laundry room had pretty, well-formed butts just like the blond Baby Cottage girl, and I liked to watch as they bent over to retrieve clothes from the hampers. During warm weather, the hottest place on campus was of course the laundry. That presented a delicious dilemma of grand proportions, somewhat akin to the choices of a Peeping Tom in a brothel. It was a tough job, but somebody had to do it, so I endured the sights of bouncing butts and dresses sticking to the hips of perspiring preteen and teenage girls and sweated though the warm Spring of 1950.

At the time of her retirement in 1957, the laundry had been under the supervision of Mrs. Marvin Minor for twenty-three years. My indelible image of this kind lady was of her gnarled salt-and-pepper hair sticking to her face in the heat, as she went about her task of supervising the young girls. She always had a ready smile for me, and I never saw her yell at or in any way be unkind to the girls under her care.

With Miss Ward's permission, I explored all the rooms on the ground floor of the Industrial Building. Upon entering the large double doors at the front of the building, the entire left side of the lower level housed Mrs. Minor's laundry facility. The first room on the right as you turned right along the hallway, housed the Mattress Room, containing several high stacks of different sizes of mattresses for children, the hospital and for the staff members who resided on campus. I spent literally hours climbing the high stacks of soft mattresses, using them as trampolines, and jumping from one stack of mattresses to another.

Due to the nature of my job as voyeur errand boy for Miss Ward, most of my half day at work during fifth grade was free time. All the toys to be handed out to the 340 kids at Christmas 1949 were stored in the "Toy Room," as they were delivered to the orphanage by the various

Masonic lodges in the state. The Toy Room was located at the bottom of the stairs on the right as you entered the front doors of the Industrial Building. Miss Beulah Ward, my mom away from home, would inform me when a new shipment of toys arrived and would allow me into the Toy Room with a pair of scissors and a roll of Scotch tape. In reality, she would allow me into the toy room to play with the toys. The pair of scissors and Scotch tape were my own doing. The Toy Room was off-limits to children who worked in the Industrial Building.

Anyway, by early December 1949, the entire floor of the Toy Room was filled with more than a thousand brightly-wrapped Christmas presents. Using one sharp point of the pair of scissors, I carefully cut a section of the wrapping paper about three inches square, then gently lifted the flap of the paper. Finding a present for a girl, I carefully taped it shut. Upon discovering candy, I ate it, usually that same day. No, usually that same minute.

On finding a boy's present, I opened the present, played with it until I tired of the game or toy, then re-wrapped it as best I could. It was fun. One big Christmas, all month long. And I had at last discovered the true identity of Santa Claus-he looked an awful lot like . . . Miss Beulah Ward.

Thus any boy at Oxford Orphanage who opened his gifts on Christmas 1949, Little Orphan Al knew what you received because I had already opened the present, played with it, grew tired of it, and re-wrapped it (as best I could). So there, I confessed. Now, after harboring my secret for more than half a century, I feel relieved. Confession is good for the soul. However, while we are in the confession mood, there were minor exceptions to the disposition of the boys' gifts as related herein.

Life Savers were sold in the form of a two-page "book," to be used as Christmas gifts. You opened the "book," and the left and right "pages" were stacks of rolls of multi-colored Life Savers. They made nice Christmas gifts. However, none, nary a solitary one, was passed out to the boys at Christmas 1949. I ate every last one of them.

One day I opened a somewhat small box, thinking it to contain candy, and was quite shocked to find in the box a man's gold Bulova wristwatch. I pondered long and hard (for about eight seconds) as to what to do with "my" present. Then, I rationalized that with all the abuse I had put up with since my arrival at Stalag Oxford more than two years before, I *deserved that gold Bulova wristwatch!* And anyway, if I had not kept it, probably one of the sadistic pricks who made me fight my friends would have received it as a gift.

My love of funny books that started as a youngster at the Standard Drugstore stayed with me when I went to the orphanage. So I scooped up *all* the funny books in the Toy Room (funny books were nice gifts in 1949), swiped a medium-sized suitcase from the Suitcase Room (that was its name), and literally stuffed the suitcase with new funny books.

The basement beneath the laundry room housed the football team's locker room. At the opposite end of the building, beneath the Toy Room and Suitcase Room, was the old Boy Scouts meeting hall, and at the end of that room was a bank of electrical and water pipes. I hid the suitcase filled with funny books in one of the many nooks and crannies found along the pipe alley. Over the years, I would periodically sneak down to my cache on the weekends to read and reread *my* funny books that I had *received* as Christmas presents in 1949. This suitcase filled with my funny books left the orphanage with me in February 1957.

One day I discovered among the toys a dartboard game. Miss Ward allowed me to take the dartboard and darts to the new clothes storage room on the second floor across the hall from her office. I was, of course, what jealous peers would call Miss Ward's "pet," and this kind lady allowed me to do just about anything I wished.

Miss Ward hung the dartboard on a hook on the far wall. I would stand in one of the aisles and spend literally hours throwing darts. Got pretty good at it too.

At one point, I had decided to call myself "Dartman," though I did admit to myself even then that the name "Dartman" sounded a little corny-not in the same league certainly as Batman, Superman, or Captain Marvel. Those were great names.

Tucked away in the recesses of my young mind was the creeping realization that I could not remain indefinitely under the protective wing of mine and Dalma Evans' benefactor, the wonderful Miss Beulah Ward.

Through her generosity, Dalma and I had enjoyed the freedom known by very few boys of our age, and I am certain our special Saturday afternoon outings to the Orpheum theatre, with caffeine-laden soft drinks and popcorn with Miss Ward eventually incurred the envy of the other boys in the Walker Building. Perhaps Miss Hobson recognized this, because my name began to appear with surprising (at least to me) frequency on the dreaded Saturday afternoon "Mr. Gray's List."

Now, something sorta puzzled me about that gold Bulova men's wrist watch. Try as I might, I couldn't recall ever actually possessing my very own personal, to the exclusion of all others, wrist watch before I stole some other kid's Christmas present in December 1949, because had I ever before owned a portable, carry-around timepiece, either wrist or pocket, some blue-with-envy kid surely would have asked me what time it was. And I could not recall answering Oh, it's a quarter to eight, or Oh, it's 3:15. Thus, that Bulova must have been my very first watch ever.

CHAPTER 19

The Ink Book

In the Fall of 1949, four months into my tenth year on this earth, and six months into my third year in this really, really foreign country called Oxford Orphanage, I entered fifth grade, the World of Baby Elephant, and already I did not give a happy whit for Miss Mamie Baldwin. This squat, dark-haired, captious woman with the Porky Pig facial features put me out of kilter with a mere glance in my general direction. She seemed immensely unhappy with her lot in life, acted as though teaching fifth grade orphans was but a temporary yet burdensome nuisance, addressed us in a tone singularly dictatorial, and had this strange odor about her that made you want to explain to her the basic concept of soap and its uses.

The moniker "Baby Elephant" had doubtless been attached to Mamie Baldwin years before my arrival in Hell-In-A-Small-Town-In-North-Carolina, and the appropriateness of this nickname was plainly evident; she was one of those squat, dumpy spinsters whose horizontal body dimensions had long ago caught up with her vertical, the latter not being of great numerical value initially. And in true keeping with my sine wave existence in this place, Baby Elephant's unwelcome valley had followed on the heels of the crest that was the friendly and helpful fourth grade teacher, Miss Ellie Parrish.

Before the world reached its half-century mark, I was to be humbled and assaulted by yet another orphanage staff member. It seemed at times that my chances of surviving this cavalry dwindled with each new grownup I encountered.

Having this small blimp for a teacher was akin to turning a starved pitbull aloose in a room full of thirty newborn bunny rabbits. We all feared her spontaneous outbursts of ill-temper, and tried our best not to incur even a thimbleful of her wrath. The Leonard-Stealing-My-Spelling-Book physical assault occurred in October of 1949. For the ensuing seven months, every time the dumpy Hydra approached my desk along the aisle, my eyes instinctively and defensively darted in her direction, my heart rate increased drastically and my entire body tensed, to await another attack.

Fifth grade was also the first year in which we were in school half days and worked half days. Children in grades five, seven, nine and eleven were in Section A; they attended school in the afternoon and worked during the morning. Children in grades six, eight, ten and twelve were in Section B; they attended school in the morning and worked during the afternoon.

In the fifth grade, all of us kids wrote with pencils, wearing out the lone metal, noisy, questionably efficient pencil sharpener attached to the teacher's desk in the classroom. That is, everyone except Leonard. This mostly quiet, amiable kid had a fascination with fountain pens, bordering on obsession. Trouble was, though, he seemed not to be very adept at filling it with writing fluid (what the modern world today calls "ink") and he forever had the writing fluid on his hands . . . and his clothes . . . and his desk . . . and on just about everything he touched or that wandered in his general direction.

After study hall each night, we placed our books in our twelve-inch square denim bookbags, hung the double-thickness denim straps over a hook along the wall, bathed, sat bored but respectful through Miss Hobson's reading of one of her Bible stories, then went to bed.

School had been in session about two months, when one day we went to class as usual. Came time for spelling class, and we reached into our denim bookbags and brought out our spelling books. That is, everyone except Little Orphan Al. Puzzled, I just sat at my desk, knowing Baby Elephant would be furious, but at the same time, certain I had placed my spelling book in my bookbag the previous night.

During class, it was Baby Elephant's practice to stroll up and down the aisle between rows of students, reviewing our work. She was walking up to my right side when she glanced down at my desk. No spelling book.

"Where's your spelling book!" she demanded loudly. Baby Elephant never "said" anything, or "asked" anything. Behind every utterance stood a caustic accusation.

Scared witless, I squeaked out "I don't know, Miss Baldwin." Maybe calling her by her name would soften her venomous heart. It didn't.

Baby Elephant was standing to my right. Without warning she backhanded me, knocking me clean out of my seat and into the aisle to my left, my head banging against Betty Jean Moore's desk. Dazed, my head throbbing, my vision blurring, I looked up to see Baby Elephant leaning over my desk, glaring menacingly down at me. With her fat face in the horizontal position looking down, all the weight of her heavy jowls dropped, and she *really* looked like an overweight porker. Downright scary, she was.

"Get up from there, young man," she screamed.

Slowly, I picked myself and my bruised head off the floor, awaiting another stinging slap across my face.

Terrified that the bitch was going to start flailing away at me, and embarrassed to be so humiliated in front of the other kids, I stood trembling, looking down at the floor.

"Now, you get yourself down to your cottage and find that book, and don't come back here without it, young man!" she screamed, shoving me with her hand toward the door.

Bewildered and frightened, I returned to the Walker Building, and explained to Miss Hobson what had happened. We searched the study hall, but found no spelling book. Then, at Miss Hobson's suggestion, we began searching the individual cubbyholes where we boys stored our clean clothes. Presently, I heard Miss Hobson's voice, full of excitement.

"Here it is, Alton. But just look at it!" she exclaimed.

She had found the blue-writing-fluid-soaked spelling book, with Leonard's name in it, hidden under the clothes at the rear of Leonard's cubbyhole. The book appeared as though it had been dipped in the writing fluid.

I told Miss Hobson that Miss Baldwin had slapped me and knocked me to the floor. "We'll just see about that!" she said, putting on her warm overcoat and heading, book in hand, out the front door. Miss Hobson walked with me back to school, and when she walked unannounced into the classroom, Baby Elephant looked up and saw me following after Miss Hobson, she with the blue-stained spelling book outstretched toward Baby Elephant.

Miss Hobson, however, did not address Baby Elephant. Looking past the teacher, Miss Hobson looked straight at Leonard, and said,

"Is this your spelling book, Leonard? Must be-it has your name in it."

Without invitation, I walked past Baby Elephant and took my seat, while Baby Elephant and Miss Hobson stepped into the hall. Presently, we heard Baby Elephant's voice boom out, "Leonard, bring me that spelling book!" I looked over at my absolutely terrified classmate, as he picked up *my* spelling book and walked into the hall. After a short time, he came back into the room, his face crimson with embarrassment, carrying his blue-stained book, and Miss Baldwin brought my spelling book to me and placed it on my desk. No comment. No apology. No nothing. Just placed my spelling book on my desk, without looking at me, and turned away.

Following that humiliating incident, I never again looked at Baby Elephant when she spoke to me. I always looked down at the floor, or at my book. To drive home the degree of abuse suffered by the children of Oxford Orphanage, one must remember that John Nichols School was a part of the North Carolina public school system and under the direct supervision of the Oxford City School System. Even in 1949, had Mamie Baldwin slapped a student in one of Oxford's other public schools, she would have been fired immediately. In point of fact, Mamie Baldwin's salary, just as that of the other teachers at John Nichols School, was paid by the State of North Carolina, not by Oxford Orphanage. Yet the orphanage administration, that is, Mr. Gray and Mr. Regan, tolerated and encouraged abuse of children by teachers, simply because they both knew they would never be held accountable for physical abuse of orphans.

Thus Mamie Baldwin had been granted unfettered rein to abuse thirty young ten-year-old boys and girls at her pleasure. I reasoned that if she did it once, she could certainly do it again, and I did my best to prepare for the worst. Just another day in the life of a child at Oxford Orphanage in 1949. God, I hated this place.

I was overjoyed to be finished with Baby Elephant at school year's end. Her condescending tone trailed after her like an evil shadow, just another adult unhappy with her lot in life, given carte blanche permission to damage vulnerable, defenseless, orphaned children.

Mamie Baldwin would not have dared so much as touch one of the town kids in the same or similar circumstances. Leonard panicked and stole my spelling book because he knew that had Baby Elephant walked along the aisle and noticed his blue-soaked book, she would have slapped him senseless into the aisle just as she had done to me.

However, had a town boy spilled writing fluid all over his spelling book, Mamie Baldwin would have gone to the principal's office, exchanged the student's soiled book for a clean one and returned it to him with a smile. Again, touch one of the town kids and she would not have had a job at John Nichols School come sundown.

The status of town boys and girls at John Nichols School was well-known among the orphanage children. In any given year, nearly one of four students at our school was a town student. In 1950, 312 orphans attended John Nichols School; there were also 106 town kids who attended school with us. We got along quite well with them and never resented any of them. They played football, basketball, and baseball alongside us and gave their all just as we did. And they were well aware of the physical abuse suffered by us kids at the hands of Mr. Regan and some of the teachers, work supervisors and cottage counselors. If one of the kids had been physically abused by a staff member, the other kids talked openly about the assault in class, so the town kids knew everything that went on in the orphanage. They were quite sympathetic to our plight.

As noted earlier, during my youth what we today call "ink" pens were known as "fountain pens," and the liquid used in these fountain pens was called "writing fluid," not ink. The most widely used product was Shaeffer *SKRIP* Writing Fluid, No. 22 Permanent Blue-Black. And this just happened to be Leonard's favorite.

CHAPTER 20

The Tonsil Clinic

At the time of my arrival at the orphanage in February 1947, a so-called "Tonsil Clinic" was conducted each Summer on the third floor of the orphanage hospital by Dr. B.W. Fassett, a Durham physician, and his staff.

Tonsils serve as a protection against infection, and as such may themselves become infected, often requiring their removal. If a child showed up at sick call several times with a chronic throat infection, Mrs. Tomblin placed him or her on a "tonsils list." When Summer arrived, Mrs. Tomblin would contact Dr. Fassett, and a snip-and-clip session would be scheduled. Apparently tonsils were looked upon at the orphanage almost as an annual crop.

By the Summer of 1949, and against almost insurmountable odds, I had finally made it to age 10, and was in the Walker Building. One day after lunch, Miss Hobson told me to report to the hospital. Yeah, my favorite person again, Mad Dog Tomblin.

Upon arrival at the hospital, Mrs. Tomblin gave me some clean bed clothes and instructed me to bathe and get into bed. She didn't tell me why, and I sure as hell wasn't going to ask her. Not me. Especially not after the "Second Time." The "First Time" had been my first night at the orphanage, February 15, 1947, when the Mean Old Bat had slapped me senseless because I wouldn't stop crying because I missed my mama and wanted to get the hell away from this awful place and had tried to escape from Hell Camp.

Just above the boys' first floor ward was a second floor boys' ward. Same for the girls' ward across the main hall of the hospital. One day in early Spring 1949, I took sick, for whatever reason I cannot recall. But it had to be serious, else I would not have been in the hospital. Anyway, I shared the first floor boys' ward with three other boys, one of whom was a high school boy. Just before midnight, he came over to my bed, shook me by the shoulder, and asked me . . . no, since he was in 3-B and I was only in the Walker Building, he must have "ordered" me, to take the book he was holding up to his girlfriend, who just so happened to be in the second floor girls' ward. *Only* because I was in a good mood and wanted to be helpful, I took the book, very quietly crept up the first flight of stairs to the landing, paused, then ascended the second flight.

At the top of the stairs again I paused, then quietly scooted across the darkened hallway to the girls' ward. Once inside, I whispered the girl's name several times into the pitch-black room. When finally she awakened, I gave her the book, she thanked me, and I crept surreptitiously back down the top flight of stairs.

As my foot touched the bottom step of the landing, you-guessed-whose foot touched the top step of the landing, and we literally bumped into each other on the dark landing. Simultaneously, we recoiled from the shock of the encounter.

"What!" she exclaimed in shock. Not a question. Since Mrs. Tomblin was meaner and bigger than I, I deferred the first comment to her.

"What are *you* doing here?" she screamed. Here I was caught between Scylla and Charybdis yet again. I was about to get my ass whipped, either by Mrs. Tomblin or the high school boy for telling on him, or both. So I offered the universal petrified orphan child's reply.

"Nothing."

The old bat appeared to be upset. I mean, *really* upset. Grasping a large handful of hair (mine), she brought her other hand down hard across my head (I had tried to duck) screaming,

"You little pervert. I'll *teach* you!" And she slapped me twice (or thrice) more hard across my face, all the time keeping a vise grip on my hair.

"Now you get to bed, young man, and tomorrow I want you out of this hospital. You're not sick at all."

Bounding down the stairs three at a time, I scooted into my bed and pulled the covers over my head, fearing the Mean Old Deviless would come back for seconds.

As I was hurriedly getting dressed the next morning, the high school boy came over to me.

"Sorry about that, kid. Didn't mean to get you in trouble."

"That's okay," I said. What else could I say?

"By the way," I added curiously, "what's a 'pervert?'"

"That means you're weird."

"But why would Mrs. Tomblin call me that?"

"She probably thinks you were humping one of those high school girls."

"What's 'humping?'" I asked with a puzzled expression. The high school boy gave me a quizzical look, shook his head, and answered,

"Forget it, kid."

I did. For the moment.

But, back to the tonsils tale. Anyway, early the next morning, I awakened in the ward with several other boys. But they did not feed us breakfast. Instead, Mrs. Tomblin summoned us one at a time, and I was sent to a small room that I learned later was called the Ether Room and was told to climb up onto a table and lie down on my back.

Following a few words of assurance from a very pretty blond nurse, she placed a round-shaped metal ring covered with gauze stretched inside it, over my face. Shortly I smelled something quite strange, and about the time I mustered the courage to ask what it was, the lights went out.

I awakened sometime later and found myself back in my hospital bed. My throat felt quite sore and it was difficult to swallow. The hospital girls did not serve us dinner, but later that day we were served ice cream, not as a treat but to soothe our sore throats. We ate ice cream several times over the next few hours, and the following day we were released from the hospital. Somebody told us later that the hospital girls had buried our tonsils in a field behind the hospital.

I had taken part in the annual Summer Tonsil Clinic, one of thirty-two children in 1949 to lose his tonsils. The number dwindled to nineteen in 1950, and further dipped to twelve in 1951, as infection-fighting antibiotics came into general use in the United States.

CHAPTER 21

The Year 1950

On June 25, 1950 the Korean War began with communist North Korea's surprise invasion of South Korea. The United States authorized fifteen million dollars in military aid to France to fight the Viet Minh government in Indochina. And the United States was in the grip of its worst communist scare ever, fueled by the sensational charges of U.S. Senator Joseph McCarthy that communists had infiltrated the highest levels of government. And in May 1950, Senator Estes Kefauver began televised hearings exposing organized crime in America.

Nat King Cole's recording of "Mona Lisa" sold more than three million copies when released in 1950. On the evening of January 17, 1950, seven masked bandits robbed the Brinks armored truck company of $2.7 million. On October 2, cartoonist Charles Schulz introduced "Peanuts" and Charlie Brown to the American public in seven newspapers.

In 1950, the population of the United States was 151,325,798, and illiteracy in the nation reached an all-time low of 3.2 percent.

Closer to home, that still I was referring to (un)affectionately as "this damned place," construction of the all-brick Masters Cottage to replace that "known fire hazard," the Walker Building, began in 1950. When half of the outer wall closest to the hospital had been completed, it was found to be out of plumb. Eventually, they got it right. Also, construction on the York Rite Memorial Chapel began that year. Once completed, we orphans got to hear Mr. Gray drone on for an hour of

Sunday night Vespers in a new setting. We kids would manage to ignore his phony diatribes equally at either location.

D.P. "Soapy" Peake had been an employee of Oxford Orphanage for thirty-nine years, most of that time as farm manager, when he died on November 5, 1950. Mr. Peake suffered from Marie Strumpel disease. His spine was solidified, that forced him to walk bent forward. Bob Davis, who had become dairy manager on July 10, 1950, assumed the duties of farm manager from the date of Mr. Peake's death, until January 1951, when Tom Adams became farm manager. Tom Adams immediately became the most despised grownup on campus, the antithesis of the mild-mannered, folksy Soapy Peake.

We slaughtered and dressed fifty-one porkers in December 1950, that being my first ever experience in the role of a mass murderer. I vowed it would be my last. This "harvest" yielded about 13,000 pounds of pork. That year, the farm received a brand new DC-3 Case tractor and harrow, and the orphanage traded in Mr. Gray's automobile. The cost of the new car was $2,125.84. The trade-in value of Mr. Gray's old car was $906.26, so for the net cost of $1,219.58, Mr. Gray began tooling around in a shiny new Buick.

The farm retained its ten mules in 1950; the dairy herd consisted of forty-six cows, twenty-five heifers and two bulls, Ace and Victor. As of that year, the five colored men who toiled as farm hands alongside the farm boys had worked for the orphanage an average of twenty-eight years each.

As of January 1, 1950, there were 317 inmates in the orphanage. By December 31, 1950, the number had decreased to 310. This was my third year of internment, and my callow mind had not given up hope that any day now mama would come and get me. Surely my time here was limited, and she was just working out the details of my release. Of this I was certain. No doubt about it. Had to be. "Real soon."

Of the 317 children in the orphanage in 1950, only 22 were true orphans (both mother and father deceased), 70 whose mothers had died, 166 whose fathers had died, and 59 who had both parents living. Thus there were 37 more children with both parents living than there were true orphans. Only ten percent of the children were of Masonic parentage.

Of the 310 students remaining at year's end, 147 were boys and 163 were girls. Eighteen high school seniors (nine boys and nine girls) graduated in 1950. Of this group, nine entered college, business school or nurses' training, and nine became employed. In addition to the 310 orphanage children, more than one hundred "town" boys and girls attended John Nichols School. Thus, about every fourth child was not an orphan.

The kind and ageless Mr. Hill had retired as Shoe Shop supervisor, and Wade Gregory took over as supervisor for the remainder of the year and for many years to come. When the boys from the Walker Building moved into the new Masters Cottage, the Walker Building was converted into apartment housing for staff members, and Wade Gregory and his lovely wife were among its first tenants.

The sweet, dear, and gentle Miss Nannie P. Bessant, who had served the orphanage since April 1, 1918, retired on August 31, 1949 as the Hostess of the Main Building. Everyone loved Miss Bessant, who was just about as tall as we Walker Building boys, and Miss Bessant had nothing but kind words for all us kids. She died on April 23, 1950, and I missed her kindness for many years.

Also during 1950, fourteen students were "taken from the orphanage by relatives," one teenager was sent to a training school, six ran away, one was expelled, and seven were "discharged for other reasons."

A most disturbing statistic here is that in 1950, a total of twenty-nine children left the orphanage who did not graduate, while only eighteen children graduated.

Now the number of applications for admission approved during the year was fifty. These fifty children were approved based on a total of 398 (yes, 398) visits to homes for the purpose of investigation. Thus, the orphanage administration, aided by the caseworker Miss Eunice Broadwell, determined that fifty children were in desperate need of a home and care that they were not receiving in their present environment. Yet, during the same year, twenty-eight children left the orphanage to return to the same kind of life (one was sent to a training school) that orphanage administrators had determined was detrimental to their health and welfare.

The obvious question central to this great disparity in the number of children "going to relatives" and those who graduated is why? Based on my in-depth telephone interviews with twenty-one of the children in the former category, the overriding reasons for relatives removing children from the orphanage were 1) physical abuse at the hands of orphanage staff members and teachers, and 2) physical abuse and threats of same by older children.

What happened to those twenty-one children returning to relatives? Only four of the twenty-one graduated from college. Nine of the twenty-one have experienced divorce; none of this group attended college. Of the twenty-one former students whom I interviewed, there were eleven boys and ten girls.

I had several girl friends while at the orphanage. One of the first girls who gave me a funny feeling in my groin was brutally beaten with a board by one of the cottage counselors when she was thirteen years old. She and her younger brother were shortly thereafter "taken home by relatives," and I never heard from her for several years.

In August of 1957, the Summer after graduation from high school, I was visiting Red Albertson, who also was from Kinston, and who had taken a job in a small town near Fayetteville, North Carolina. On my drive back to Kinston, I recalled that the girl in question lived in a small town I happened to be passing, one of those numerous spots on a rural road that you will miss if you happen to yawn while driving through.

I stopped at a filling station (that's where you filled your car up with gas) and asked the full-serve gas station attendant where the family lived, calling the girl and her younger brother by name. The man directed me to the house at the edge of town.

Only it wasn't a "house." It could at best be described as a hovel, little more than a shed, with a flat tin roof, the outer walls covered with roof shingles and linoleum flooring. The girl's younger brother, whom I had known quite well because he was the same age as my younger brother Pete, who was four years my junior, was sitting on a low stoop in front of a broken screen door. He saw me as I got out of my car, and rushed toward me sporting a wide grin of recognition.

The poor boy probably had not had a bath in weeks, and his front teeth, almost brown, likely had not felt a toothbrush since he and his sister left the orphanage. I almost cried at the sight of his dirty, undernourished body. The first things he asked about were his friends at the orphanage, specifically calling them by name. I chatted with him for about fifteen minutes; he was so happy to see me.

The boy informed me that his sister was not at home, that he did not know when she would return that day. I could only visualize the state of her health, and after I reluctantly climbed into my car and headed back on the road to Kinston, could not control the flood of tears.

Two days later I packed all my belongings into my black two-door 1951 Chevrolet Powerglide that I had purchased with four hundred dollars of the money daddy had left for me in the Kinston First National Bank, and headed off for Berry College in Rome, Georgia, to study physics and mathematics. I never again heard from that beautiful, warm, sensitive girl or her younger brother.

CHAPTER 22

My Move From Walker Building to 1-B

By the time I moved from the Walker Building to 1-B in June 1950, I believe I had made Mr. Gray's List an unprecedented seventh time. I had lived in the Walker Building for two years, through fourth and fifth grades, and I felt a lot like my hero Lou Gehrig, except that most of my luck had been bad.

So what did I take with me when I moved from the Walker Building to 1-B, except my worn-out toothbrush and clothes? Mainly confidence. Not cockiness or mouthiness; no, Coley Lee had already cornered that market. The smart-mouthed little bastard had been an inspiration to all of us lily-livered scaredy-cats. But my outlook on corporal punishment luckily had evolved from stark fear at my first flogging at the hands of Old Man Gray, to a smug confidence that I had outsmarted the pseudo-saint with my extra padding, pride in myself that I had possessed the intrepidity to chance it; downright relief at not being discovered.

Because of the unfortunate fact that my physical and emotional well-being during my fourteen months in the Baby Cottage hinged quite precariously on the whim and caprice of two teenage orphan girls and Miss Warwick, I held the singular kindness bestowed upon me by Miss Beulah Ward together in the same fragile spot in my heart as Ann's compassionate and protective care during my stay in the hospital.

By this time however, thanks to my "five-shorts padding" solution, my name being called by Miss Hobson after dinner on Saturday to "go to see" Old Man Gray did not evoke the same degree of diarrhea-producing debasing terror in my still-racing heart as on previous encounters, and as time passed my palms barely sweated as I stood before the supercilious sonofabitch awaiting the brief lecture on duty, responsibility and the dire and certain consequences of "talking back to" or "sassing" Miss Hobson, followed immediately by the inevitable command of "bend-over-and-grab-your-ankles" wasp sting strikes of the child-abuser's board.

My young spirits were buoyed doubly by the fact that, at least until now, not only had I outsmarted the sadistic bastard, without doubt an enviable accomplishment at such a young age, but that I had succeeded in convincing the Saturday afternoon "regulars" on Mr. Gray's List, Coley Lee, Newton, and Blockhead, and the random unfortunates-of-the-week, needed to make the trip worth Mr. Gray's time, that my butt was as sore as theirs immediately following Mr. Gray's Physical Abuse Hour.

Thus save for the normal apprehension associated throughout life as one goes from being a big fish in a little pond to being a little fish in a big pond, my move from the Walker Building to 1-B in June 1950 was not all that traumatic. And anyway, I had never felt quite that safe in the Walker Building following the fire-in-the-wall scare of the Winter of 1948.

Life at Oxford held a certain sense of wonder and anticipation. Each move to a higher cottage presented a different set of both opportunities and tribulations, (very) low peaks and (cavernous, foreboding) valleys of responsibilities and adventure.

Such was the case in my move from the Walker Building to 1-B, the first boys' cottage; yet at the same time each move "up" was met with a sense of loss for the simpler days of less responsibility.

An irresponsible child will not overnight by some miracle blossom into a responsible adult. It simply does not happen. A former Oxford orphan is by definition a "responsible" adult. He or she may not handle responsibility particularly well, but each of these former orphans, if he or she made it at least into high school as a "sylum dog," had the concept of responsibility drilled into him or her to the point that it was an integral part of the child's mental makeup.

While in the Walker Building, I would find myself just staring off into space, searching, I am sure, for a better place than this, a happier place, a more contented time from my young past; searching for my daddy, and Bill, and Kenny, and Doc, and J.B., and Pete, and mama. I missed them terribly, and constantly, but when I was subjected to punishment, physical or mental, it only worsened, and I just wanted to shut out the hurt, the animosity, the harsh, uncaring grownups in my new life. But they were always there; these unwelcome and feared fixtures in my daily existence just would not go away. Even as an eleven-year-old, it did not require a great deal of nous to fathom that a childish exuberance oftentimes disguised our Stepford existence in this confined little world.

Mrs. K.P. Robinson was a spinsterish old biddy who appeared as though she came with the fifty-three year old 1-B cottage over which she held reign. She would best be described in a manner similar to that of Mrs. Warwick, that is, a cottage "grandmother" rather than a cottage "mother." If you can visualize the cartoon rendition of a proverbial Halloween witch riding a broomstick, you have the best description of Mrs. Robinson. Behind her back, we called her "Witch" Robinson. She retired in 1957, the year I left Oxford, after serving as cottage (grand)mother of 1-B for many years.

For the most part, Witch Robinson was a harmless old fuddy-duddy, whose seemingly permanent scowl concealed a reasonably fair heart. She never harassed me while I was under her supervision, and if she had been prone to seek out troublemakers, she would have snatched me up in a blink.

Consciously determining not to get on either of Witch's "bad" sides from the outset (most cottage counselors had no "good" side), and not being certain whether she enjoyed a similar child-maiming referral arrangement with Old Man Gray (unfortunates on the Walker Building "list" were bruised, buffeted, beaten, and berated at one o'clock each Saturday afternoon-was the 1-B "list" scheduled for two o'clock?), I resolved even before my arrival at 1-B to stay the hell out of the scary old biddy's way. I was admittedly, at the time, still a shade shy of being dirt-clod stupid, but I was soaking up like a sponge all the survival techniques I could.

At Oxford the administration (Gray and Regan) granted the cottage counselors a great deal of really weird, quite idiosyncratic latitude in supervising the children under their care.

This uniform lack of uniformity in discipline and procedure meant that a child might get away with certain questionable conduct in one cottage that would not be tolerated by the new cottage mother when the boy "moved up" to his new home.

One of the strangest house rules in any cottage was the 1-B cottage mother's rule concerning brogans, or just "brogues," the ankle-high brown leather work shoes that we boys wore every day except Sunday. When a half dozen of us newly-minted eleven-year-olds moved up from the Walker Building to 1-B in June 1950, we clomped up the steep rear concrete steps to the main (study hall) level and entered the hallway, where we then quite innocently clomped with our well-worn brogues into the study hall, where we sat to await the appearance of Witch Robinson.

Presently the scary old biddy appeared in the doorway, and as soon as we half-dozen attempted (meekly and fawningly) to make eye contact with our new "mother," she made "eye contact" with something on her just recently buffed, shined and polished floor, her gaze scanning quickly six pairs of well-worn, mud-stained brown brogans.

"What are you boys doing with those brogans on in this house?" she demanded, her voice rising sharply to where it took on a really high-pitched shrill by the time it arrived at the question mark.

No answer. But then again, it was a very difficult question, once we thought about it for a moment. This was my third cottage counselor in as many years, and this old bitch was starting out our relationship on par with the previous duo of blue-haired aging dimwits, who themselves had been strange beyond reason. Asking rhetorical, unanswerable questions that in reality were thinly-disguised accusations, all the while looking from one addle-brained child to another as though expecting a rational answer to their quite irrational queries.

Embarrassed, and at the same time filled with unease and apprehension, our tremulous and unsteady gaze alternated between that certain unfixed fixed middle distance near the floor and a similar spot toward the ceiling, but none of us could locate the elusive answers in either of these transitory locations. But we continued to bob our vacuous heads up and down, searching just the same.

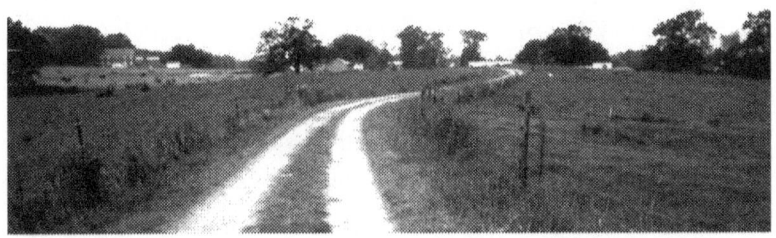

The Farm Road. Looking back toward main campus. Approximately a mile long, this picturesque, ageless artery had more curves than a rattlesnake.

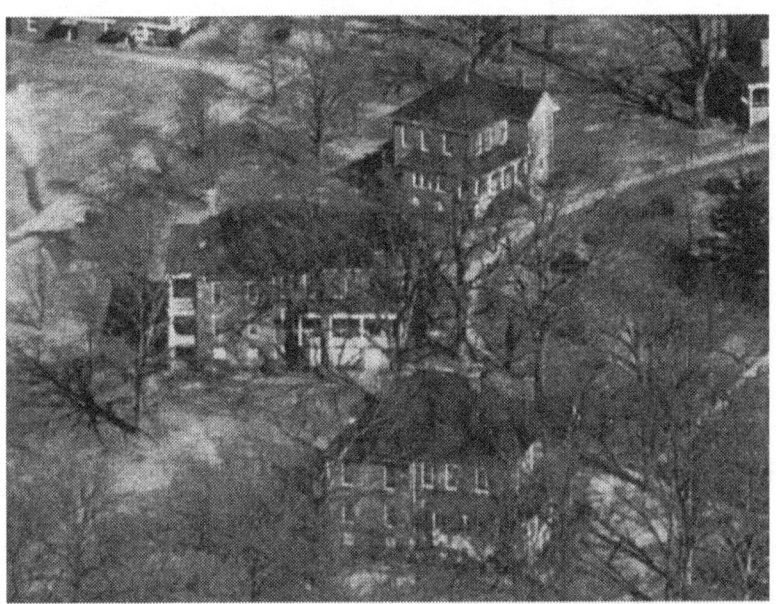

1951. Three of the boys' cottages. From top to bottom: 2-B, 3-B, and 4-B. "Dabs" battleground and school are in upper left.

Experience during those early years of confinement had taught me that, at Oxford anyway, the proverbial "voice of reason" likely had not been heard for decades. And this instance brought no exception to the norm.

"You boys will not wear brogans in this cottage," the caustic admonition continued. "Not in this study hall, not in your rooms, not even in the basement."

And as the grouchy old fart paused "for effect," Bobby Lee, either not understanding her instructions, or not knowing a lot about cottages, asked innocently, "What about the downstairs, Mrs. Robinson?"

Puzzled, Mrs. Robinson just stared at Bobby Lee. We other boys just stared at Bobby Lee. Nobody said a word. The proverbial "pregnant pause."

After a moment one of the newcomers whispered in Bobby Lee's direction, "The basement is the downstairs, you idiot."

Then I asked, quite innocently, "But where do we keep our brogans, Mrs. Robinson?"

"Underneath the back porch," she replied, then added, "And I want the shoes neatly arranged."

"What if it's raining or freezing outside?" I asked, half expecting a reasonably logical response, but being disappointed yet again.

"Well, what *if* it's raining or freezing outside?" came her mocking repartee. "You will *not* bring your brogans into this house. Do you understand?"

Five-sixths of our group answered with the respectful "Yes, ma'am." But Bobby Lee just refused to give up. Breaking the chain of obedient "Yes, ma'am," the little pest asked, "What about our socks, Mrs. Robinson?"

Anyway, 1-B was the only one of the eleven cottages on campus that for years never had been trod upon by shoes, not even in the basement (nor even downstairs).

Rain or shine, below freezing or ninety degrees in the shade, we took off our brogues (socks were allowed) prior to entering any part of the cottage. No former 1-B boy will ever forget walking out the basement door and slipping his warm feet into damp, freezing brogans during a

January snowfall or ice storm. And we hated the scary old witch for her callous and insensitive treatment of us boys.

In the cottages, the seven-to-nine o'clock nightly study hall was monitored personally by the cottage counselors. The "quiet" rule prevailed, so each boy did his own homework. Because talking during study hall was strictly prohibited, if a child needed assistance in his studies, he waited until study hall was over to get help from his classmates or older boys.

In the Walker Building, 1-B and 2-B, study hall was followed immediately by "bath time," in which we boys crowded en masse into the large gang shower area, the showers remained on for the entire time, and the bars of soap were passed from one boy to another.

While in the Walker Building, Miss Hobson did not supervise bath time. When I moved "up" to 1-B in the Summer of 1950, however, I noticed that Witch Robinson nightly observed us youngsters bathing. Although at that young age we all assumed that the only function of our weenies was to do pee, some of us nevertheless felt self-conscious washing our private parts before this audience of one old biddy, who nightly stood like a palace guard at the entrance to the shower area, silently gawking at our nakedness.

Some of us preteen boys were more sensitive than others to our nakedness. Upon entering the shower area, the more self-conscious among us would quickly position ourselves as best we could, closer to the far shower wall, so as to create human shields between ourselves and the granny voyeur. At times, however, the pushing and shoving to escape the intrusion into our state of nature resembled a pack of white rats scrambling to escape a burning building.

One of the saddest days at Oxford was the last day of school each Spring. That was the day several of the kids learned, as did several hundred other children, that these few would be required to repeat the following year the same grade they had just completed.

It was easy to spot these unfortunate children-they were the ones who showed up at dinner with tears streaming from red eyes and flowing down puffy cheeks. It was a stigma almost impossible to lose.

CHAPTER 23

The Korean War

It goes without saying that we orphan boys growing up during the '40s and '50s were products of our times and our environment. Even as a child, I knew what a "Kraut" and a "Jap" were, and I could find Germany and Japan on a map of the world with which my daddy used to follow the progress (at least most of the time, anyway) of the war.

I was five years old when the Americans stormed ashore at Utah Beach on D-Day, June 6, 1944, and was about to start first grade as a six-year-old the following Summer, when the crew of the *Enola Gay* brutally introduced the world to the atomic age at Hiroshima.

However, despite the periodic nighttime blackout drills, and the mild (to me, at least) inconvenience of wartime rationing, I was for the most part untouched by the war. I was bright enough even then to look at the map of the world and reason that in order for the Krauts or Japs to get to 208 East Bright Street, they had to come an awfully long way, and anyway, my ace-in-the-hole was my daddy, who carried his glistening .38-cal. pearl-handled revolver hanging over the lip of his right back pants pocket. That big map of the world, my daddy, and his .38-that's all the security I needed. I felt infinitely safe.

However, the Korean War was another matter indeed. I had just turned eleven when on June 25, 1950 the North Korean communists launched their surprise attack against South Korea across the 38th parallel.

Fortunately, I had survived Baby Elephant's fifth grade only once being slapped out of my chair, and was moving up to 1-B.

Each cottage received daily a copy of the Raleigh *News and Observer* or the Durham *Morning Herald*. Many of us read the funnies every day, and Bill Herrington and I made sure we got the front section of the paper. We read and discussed world events, and both of us were fascinated by the news that the United States was engaged in another war.

The words "communism," "gook," "Reds," "North Koreans," and "chinks" crowded their way into our daily vocabulary. We learned that "South" was good and "North" was bad (just like the Civil War), that "communism" stood for aggression and oppression, and that "gooks," "slopes," and "slants" from North Korea were subhuman, immoral, and downright ornery. Cast in a 1943 B-western, these yellow-skinned aggressors would have been assigned the roles of Injuns, stagecoach robbers, or sundry desperados and no-gooders.

Some of us boys in 1-B and 2-B spoke quietly about the war and even our possible involvement in it. When the Korean War broke out in late June 1950, I had just turned eleven and was beginning my education in life at the orphanage dairy.

Bill Herrington and I followed the ever-changing, see-sawing battle lines drawn on the war map that was a permanent fixture on the front page of the daily newspapers. During that period, my mood tended to fluctuate with those battle lines, and if one day the line swooped too far to the bottom of the page (South), I prayed (hoped) that the next day I would find it had headed back to the top (North). And for the first year of the Korean War, the battle line resembled a darn yoyo.

Odd thing about this thing called "war." Doesn't take a military strategist to figure out when the darn thing's gonna start. When it's gonna end? Now, that's a different matter indeed. Yessireebob. Smartest man in the world can't tell you when war's supposed to end. As I turned fourteen on April 30, 1953 and started high school a few months later, the Korean War was still going full steam. Americans were being killed by the thousands. American boys only a few years older than I. Damn right I was worried. And I thought a lot about my future because in just a few short years, "future" would segue into "now."

More than a few boys in 4-B and 3-B were reading the daily headlines in the Durham and Raleigh newspapers, and talking openly about the war. Sure made believers out of a lot of us. The war had been raging for three years, and I hadn't read anything about those dirty rotten pinko commie gook bastards waving any white flags yet. It wasn't that I worried my *country* was in peril; no, even as a youngster I believed that the United States was forever. However, I was at that time greatly concerned that my *life* might be in danger. My paladin during World War II, my daddy, would not be around to protect me. And suddenly the map of the world had shrunk so that, lo and behold, Korea was only a handspan away from Oxford Orphanage.

When in July 1953 we received news that the Armistice had been signed and the fighting had finally ended, not in glorious victory but in a costly stalemate, about sixty anal sphincters in 3-B and 4-B began to slowly relax. Nobody called for a victory celebration, and nobody voiced his relief openly, but the feelings of elation were present nonetheless.

My political conservatism was molded as a youngster in 1-B and 2-B, spurred on by a real fear of communism enslaving the population and the puzzlement I perceived as a weakness on the part of the United States that a great nation that not once, but twice had saved the world from German and Japanese aggression could not go over and stomp hell out of such a small aggressor. This experience and the perceptions gleaned therefrom led me early on to the conviction that even as a democracy, and even as large as is the United States, the foremost duty of the American government is to ensure the defense and military preparedness of the nation.

The Korean War affected in no small way life among the older boys at the orphanage. It was a well-acknowledged fact of American life that the ranks of the infantry, the foot-soldier most in close combat with the enemy during war, would be composed of (just as during World War II) the nation's lower socioeconomic class.

To appreciate the older boys' preoccupation with their mortality, one has to look no further than the John Nichols School's high school yearbook, *The Log.* The inglorious Korean War began with communist North Korea's lightning invasion across the 38th parallel on June 25, 1950, that quickly began decimating South Korean President Syngman

Rhee's ragtag South Korean Army. Elements of the poorly equipped and badly under-strengthened U.S. Occupation Army in Japan, rushed to the front piecemeal, fared no better than the inept South Korean Army.

On August 12, 1950, at the still innocent young age of twenty-two, the first former orphanage student lost his life in the war. *The Log* of 1951 contained a memoriam to Sam "Greek" Winfield, who came to the orphanage from Leechville, North Carolina, on August 30, 1939, just four months after I was born, and graduated in 1948, when I was just moving from the Baby Cottage to the Walker Building.

When the Korean War erupted on June 25, 1950, I had just started working at the dairy. Sam was a corporal in a tank battalion stationed with the U.S. Army's 25th Division, enjoying posh occupation duty in Japan. He was one of thousands of ill-trained, equally ill-equipped young Americans of the 25th Division rushed to the front in desperation, arriving in Korea on July 10, 1950.

The 25th Division held its defensive positions in the center of the country until July 30, 1950, before being compelled to retreat southward. By August 12, 1950, the 25th was desperately clinging to life along the infamous "Pusan Perimeter," the American Army's "do-or-die" southernmost toehold on the Korean peninsula. It was in this godforsaken hell that Sam lost his life.

Sam's death on a faraway battlefield had an immediate and sobering impact on the older boys at the orphanage. The year Sam graduated from high school (1948), the boys in the class of 1950 were Sophomores, and those in the class of 1951 were Freshmen. They knew Sam as a brother, as a classmate, and as a teammate on the football field.

Suddenly word came that Sam had been killed on some distant battlefield, a place called "Korea," and the realism of war and death came home to roost at Oxford Orphanage. War is not akin to playing a football game, there is no "time out," and you never know when it will end. In addition, Sam was not the only former orphan to be sent to Korea or to be drafted into the service during that war.

To mention only a few, Dan Braswell, who graduated in 1949, served in the U.S. Army from 1950-1953. John Wiley, also in the class of 1949, served in the U.S. Air Force from 1950-1954. And Robert Forbes, who later became an attorney, served in the Korean War as a paratrooper and Ranger.

The high school yearbook, *The Log*, customarily noted beneath the photo of each graduating senior, the life aspirations of the boy or girl. This format changed in 1953, and listed below each graduate's photo were items such as "Ambition," "Pet Peeve," "Favorite Pastime," and other trivial silliness. Bobby Ray Boyette, who was always a good friend and on whom I could rely to "take up" for me when I was younger, listed "At the Rainbow's End," the notation "A Draft Notice." Javon Lee Frye, another good friend and advisor (read that "protector") stated that his "Ambition" was "All Nations at Peace."

At "town boy" Billy Parrot's "Rainbow's End," he wished for a "4-F Card from the Draft Board." And my friend Billy Willis' "Ambition" was "To Leave Korea With No Holes," and at his "Rainbow's End" were "Discharge Papers." No need to wonder what these boys had on their minds most of the time. And to all those pretty girls who graduated between 1951-1954, who thought the boys were not paying enough attention to them-they weren't.

Nine years later, as the feature writer for the daily newspaper, *The Pacific Stars and Stripes*, I stood with fellow journalists, peering through an open window of the baby-blue quonset hut in which were gathered negotiating teams of communist China and the United Nations. As I witnessed that day the seemingly endless argumentative harangue of the Chinese general and the all-too-evident impatience of his counterpart, U.S. Major General Joseph Gill, I could not help but think of Sam Winfield, and reflect on the idiocy of war and the futility of Sam's death.

Two months later, I was accepted into U.S. Army Intelligence and sent to the Defense Language Institute in Monterey, California, for a year to study Korean. Upon graduation from the language institute, I underwent months of training at the U.S. Army Intelligence Center at Ft. Holabird, Maryland, then was stationed in Seoul, Korea for a year and a half as a prisoner interrogator, Korean linguist, and intelligence analyst. This experience solidified my anti-communist fervor for the remainder of my adult life; however, the seeds of my strong political beliefs were sown as a 1-B preteen in a sleepy Southern town.

CHAPTER 24

The Dairy and Bob Davis

Damn! Double damn!! I couldn't understand even one single solitary word he said. He may as well have been speaking Arabic. "He" was Bob Davis, whom we boys addressed quite respectfully as "Mr. Davis." The time was July 1950. I had just completed fifth grade, was two months into my eleventh year of life, and had been in 1-B just long enough to understand why the cottage counselor, Mrs. K.P. Robinson, long before had been tagged with the moniker "Witch." And after more than three years in "This Damn Place" I was still asking myself "Why me?" and still not coming up with a logical answer. And I still missed my daddy terribly.

Work assignments and moves to higher cottages ("higher" in terms of age and grade level) were made the first week in June each year. High School graduation in May had opened up living spaces in 3-B and 4-B (recall that the highest boys' cottage was 3-B, not 4-B) and boys were moved up accordingly. Same for the girls' side of the campus.

Witch Robinson had notified us of our new work assignments, and I had been instructed to report to the dairy the following morning at 8:00 o'clock. I had just turned eleven, and like Arnold, Frank, Coley Lee and Butch, was oblivious to the "fate" awaiting me. Little did I know that this chance work assignment would signal the beginning of my real education in life, one that would become the instruction ground for the emergence of the conniving little nonconformist shit I was to become.

..

Our first few weeks at the dairy were spent in limbo, with seemingly no grownup really to direct our initiation into dairy life. Little did I realize that within two weeks I would find myself floundering in a wagon full of fresh cow manure and slowly picking myself up, dazed and confused, off a concrete floor after having been kicked unceremoniously against a white-washed concrete wall, all for the pleasure of some really sicko stupid-assed Big Boys. Goddamn cow just about killed me, and they just laughed.

But on a bright Summer morning Butch, Arnold, Coley Lee, Frank and I stood, amazed and dumbfounded, looking up expectantly into Mr. Davis' face, shifting our weight from one foot to the other, and back again like we were five human skinny-assed pendulums, or is it pendulae, or pendula, trying our damndest not to burst out laughing. We new boys had worked at the dairy for only a few weeks before Mr. Davis became Dairy Manager, or as was his official title, "Dairyman." I used to picture Mr. Davis with a large yellow "D" emblazoned across his chest, somewhat akin to the manly "S" that my hero had stitched onto his blue suit.

"My nae i Mi-er Da-i," he began.

"Na, di i wa i wan yu boy dur do. Um ur oo rill urh in dur mur-nin, dur uh-ur rill urh in dur a-ur-noon. U uneran?"

The end of this meaningless gibberish carried a rising inflection which, perceptive and intelligent little bastards that we were, we took to mean perhaps that he was asking us a question?

But none of us moved. None of us answered. And if one of us had even snickered, he would probably have killed us all then and there. Instead, we four thoroughly confused orphan kids just stood there, nervously shifting our weight back and forth, gazing first up at the stern-faced Dairyman, then quickly redirecting our gaze purposely and quite determinedly at a spot in the famed "middle distance." Small orphan kids should all be thankful to God for inventing the middle distance. It is the orphans' ultimate crutch. I think it made all of us a little crosseyed.

Bob Davis was born in Dickerson, a spot on a Granville County road about three miles outside Oxford. He attended North Carolina State College in Raleigh, and in 1948 became the farm and dairy manager at Nazareth Orphanage in Rockwell, North Carolina. However, Mr. Davis wished to manage only a dairy. In 1950 Oxford Orphanage offered Mr. Davis the position of Dairyman, with a higher salary, and the move would put him closer to his hometown.

Thus on July 10, 1950, at the young age of 26, Bob Davis began his new duties as Dairy Manager, as we called him. I had been working at the dairy for only a few weeks when I stood in childish, gawking awe at the stern-faced, tongue-tied young dairyman, biting my tongue to keep from laughing out loud at his dyslexic attempt at communication.

D.P. "Soapy" Peake had served as manager of the orphanage farm for 39 years by the time Bob Davis came to the orphanage on July 10, 1950. So I had worked for Soapy Peake for about a month before meeting Bob Davis.

Edwin G. Kerr had been dairy manager since December 1, 1947, having replaced Thomas Hugh Cameron, who died on August 31, 1947. Mr. Davis succeeded Mr. Kerr as dairy manager on July 10, 1950. Four months later, on November 5, 1950, Soapy Peake died, and in January 1951 Thomas R. "Tom" Adams became farm manager. The sadistic sonofabitch!

So the four of us just stood in silence while Mr. Davis continued to (mis)articulate meaningless instructions. He pointed toward the dairy directly behind us, and uttered (to us, at least) unintelligible sounds. He waved his hand in the general direction of the Green Barn, that housed the young calves, and made what seemed at the time and every time thereafter to be the same unintelligible sounds. Odd thing is, it was as though he expected five eleven-year-old dumbass kids to understand his incoherent open-sesame patter. No way in hell were we youngsters ever gonna fathom this mumbo-jumbo rigmarole.

Eventually I broke the Bob Davis Foreign Language Code. A reasonably accurate phonetic equivalent of the foregoing inarticulate mumbling would appear to be:

My name is Mister Davis. Now, this is what I want you boys to do. Some (um) of you will work in the morning (mur nin), the (dur) others will (rill) work in the afternoon (aurnoon). You understand (oo unerand)?

Mr. Davis' speech impediment prevented him from pronouncing his consonants, such as d, k, s, t, and p. Good thing God blessed the

English language with at least a smattering of vowels. It was as though we five addle-brained kids were witnessing a monodrama of grand dyslexic proportions.

The dairy, and the part of the farm that housed the herd of fifty cows, was laid out as follows. At the head of the long, wide concrete driveway that ran sloping toward the main dairy barn, the small milk processing building we called the Little Dairy, and the two huge silos, each holding seventy-five tons of silage, that served as solid, unflinching sentinels guarding the complex, sat the Mule Barn, that in 1950 housed the farm's ten mules. Big old monsters they were.

The walls of the Mule Barn were constructed of unpainted concrete blocks that in those days we referred to as "cinder block," supporting a half-round roof made of corrugated metal, somewhat like an Army quonset hut. The dairy owned one of the ten mules, whose name was Bell. This huge brown animal had only two jobs. One task was pulling the milk wagon to the main campus kitchen, Baby Cottage and hospital twice each day, after the early morning and late afternoon milkings.

Bell's other job was pulling the cow manure wagon to the field once the wagon became full, while we boys walked behind, dragging the fresh cow manure off the back of the wagon with shovels or hoes, to use as fertilizer.

Adjacent to the Mule Barn in the direction of the farm stood the Green Barn, used to house the young calves, and as a birthing barn, where pregnant cows could give birth and stay with their younguns for the first few weeks of life. The Green Barn was larger than the Mule Barn, and was constructed of wood with a sloped roof.

Adjacent to the Green Barn toward the farm proper was the monstrous Long Barn, that was much longer than the Mule Barn and Green Barn, and much taller. This enormous wooden structure was surrounded by a large outside area enclosed by a cyclone fence. During the Summer the expansive loft was filled with hay from the cuttings of tens of acres of alfalfa.

In the dead of Winter we could not let the herd of fifty cows out to pasture, so we housed them in the Long Barn. The two hundred foot long by eighty foot wide Long Barn had a ground level that housed the herd, above which was the massive hayloft, running the full length of the structure.

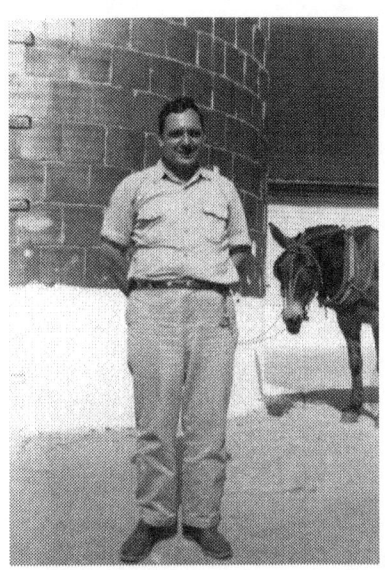

1950. Bob Davis, Bell the mule, silo and milking barn.

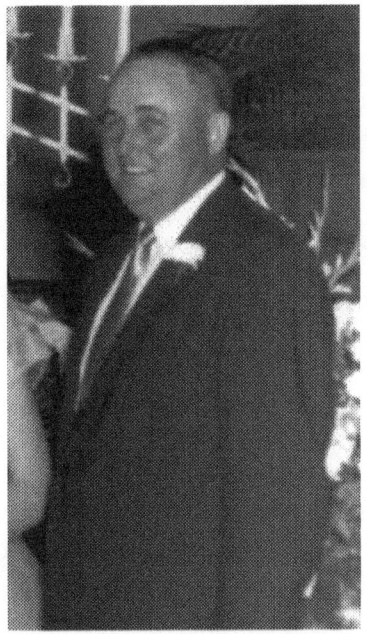

Tom Adams, Farm Manager.

In addition to the front and back sliding doors, the Long Barn contained 12 square openings on each side, for cross-ventilation. On both sides of the barn, against the walls, were wooden slatted bins, open at the top and sloped toward the wall at the bottom. Hay was dropped down from the loft to these hay bins through openings along the walls. We boys spent many hours swinging by ropes from the rafters and landing on the soft hay below.

Operation of the "Little Dairy"

Conception in a cow triggers the development of the milk-producing tissue, but the actual secretion of milk from the udder begins only at the time the young cow's first calf is born, a procedure known as "birthing." The term used more commonly in some regions of the United States for this event appears to be "calving," although I never heard this term used in that context at the orphanage dairy. We just called the fascinating event "birthing."

After the cow's first calf is born, and the cow becomes pregnant with her second calf, the cow will "run dry" for a month or two preceding this and future birthings.

Prior to actually milking the cow, the milker had to wash the cow's udder and its four appendages, the tits. Then the boy would place the stool, always on the cow's right side (horses are mounted from their left side; cows are milked from their right side), sit on the stool and milk the cow. The tops of the round metal milk buckets were two-thirds covered, with an oval opening for the milk to go in. Each bucket held about thirty pounds of milk.

Although Mr. Davis of course frowned on the idea of us kids riding the cows, it was really a lot of fun. So if you are mounting a cow, do you approach from the left (mule-mounting) side, or from the right (cow-milking) side? Apparently the action, and not the animal, controls the situation. Thus we milked the cows from the right side, but still mounted the beasts from the left side. It's something to which we never gave any conscious thought-that's just the way it was done.

During my first two years at the dairy, we milked the cows by hand twice a day, at around five in the morning and around three-thirty in the afternoon. After the first two years on the dairy, we used them there newfangled milking machines. Turned out to be more bother than anything else; didn't save a minute of time, and it was really more work for us boys to monitor the machines and keep them washed out.

After milking the cow, the milker weighed the milk on the scale that hung from the ceiling near the side door, and recorded the milk weight in pounds, on a chart on the wall, beside the cow's name. A "good" cow could produce about twenty-five pounds of milk at a milking, or about fifty pounds a day. However, we had some cows that produced consistently sixty-five to seventy pounds of milk daily.

The orphanage herd consisted solely of the Holstein-Friesian breed, that we referred to simply as Holsteins. These monster black-and-white milk factories "give" (produce) more milk than any other breed, and the average butterfat content is 3.7 percent. However, the protein content, at 3.23 percent, is the lowest of the major breeds. We had at nearly all times forty-six cows producing milk on the dairy.

After weighing and recording the weight of milk, the milker carried the bucket of fresh warm milk across the wide concrete plaza to a smaller building we called the Little Dairy. Located just inside the door were three steps leading up to a platform, to the left of which was a long rectangular stainless steel vat, covered with several layers of cheesecloth, stretched tightly at the top rim.

Once standing on the wooden platform, the milker poured the fresh warm milk over the multi-layered cheesecloth strainer covering the rectangular stainless steel vat about three feet long, one foot wide and one foot deep. This first metal vat was constructed about five feet above the floor. This initially strained milk from the first vat flowed from the bottom of the vat, through a pipe in the wall and into the adjacent "Aerator Room," where it flowed onto and through a second series of cheesecloth layers into an identically shaped vat.

From the bottom of this second stainless steel vat the milk flowed into a long trough containing tiny holes along the length of the bottom. The still-warm milk passed through these tiny holes, where it rippled down both sides of the "aerator," a strange-looking contraption resembling two corrugated metal washboards placed back-to-back.

According to Mr. Davis, the inside of the top half of the sealed aerator contained cold well water, that "knocked" some of the cow's heat off the milk as it rippled over the aerator's double-metal surfaces. The bottom half of the aerator contained a coolant, Freon, that cooled the milk to the required fifty degrees Fahrenheit (ten degrees Centigrade) required to preserve the milk until we delivered it to the orphanage kitchen, Baby Cottage and hospital.

The ice-cold milk rippling down the aerator flowed into one of two sizes of milk cans. The dairy always produced more milk than needed for the orphanage staff and children. The three-and-a-half gallon cans were transported to the kitchen on the milk wagon. The five-gallon cans of milk were picked up (at the morning milking only) by a delivery truck from Pine State Dairies. In 1951 we sold a surplus of 2,820 gallons of milk to Pine State Dairies, and the children and staff consumed more than one hundred gallons of milk each day.

The aerator coolant caused milky ice crystals to form at the base of the aerator. We kept large metal drinking mugs in the Little Dairy, and when thirsty, especially on hot Summer afternoons, a foam-filled cup of ice-cold milk was the best treat of all.

Pasteurization is a process in which raw milk is heated in order to destroy pathogenic microorganisms. Homogenization is a process in which the fat globules of milk are broken up in order to prevent cream in the milk from rising to the top of the milk can. Our milk was neither pasteurized nor homogenized. This was not considered a cause for concern, according to Mr. Davis, because most of the milk produced at the dairy was consumed by the children and staff that same day, or sold to Pine State Dairies, and the milk was tested monthly by certified inspectors from the state DHIA (Dairy Herd Improvement Association).

However, lacking homogenization, by the time we delivered the milk containers to the kitchen, the thick cream had already begun rising to the top of the cans. This cream was ladled off the top of each milk container by the kitchen girls, and used as cream for coffee for the staff, and in preparation of ice cream and other foods.

Showing Calves

In 1951, my second year at the dairy, Mr. Davis allowed six of us boys to have a 4-H Club project. We each selected a calf from the beef cattle barn, and in our free time, we washed, walked, currycombed and pampered our calves. We kept our calves in the Green Barn.

Being the smallest of all the dairy boys, I was thrilled that Mr. Davis allowed me to show a calf, and I still don't know which of us led the other around the show ring. Anyway, it was a means of escape from the dairy scutwork for Ersul Sowers, Frank McMillan, Boney Wyatt, James Strum, Butch Mitchell and me.

We entered our calves in the Eastern Carolina 4-H Club district show, winning two first place and four second place prizes. Four of us took our calves on to the North Carolina State Fair in Raleigh, and for a week we stayed at the fair grounds, sleeping on the hay next to our calves at night. The stupid older boys, Boney and James, spent their money in less than an hour, and took money from us younger boys, and "somehow" (I'll never tell how) after we returned from Raleigh Mr. Davis found out about it. The next year, in 1952, we again went to the state fair, and this time Mr. Davis kept our money, and we asked him for some when we needed it. If the thieves who took our money in 1951 had found out who told Mr. Davis about it, they probably would have killed me, er, rather, him.

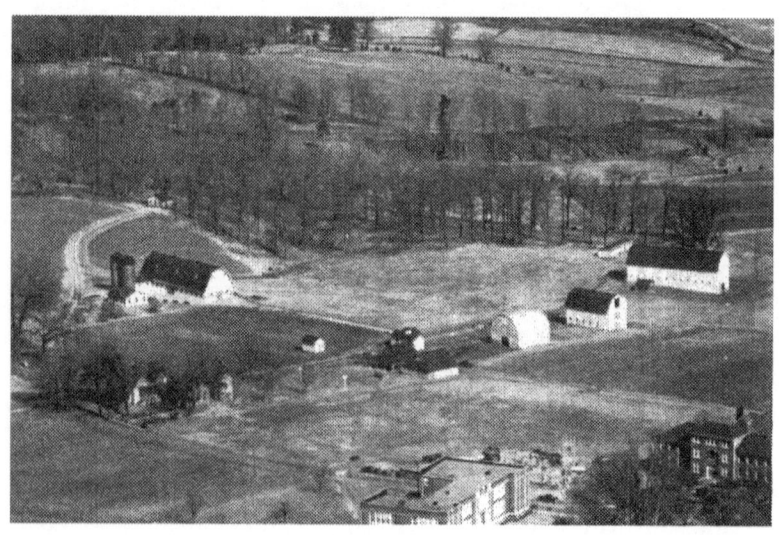

1951. Dairy Complex. At far left: milking barn, silos, and Little Dairy. Path behind dairy leads to bull pens and covered stalls. Structures from center to right: Corn crib and tool shed, mule barn (concrete block and Quonset roof), Green Barn (calves and cats), Long barn, and small enclosed, and covered calf-weaning stalls.

CHAPTER 25

Bringing in the Cows

We walked out the basement door of 1-B into the muggy moonlit heat of that early June morning. We were the first movers on campus, the boys who brought the campus to life each day.

"I'm gonna help you this morning," said Robert, heading away from 1-B, across the campus toward the farm. I followed.

"I had one of the other boys wake up everybody else. It'll take about an hour from the time I wake you up until you get the cows in so we can start milking."

"How long have you been on the dairy?" I asked, trying to make conversation as we crossed the expansive dew-drenched ball field and approached the "Tool Shed" and "Corn Crib" that marked the near edge of the farm.

"I been here going on three years now," he answered. "What grade you in this coming year?" he added.

"Sixth," I responded.

"I'm in eighth. You'll stay on the dairy for about three years, just like me. You'll go get the cows for about a year, and do all the shitwork around here." I didn't like the sound of that. And in the coming weeks I was to learn firsthand the meaning of his term "shitwork." In the darkness we passed between the tool shed and corn crib on our left, and the Mule Barn on our right, and at that point the narrow tar-and-gravel one-lane road leading from the farm to the campus proper ended. The road from that point to all areas of the farm was dirt, the one exception being what amounted to a wide concrete driveway that sloped from this intersection down to the cavernous dairy and the adjacent smaller milk processing structure, the aforementioned Little Dairy.

We walked down the concrete driveway to the left side of the huge wooden gambrel-roofed milking barn, where Robert slid open a large door that hung by metal rollers resting on a metal slide attached to the barn wall above the door. There were four such massive doors, one on each side of the rectangular structure.

Robert flipped up the handle on a large gray electric switchbox attached to the wall, and the interior of the yawning barn instantly was flooded by blinding light from a battery of long winking fluorescent bulbs. I had no way of knowing at that time that this monolithic structure was to become the focal point of my education in work ethic and sense of responsibility that has guided the last fifty years of my life.

To a young eleven-year-old city boy, cows were fascinating creatures. That first morning I helped Robert "bring in the cows," I stood transfixed at one end of the barn as the huge animals lumbered in single file through the wide doorway, and it appeared to me that each cow knew exactly where to go.

The large milking barn, that we called simply the "dairy," was divided by two aisles, a long one and a short one, intersecting in the center. This divided the barn into four sections, with each section holding about thirteen cows. The barn was a stanchion barn; when the cow stepped gingerly over the drainage gully, she moved forward and her head and neck went into a two-piece metal stanchion, that I then clamped at the top to secure the cow.

After a few days it came to me that each cow actually did have her own place in the barn. I was dumbfounded. The first cow would enter the completely empty barn, go to the correct one of the four sections, and enter the exact same stanchion as she did twice a day, every day. Uncanny. Amazing.

Occasionally, I observed with some degree of puzzlement, a cow walk behind another cow already in a stall, pause, then butt that cow with her head from behind, pause, and when she got no reaction from the cow she had butted, would then find an empty stall nearby.

The act reminded me of an older boy who, without comment, would push or shove a younger boy, for no other reason than to remind the younger boy of his "place." I asked one of the older boys why one cow butted the other, and he explained that the first cow in had misjudged and had taken the stall belonging to the second cow. Amazing!

Each cow had a name-Betsy, Mary, Joan, Polly, etc., and within a month or so I had memorized the name of each of the forty-six bovines and could recognize her on sight. If cows were missing I could tell which ones were not there just by a process of elimination.

The older boys milked the cows by hand, each boy milking six or seven cows at a session. As soon as I brought in the cows and secured each in her stall, I located a wheelbarrow and began feeding the cows, that in Winter consisted of a heaping mound of silage from the two massive silos, covered by bran.

The bran came in one hundred pound tow sacks (we boys would have spelled the word "toe") that were stored in the massive hayloft above the dairy milking floor. When the bran was delivered from Statesville Milling Company (in 1951), or from Farmers' Exchange (from 1952 on), little skinny-assed Al had to carry these hundred-pound sacks of bran up the steep flight of stairs just like the older boys.

The Milling Company/Farmers' Exchange prepared the bran to Mr. Davis' specifications, that consisted of a formula of corn, oats, molasses, soybean meal and minerals. These sturdy bags were sewn with heavy string across the top by use of a serger, or a sewing machine. If you loosened just the correct loop on one end, the string unraveled easily. We boys were very careful opening the tow sacks, because Mr. Davis was kind enough to give us kids all the money he received when we returned the sacks intact to the supplier.

The milking herd at the orphanage consisted entirely of the Holstein-Friesian breed, that we knew only as "Holsteins." Holsteins "give" more milk volume than any other breed of milking cow, and the amount of milk this breed produces is great when you consider that these animals are fairly low-maintenance. The main sustenance for cows at the orphanage was pasture grass, that was quite abundant on the sprawling three hundred fifty acre (more or less) farm. Large areas of the land were planted in alfalfa, and when harvested as hay and stored in the expansive hay lofts of the Mule Barn, Green Barn, Long Barn and Farmers Barn, more than supplemented warm-season grass as roughage. The two enormous silos that stood like towering somber sentinels over the dairy milk house and the Little Dairy, were filled with silage, consisting of chopped-up corn stalks, during the Summer, to supply green roughage during the cold Winter months, and molasses-enriched bran was fed to the herd at each of the two daily milkings year round.

In 1950, the year I began working at the dairy, the herd consisted of forty-six milk cows, twenty-five heifers and two enormous bulls, Vic and Ace. Twenty-nine head of the herd were registered Holsteins. The hay crop that year was one of the best in years, and more alfalfa was harvested than needed. The rolling permanent pasture was reseeded that year in Ladino Clover and Kentucky Fescue.

CHAPTER 26

World Champion Cow-Caller

A few weeks after beginning work at the dairy, the job of bringing in the cows fell on my skinny shoulders like a ton of bricks! On my first night as the boy who brought in the cows, I observed with keen interest that Robert began "calling" the cows at about the time we started down the long, sloping concrete driveway toward the dairy.

Calling cows is itself an art, and by the very definition of the word "art," being "skill" or "craftsmanship," some are naturally better at it than are others. I would be terrific (or so I believed) and thus reasoned (with sound logic) that if the cows could hear and respond to Robert's weak but steadily ascending succession of soprano o-o-o-o-o-O-O-O-O! that he began at the top of the concrete dairy driveway, surely these same dumb animals could instantly recognize and thus heed my thunderous, all-caps OOOOOO-OOOOOO-OOOOOO!!!! and in order to further impress (both the cows and) my co-workers, if I started calling the cows the moment I reached the edge of the baseball field, while still well on the main campus, I would have about a four hundred yard head start on every other far less intelligent orphan cow-caller who ever plied his trade. Students and staff alike would be remarkably impressed by my knowledge, intelligence, and animal husbandry prowess, my cow-calling fame would quickly spread far and wide, and I would have attained the universal orphans' elusive but much sought-after prize-Recognition for a Job Well Done! My little skinny chest swelled with pride. I would be "in" with the Big Boys.

I hardly slept the following night, and when Robert rousted me out of my bunk at 3:30 a.m., I already had on my clothes and brogues. While Robert went to awaken the other dairy boys, I headed for the dairy-and fame and glory! Aiming to be the very best, I began my cow-calling at the near campus edge of the baseball field, located between the Walker Building and the hospital. My stated purpose was to contact forty-six sleeping cows located a half-mile away, and I was certain my manly, authoritative voice would surely accomplish this result. I recall thinking that I might even be too good, and the cows possibly could be waiting at the dairy for me when I arrived, bursting with respect and admiration.

However, my grandiose scheme failed to account for one small, eentsy-teentsy little problem. At the time I began calling the cows, I was only about thirty yards from the hospital to my right, with the Walker Building down aways to my left, and not too far away (quite close, really) were the residences of the (sleeping) Tom Adams and his (sleeping) wife, and the (sleeping) Mr. & Mrs. Eben McSwain. And not far behind me were the (sleeping) boys and cottage counselors of the four boys' cottages, and the second floor Business Office residences of the (sleeping) Coach Gabe Austell and his (sleeping) wife and children.

However, because we of superior intellect and foresight, in search of personal fame and fortune, often are oblivious to the rights or even the existence of those mere mortals around us, I was totally unaware of any living creatures save myself and my forty-six soon to be appreciative cows. So I just kept on calling my herd. And I was really loud.

And as I had predicted, my wonderful theory of cow-calling worked! I met the first few cows approaching the dairy barn in almost a dead heat, and the forty-six awe-struck bovines were all in and stanchioned long before the first milkers arrived.

All went well until about mid-morning, when Mr. Davis approached me while I was busy scrubbing milk containers in the Little Dairy. Quickly drying my hands in case he wanted my autograph, I suddenly noticed that he was not smiling, nor did he appear to be about to extend his right hand in a congratulatory handshake. In fact, because I had by that time an overabundance and then some of the knowledge of the various moods of the staff and teachers at the orphanage, I noticed that he did not appear to be in a very good mood. And thinking back on that moment at a later date, I seemed to recall he was really, really unhappy about something.

Because repeating what Mr. Davis really said to me would involve a whole slew of agitated vowels and veritable dearth of consonants and would have to be translated from Davis-speak anyway, the gist of the visibly upset dairy manager's incoherent babblings was that Coach Austell, Mrs. Tomblin, Miss Hobson, Mr. McSwain, Mrs. Dye, Witch Robinson and Tom Adams had already called Mr. Gray to complain about that stupid, totally inconsiderate kid who was yelling and waking them up at 3:30 in the morning.

However, greatness and remorse being incompatible traits, without apology I defended my right to call my cows from the populated edge of the campus. Mr. Davis countered that if he received another complaint from Mr. Gray, it might not go well for me. Thus after a great deal of wrangling and posturing, vacillation on his part when matched with grim determination on my part To Do The Right Thing, and because of my magnanimous ability to compromise and thus allow the dairy manager to save face, we reached an agreement, of sorts, as follows. I agreed to wait until I had at least reached the corn crib/tool shed before beginning my masterful cow calling, and he and/or Mr. Gray and/or Mr. Regan would not inflict upon my frail being grievous bodily harm. I had learned painfully by the age of eleven, that negotiations with the orphanage staff involved a certain degree of give and take, with me agreeing to "take" whatever the insensitive, bottom-feeding grownups had to "give." Amazingly, the concept of self-preservation is one easily assimilated by disadvantaged and oppressed preteen orphans.

But suffice it to say that for now I was the best damn cow-caller in the state of Nauthcalana. If you don't believe it, just ask Mrs. Dye and Witch Robinson and Mrs. Tomblin and all the boys in 1-B and . . . .

CHAPTER 27

Mules, The Milk Run, Bridling Bell

Beasts of burden on the orphanage farm included about thirty boys during the Winter, and nearly double that figure during the Summer truck farming season. Oh, and there were also the ten mules. Oftentimes the four-legged animals fared better than the two-legged toilers. Strange as it may seem, somehow I never observed Tom Adams slap one of the huge mules across the face with his bare hand, while admonishing the mule "I know you didn't say anything, but you were thinking dammit."

Throughout the South, the mule appeared to be the choice of labor for such work as plowing fields and pulling wagons. I left the orphanage in February 1957, and following my first year in college, in the Summer of 1958, I worked out West as a wheat harvester, traveling extensively through northern Texas, then Oklahoma, Kansas, Nebraska, Wyoming and Montana. This is what the locals called "following the wheat," or "following the harvest," because the wheat in those states ripens as you travel north toward Canada during the Summer. I observed that the farther north we went the more the mule was replaced by the horse for such work.

Sturdy as an Arizona boulder, yet docile as a newborn kitten, the large mules on the orphanage farm were as dependable as the rising sun, their temperament remaining as constant in a scorching August sun as in a freezing January rain. Low maintenance workers, the ten farm mules subsisted mainly on hay and corn. To my utter amazement, I discovered that a mule will eat the corn off the cob, spitting out the cob. So we didn't have to shell the corn, but shovel the shucked ears from the corn crib into hampers, carry it to the mule barn, and dump it into the feed trough.

The "Dust Bowl" covered a section of the Great Plains that included parts of Colorado, Kansas, Texas, Oklahoma and New Mexico. At the end of World War I millions of acres of that area's vast grassland were put under the plow in order to grow the aforementioned "amber waves of grain."

Following years of overcultivation, combined with poor land management in the 1920's, the region suffered a severe drought beginning in the early 1930's that lasted several years, and the exposed topsoil was carried off by strong Spring winds.

In a concerted effort to save the animals from certain starvation, entire herds of range cattle, sometime erroneously called "steers," were rounded up and shipped eastward by train, and some of these longhorn "beef cattle" were transported to Raleigh and eventually from there to Oxford Orphanage.

A large section of pasture was fenced in down past the hog farm, and eventually a small barn was constructed. The names "beef cattle pasture" and "beef cattle barn" stuck, became commonplace on the farm and dairy, and that is what these animals were called at the time of my arrival at the orphanage in early 1947. According to Mr. Davis, he preferred the simple descriptions "heifer pasture" and "heifer barn," but went along with tradition, referring to the heifers as "bee adda" (beef cattle) and the heifer barn as the "bee adda arn" (beef cattle barn).

Following weaning, male calves were driven to the beef cattle pasture, where they remained until they were sold. When the alfalfa fields were cut, sufficient hay was harvested and stored in the beef cattle barn for Winter use, and this supply was replenished as required, from the huge stocks in the Farmer's Barn over past the Thousand Dollar Spring, or from the Long Barn.

After weaning, the female calves were housed in the Green Barn during the Winter months, and driven to the beef cattle pasture to herd with the male calves during the warm season. The budding horns were snipped from both male and female calves, to prevent them from goring one another.

The mule used by the dairy to pull the milk wagon twice daily and to pull the manure wagon through the plowed fields several times each week, was named Bell. My first week on the dairy, Robert had talked me through what at the time seemed an immensely complicated procedure for bridling Bell and harnessing her to the shafts of the milk wagon, then immediately informed me that 1) this was to be one of my duties each morning, 2) this was the only time he would show me how it was done, and 3) it would be my responsibility to ensure Bell was ready to pull the milk wagon the moment the ice-cold cans of milk were loaded aboard the wagon.

The unhomoginized, unpasteurized but twice-strained and ice-cold milk filling the three-and-a-half gallon sized cans that had just flowed gurgling over the aerator, where it had been cooled to less than fifty degrees Fahrenheit to prevent spoilage, sat waiting for the arrival of Bell and me. Robert told Frank McMillan to help me, because Frank was more familiar with the milk route, so off we rode, two preteens on a mission of great importance, our precious cargo of cold milk cans sweating in the heat of an already muggy June morning.

Up the concrete driveway from the dairy barn we went, Frank and I astride the great brown beast, past the mule barn on the left and the corn crib and tool shed on the right, and headed up the steadily rising slope until Frank, sitting in front of me, pulled gently on Bell's reins and delivered the universal mule-halting command, "Whoa, whoa Bell!"

"The hospital gets one can," said Frank, and each of us grasped a handle of one of the milk cans and trudged up the concrete driveway that circled the hospital.

Lugging the heavy milk container up the concrete steps at the back of the hospital, we opened the door to the kitchen, where the housekeeper greeted us with a warm smile. She had just finished toasting and buttering bread for the hospital breakfast, and offered Frank and me some strawberry preserves on toast, that we scarfed down, thanked the kind lady, and were on our way.

Next stop was the dining room-kitchen. Anyway, the three-and-a-half gallon milk containers were quite heavy and cumbersome, to the extent that each of us grabbed a handle of the substantial can, and began to lug it up the steep stairs one at a time, both cans and steps. One at a time, that is.

Halfway up the stairs with the third can, with me holding the can's handle in my left hand and Frank with his right, suddenly the can of milk felt approximately twice as heavy as it should. Glancing quickly out of the corner of my left eye, I observed that Frank's right index finger was thrust to a depth of about the second knuckle up his right nostril, and he was rummaging about inside his sameside nasal cavity as though he were attempting to locate a swiftly darting object, like a butterfly or something.

"What the hell're you doing, Frank?"

"Sorry," replied my explorer friend, who quickly grabbed his side of the milk can handle, the weight abruptly decreased by about fifty percent, and we continued our ascendancy of the steep gray stairs, both of us shaking our heads, I in utter disbelief and Frank because he often shook his head, a "John Williamson" act that we youngsters referred to as "wagging" one's head. I recall wondering if Frank's elevator really reached the top floors.

I must have been the dumbest kid who ever worked for Bob Davis. At times I thought I was the dairy Designated Scullion, that is, Mr. Davis' permanent "volunteer" and the older boys' gofer, as in the expression "gofer this and gofer that."

Mr. Davis was always asking for volunteers. And every time he did, the other boys would immediately look as far away as their goldbricking eyes could reach, and stupid Little Orphan Al would just as immediately make eye contact with Mr. Davis. Since I was the only kid who ever even indicated I had heard him, he somehow always took that to mean I was interested in whatever scutwork he wanted somebody to do.

Scents, smells, odors and aromas are catalogued in our life's filing cabinet just as are visual experiences. One of the sweetest olfactory indelible impressions is that of the smell of the orphanage kitchen coming in the second-floor outside door on a cold Winter's morning. No dairy boy will ever forget it. The welcome aroma of pans of melted butter greeted Frank and me on that first morning's trip to the kitchen.

The kitchen girls, mostly preteen and teenagers, did not butter each piece of bread using a butter knife. Rather, the pure U.S. Grade A surplus butter was melted in large metal containers, then liberally basted onto each slice of orphanage-baked bread, and placed in the large ovens on large metal sheets. Thus each piece of toast probably contained a good part of a third of an ounce of pure butter.

I would have given Frank's right arm for a few slices of that golden toasted bread, but I didn't have to. After we carried what seemed like 725 milk cans up that long flight of stairs (but was at the most only ten or fifteen containers) one of the younger girls thrust three pieces of toast at each of us, we mumbled "Thank you," and out we went. Frank and I sat on the gray wooden landing and relished our reward. The rest of the day could take care of itself.

Sleep did not come gently that following night. My fitful thoughts were of Robert's admonitions about my new responsibility concerning Bell and the milk wagon, making the already warm night's sleep difficult at best.

Robert had spat out the parts of the bridle so fast, and the entire procedure was completed in an instant. How was I to remember these details? Would the huge animal hold still while I fumbled about with her harness? How would I tell which one of the ten mules was Bell? Would she come dashing out of the Mule Barn when I approached calling her name? What if I bridled the wrong mule, and all the Big Boys laughed at me? What if I failed in my attempt at my new job as "bridle boy?"

I awoke at 3:30 that morning feeling very inadequate indeed. But with no way out of my responsibility, I decided to do the best I could, and looking back on that morning, I'm certain I approached the dairy with mixed feelings of inadequacy (one part) and pride (one part) in refusing to tell Robert that I had not understood a single word of his instructions, and could he be ever so kind as to demonstrate that "bridling" business about a dozen or so more times?

After "bringing in" the cows, as it was called, I hurriedly set out for the Mule Barn, reasoning the quicker I got there the more tries I would get to figure out this stupid bridle business.

As I reached the top of the long concrete driveway leading from the dairy to the farm buildings, I began calling "Bell, Bell, Bell, here girl!" until as I approached the Mule Barn I spotted the one lone mule emerging slowly from the darkened interior of the barn and begin approaching me.

Good! First round to Little Orphan Al! Taking Bell's bridle from the rack on the inside barn wall, I cautiously approached the gentle monster. She did not back away or turn. I determined the best approach would be the logical one. But what was logical to an eleven-year-old city kid who had never until the day before even touched a bridle or a mule?

What was the order of bridling a mule? Do I pull the leather thingy over her ears, then stick the metal thingy in her mouth? I tried it that way, but somehow the whole leather thingy kept slipping off her ears. No, this couldn't be right. Let's try it in reverse.

So, throwing the cumbersome leather bridle and assorted leather straps over my narrow shoulders, very cautiously I began trying to work the metal piece into her mouth. This metal thingy I learned later, is called the "snaffle," or "bit." It consists of two short metal bars jointed at the center.

The outer end of each bar is attached to a metal ring on each side of the big animal's mouth, to which also are attached one end of each rein and the bridle proper. So far, so good. Now, if I pulled the bridle up, I could place the leather straps (the headstall) over her ears. Not too difficult. I felt a sudden sense of accomplishment, if I could only figure out the rest.

Once the straps were in place over Bell's ears, I then buckled the leather straps (the throat latch) under her chin, which secured the bridle firmly on the big mule's head. The "browband' and the "noseband" sorta fell into place where they should. Mission accomplished! I was a raving success.

Cautiously picking up the dangling reins, I led the lumbering brute to the side of the watering trough in the center of the barnyard. Balancing myself on the side of the well-worn wooden water trough, I sprang onto the old girl's back. Gosh, I sure was high up. A mule seems about twenty feet high when you're sitting on her back.

Once seated securely, I leaned forward, grasped a rein in each hand at the point where the reins were attached to the metal ring on each side of Bell's mouth, dug my tiny eleven-year-old's leather brogues into the big creature's sides, pulled on one rein and then the other (like all experienced cowpokes, or rather, "mulepokes" do) and made clucking sounds in an attempt to coax the big girl forward. But before climbing onto her back, I had held the reins and pointed her in the general direction of the dairy barn, just to hedge my bets a little. In other words, I reasoned, if I did get her going at all, she at least would be headed in the right direction, and I needed all the help I could get at the moment.

Some tasks in life are best learned by observation, by copying what we have seen, by following an example. This bridling business happened to be just such a task. The procedure I was following, I realized at a later date, was subconsciously the routine I had observed used so successfully by Sunset Carson, The Lone Ranger, Hopalong Cassidy, Roy Rogers, Buster Crabbe, Johnny Mack Brown, Lash LaRue, Gene Autry and others of my heroes in dozens of wartime Saturday matinee B-westerns, in the pitch-black Paramount picture show on Queen Street in Kinston.

And to my utter amazement, it worked for a little half-pint orphan with Bell, just as it had for Roy and Trigger, The Lone Ranger and Silver, Gene and Tony. I was in good company!

My lifted spirits actually caused a brief moment of lightheadedness, for this was truly the first time since my arrival at the orphanage three years earlier that I felt like I was in charge of something. Sitting high in the air astride Bell, I experienced a sudden surge of confidence. I was (or at least it appeared to me) in total control of this huge creature, and just by bumping her sides with my leather brogues, pulling the metal bit left and right with the reins, and copying my good friend and fellow cowboy Gene Autry, I said loudly, "Dig dirt, Bell!" and off we headed toward the dairy . . . at the big mule's own plodding gait.

But even in my moment of personal triumph, as usual some scumbucket Big Boy was determined to pee on my parade. As I passed on the farm side of the small tool hut at the head of the dairy driveway, I was so impressed with my "bridling" success that I did not observe movement off to my left, so in good spirits I paraphrased my cowboy hero Gene Autry, and commanded loudly, "Dig dirt, Bell. Dig dirt, old girl!" and was about three bars or so into *She'll Be Coming Round the Mountain*, when I was almost startled off "Tony" by Jack Barger's derisive comment, "What's this 'Dig dirt' shit, kid?" And then the sorry bastard added, "Who you think you are, kid, Gene Autry or something?" And off the idiot went down the driveway, disappearing through the door at the front of the dairy, chanting loudly "Dig dirt Tony. Dig dirt, Bell."

Once the dirtbag older dairy boys started on you, they never let you go. So for the next week or so I had to put up with "dig dirt" hoots and hollers. Insensitive pricks! But it worked. You can bet your cowmanure-soaked brown brogans that three words nobody ever heard from me again, not ever, were "Dig dirt, Bell." Talk about stifling creativity! Those lowlife older dairy boys were creativity-stiflers extraordinaire. They had a veritable lock on the art. Bumpkins. Goddamn Yahoos.

Bell was a friendly, lovable, docile creature, though occasionally if you stood too close to her head and just happened to be looking the other way, she would sneak a nibble at your skinny bare arm. So we stupid "new" dairy kids learned quickly to keep our distance.

During the Winter months, when the temperature dipped below the thirties, or if it snowed or there was ice covering the long concrete road leading from the dairy barn up to the farm and campus, Bell was relieved of her duties. If there was any doubt, we left her in the mule barn, because we could not chance her slipping on the ice or snow and breaking her leg.

Thus in very inclement weather Frank McMillan and I, as the milk delivery boys, had to take hold of the milk wagon shafts and become jinrikisha ("ricksha") drivers for the milk run. Frank and I would slip and slide and occasionally lose our footing and hit the icy road. However, unlike the two of us, Bell could not easily be replaced. Or so Mr. Davis must have reasoned.

Frank and I used to have contests with the milk wagon. Once we delivered the milk to the hospital, Baby Cottage and kitchen in the morning, we ended up with a milk wagon full of empty milk cans. We would unharness Bell and return her to the Mule Barn, and one of us, grasping the wagon shafts, would run down the dairy driveway at breakneck speed, and see who could make the sharpest turning radius and stop in front of the Little Dairy without losing any milk cans.

CHAPTER 28

And What is This Knob
Marked "V-HOLD" For?

Bill was leaning forward in the pew just in front of me, craning his neck, weaving his head from side to side, trying his best to see around the head of the boy leaning forward and half standing, as though a horse chafing at the bit, in the pew in front of him, in turn weaving his head from side to side. And so on, and so on, throughout the length and breadth of the ancient chapel that was the beautiful centerpiece of the stately Main Building.

"Down in front!"

"Shut up, I cain't hear!"

"Shut up yuself!"

"Make me!"

"Cain't see through muddy water!"

These and other irritable, very loud whispers rippled throughout the assembly of more than three hundred fifty orphans and staff on that historic, sweltering early evening in late August 1950. At the age of eleven I sat mesmerized, gawking in utter amazement, at something none of us had ever before experienced, a veritable phantasmagoria, a unique mixture of movement, light and sound being emitted from a small black box resting atop a large wooden table on the stage at the front of the chapel.

We all had been assembled at the chapel on that hot Summer evening to watch our first ever "television" program. In the yet stifling heat of the muggy August evening, three hundred fifty pairs or eyes of all ages stared, singularly impressed and infinitely intrigued by the chorus of "Fred Waring and his Pennsylvanians," and interspersed among lyrics, ditties and ballads we became thoroughly impressed forever by the merits of various soap powders, toothpowders and double-edged safety razor blades, products, I naturally assumed, that were used daily by Fred and his bouncing band of merrymakers, and being commonly found in every home in America. No doubt about it. Had to be.

My favorite song of all time is still *I'll Be Seeing You*, and Fred's group more than did it justice. Back then songs told stories, and we could hear every word of the song. The wartime years had given birth to a distinctive style of musical impression, centering around loss, longing, sacrifice and hope, and this genre of music carried over into the postwar years of the late forties and early fifties. The word "nostalgia" evokes different memories in people. To me the word always has been synonymous with the forties.

Prior to that memorable night, we had never even heard the word "television," and the phenomenon quickly became a welcome diversion from my seemingly neverending longing for my pre-orphanage security and family love.

In 1950 there were more than one hundred series that had run on radio for ten years or longer. But don't stand in the way of progress. And television was certainly progress. Figures don't lie. By 1953 there were more than one hundred television stations in the United States, and radio and picture shows began to lose millions of dollars to the new kid on the block.

Milton Berle, the popular vaudeville and radio comedian, became emcee and main attraction of the immensely popular Tuesday night Texaco Star Theatre on NBC. By the end of 1952 there were more than nineteen million television sets in the United States, and more than ten million of these sets were tuned one night each week to the ever-popular I Love Lucy comedy show.

As a foggy-minded youth, one of my favorite radio dramas was "The Shadow." My obtuse and abstruse peers in the Walker Building and 1-

B knew of my good friend Lamont Cranston as merely a conceited, indulgent rich man, playing grabass with (if her sexy voice was any indication) the strikingly beautiful, voluptuous Margo. Because Margo was trapped inside the little radio box and I couldn't see her, I envisioned her as looking an awful lot like my first grade teacher, so I called her Margo Wellbuilt.

However, only a few of Lamont Cranston's extremely small-diametered circle of friends (a group that included Little Orphan Al) knew the central character's true identity. And just to assure The Caped Guy that I could indeed keep a secret, I divulged his true identity to only about fifty or so of my close-mouthed friends in the Walker Building and 1-B. Those other three kids just couldn't keep a secret.

The half-hour radio thriller opened with the hushed voiceover announcing "Who knows what evil lurks in the hearts of men? The Shadow knows." The secret shared by Lamont Cranston, Bouncing Butt Margo Wellbuilt and I was the evil that lurked in the hearts of the Band of Abusers of Younguns at Oxford Orphanage.

I tried to get in touch with my friend Lamont Cranston. One day I sneaked into the second floor hallway of the Business Office, where a community phone rested atop a small table, and asked the operator for a Mr. Lamont Cranston. She said she had a John Cranston in Oxford. Must be Lamont's relative. So I called the number, and a man told me, upon my inquiry as to whether he was related to Lamont, to "get off the goddamn phone, kid, and if I ever catch you, I'll wring your goddamn neck." So I guess The Shadow didn't live in Oxford, North Carolina after all.

Life at the orphanage was abruptly and forever changed by television. All of a sudden our Saturday afternoons were spent watching college football games, and we spent less time roaming the woods or playing choose-up football games on the large practice field between the school and the football stadium.

A few of us 1-B and 2-B boys were watching a football game the first weekend the lone black-and-white was resting on the table in the chapel, when suddenly without cause the picture started rolling a mile a minute, like there was a mad organ grinder inside the black metal box. We kids just looked at each other rather stupefied (we did that a lot before television, too), so I approached the front of the set and played with the few knobs at the bottom of the runaway screen. No results.

Then I went around to the back of the metal black box, bent down and, looking closely, noticed two twist-knobs, one marked "V-HOLD" and the other "H-HOLD." Fine tuning the "V-Hold" knob caused the speeding picture to slow down and eventually, bracketing it in as would the captain of a destroyer chasing a U-boat in World War II, I finally got the speeding picture to slow down and stop, and we kids then and there became certified television repairmen. What a thrill! Something else we could control in our little world.

After a fashion we mastered the technology of harnessing the cantankerous "H-hold" knob, and following a great deal of instruction, Van, Bill and I taught Coley Lee and Blockhead how the "VOL" knob functioned.

For quite awhile the only television set on campus was the lone box resting on the stage in the Main Building chapel. The big event of the week occurred every Wednesday or Thursday night (I forget which) at 7:00 o'clock, when the student body and any staff members who dared to brave the sweltering heat of the Summer evening, assembled in reverence to watch "Fred Waring and His Pennsylvanians" strut their musical stuff. It was a welcome diversion for us kids, like we had our very own miniature picture show.

A few years later, I believe when I got to 4-B, the Masons donated a black and white television to each cottage, and during the week after study hall ended at 9:00 p.m., we boys would watch shows like *Man Against Crime*, starring my favorite actor at the time Ralph Bellamy.

Possibly the earliest recorded "T.V. Widows" in the United States were the 3-G and 4-G girls at Oxford Orphanage. All us boys loved football, and on Sunday afternoon in the Fall we were glued to the "box" to find out which professional football team was pulverizing the hapless, inept Washington Redskins that day. Courting the 3-G and 4-G girls was not on the Sunday afternoon agenda.

During the school year, after study hall ended at 9:00 p.m., as a break we 3-B and 4-B boys would trek to Red's Three Way Stop at the north end of the campus, for a Chattanooga Moon Pie and an RC Cola. One night in 1955 a few of us 4-B boys were walking along the sidewalk just north of Red's, when our attention was drawn suddenly to a dancing array of colors being emitted through the shrubs from inside a house.

One of the brave among us told us to wait on the sidewalk, and he crept close and parted the hedges with his hands, and looking over his shoulder, I knew then and there how Lindbergh must have felt when he touched down in France. We kids were absolutely mesmerized by our first ever color television set. Before long a bunch of us teenage orphans were seated each night at around 9:15 outside the "color television house," eating Chattanooga Moon Pies, drinking RC Colas and enjoying that beautiful color television set.

At Oxford in the late forties and early fifties, styles or fads or whatever you wish to call these sudden changes in appearance, clothing or lifestyles that appear out of nowhere, last a year or so and then fade away, were not known to us orphan kids. But television changed all that, because this brand spanking new communications medium brought the outside world to us.

When Brylcream was advertised on television, as soon as I could, I hoofed it on down to the drugstore in Oxford and purchased a large tube of the greasy hair cream. In the mid-fifties the hair style among teenage boys was the "duck's ass," wherein the boy swept the hair on both sides of his head straight back, and the loose ends met at the back of the head. Brylcream made certain your hair stayed just the way you combed it. And really, all it took was a "little dab."

And then the television pitch man informed us that if you put a spot of Clearasil cream on top of a pimple, the unsightly yellow-headed blemish would just disappear overnight. Presto! Just like that. Of course, it worked in theory better than in practice. But we kept on trying.

The "test pattern," that geometric chart that appeared on the television screen to assist in adjusting reception, presented a special challenge for some of the 1-B and 2-B wizards. But we finally convinced Red Albertson and Ersul Sowers that no, they didn't have to study for the test pattern, and no, they couldn't possibly fail it.

CHAPTER 29

The Manure Wagon

One of my many chores at the dairy each morning was helping to clean the sprawling concrete dairy floor. After milking was completed, we undid each metal stanchion, thus releasing the cows, and all forty-six of the big milk-depleted bovines filed from the barn and spread out in the pasture to begin milk-making for the afternoon milking. We boys went to breakfast, after which we returned directly to the dairy.

Taking large flat shovels and a wheelbarrow, we scooped up the still wet cow manure, loaded it into the wheelbarrow, and wheeled the barrow to the back of the dairy. There a long ramp led up to a platform, into which was backed the manure wagon, that was about the same size as the milk wagon.

A four-by-four had been bolted to the far edge of the platform in such a manner that if you rolled the wheelbarrow up the ramp, onto the platform and kept going, the wheel bumped the four-by-four, and *if* at the same time you lifted the handles of the barrow, the cow manure was by its natural inertia propelled through the air and into the wagon.

But if the dumbass new kid did *not* release the barrow handles at the proper instant, the force of inertia also propelled the hapless boy into the wagon full of cow dung. Not a pretty sight. It never happened to me, of course, but I did see it a few times.

Anyway, when this preliminary chore was completed, we scrubbed and hosed down the concrete floor until it passed inspection by Mr. Davis or one of the older boys.

We four new boys had been working at the dairy for about a week, already the butt-end of mindless bull-and-cow jokes and juvenile pranks, when one morning Bill called me to the back of the dairy. Apparently there was something wrong with the four-by-four at the edge of the ramp, and he needed me to stand on the square board to hold it in place while he made repairs. And I believed him because 1) he was holding a hammer in his hand, and 2) he was a damn sight bigger than I, which in itself mandated that I believe every single word he said.

So I did as "requested," standing on the four-by-four to hold it down while Bill pounded it with the hammer, though I don't recall him using any nails, and there did not appear to be any definite pattern to his hammering.

All I felt was Bill lift my left ankle, just enough to put me off balance and, screeching and arms windmilling, back I fell into a wagon full of fresh, wet cow manure. My backside had no sooner contacted the slimy, smelly cowshit when I heard the squeals of laughter emanating from the audience-of-stupids inside the dairy, that had gathered for this humiliation of one of the dumbass "new" boys.

"Sorry, kid, my hand slipped."

But Bill didn't offer to help me out of the manure wagon. By the time I climbed over the side of the wagon, I was covered with wet, smelly cow manure, and Bill offered to hose me off. I didn't answer. I was too embarrassed, not so much of the cow manure, as being suckered into standing on the stupid four-by-four in the first place. About two percent of the time I was smarter than all the other kids around me. This was the other ninety-eight percent showing through.

I vowed I never would so humiliate any new dairy boy, and I meant what I said. A few years later, after I had been transformed into a hated and reviled Big Boy, one of the new dairy boys was little ole Robert Batchelor, my friend and classmate Arnold's brother. Robert was a good kid, and I really liked him. About fifty years later, I had a conversation with Robert, and he reminded me that his first week on the dairy, I had lured him onto that four-by-four, and had dumped him back first into the manure wagon. I simply refused to believe him.

It was in this dairy setting that we youngsters learned the importance of responsibility and the thrill of competition. You were considered smarter than the other kids if you could sucker them into falling for a practical joke. Eventually I learned not to take at face value instructions from my older dairy mates, and to mentally compute everything other kids at the dairy said to me.

After awhile we younger boys learned to take practical jokes as good-natured fun, for this was how such boyhood pranks were intended, and soon we began to plot and scheme ways to get back at the older boys, and not get thrashed for our trouble. But then again, sometimes the practical jokers went a wee bit too far, at which time they were forced to suffer the wrath of the Revenge of the Pisser.

CHAPTER 30

Little Orphan Al's Revenge

Bobby taught me how to milk cows. The dumbass. Tall and gangly, with thinning brown hair, except in the dead of Winter Bobby went everywhere with his pantlegs rolled halfway up to his knees.

As part of my ongoing indoctrination into dairy life, one morning after I had herded the cows into the barn for milking, and had fed all forty-six of them, Bobby called me over to where he was milking a cow.

"Come on ova heah, and I'll teach yu how to milk a cow."

"Might as well. Got nothin' better to do right now."

Unbeknownst to (naïve, really naïve) me at this point, the orphanage dairy apparently served as the headquarters of the most ingenious and evilminded practical jokers south of the Mason-Dixon line, and grist for this ever-revolving mill of neverending personal humiliation just happened to be the "new" boys.

Apparently the Summer of 1950 brought a bumper crop of us stupid new boys to this house of laughs. What the devious practical jokers did not count on, however, was the Revenge of the Pisser. But first to get on with our milking "lesson" that Bobby was so eager to offer me, and in my greenness and innocence I was so eager to accept.

As I approached Bobby I observed the cow he was milking had some sort of shiny metal clamp-thingies attached tightly to the backs of her legs. That must really hurt, I thought.

"Why does she have those metal things around her legs?"

"Oh, some of thu cows are old an cain't stand up straight when you milk 'em," he-lied-and-I-believed-him. Come to think of it, compared to some of the cows in the barn, this one didn't look "old" at all. But if Bobby said it, and appeared as sincere as he did while saying it, then it must be true. Stupid kid.

Bobby pulled the milk stool up close to the side of the cow, and sitting down, turned toward me.

"Yu cain't (that's "can't" to the rest of the educated free world, "cain't" to Bobby) sit up straight 'n milk a cow. Cain't get no levrege."

Whatever that is. Must be important, though. I'll have to look it up.

"Yu gotta hunch yur shoulders ova, an lean inta thu belly," he said, indicating a point just where the cow's thigh met her body.

"An berry (try "bury," Bobby) yur head inta her side."

He demonstrated. I observed.

"Then yu rest yur elbows on yur knees, so's yur arms won't git too tard."

He demonstrated. I observed. What's "tard" anyway? I'll look it up.

"Now, git real close, so's yu kin see whut I'm doin."

I got real close. To observe.

Bobby reached down, grabbed the end of the cow's tit, and jerked lightly.

"Yu cain't do it this way. Yu gotta grab th tit first up close to thu 'bag' (which normal people call the 'udder') then squeeze here first, an then squeeze yur otha fingas, yur little finga squeezin' last. Now git closa an I'll show yu how it's done."

I got closer as directed. Seemed awfully close to me. But what did I know from nothing?

By this time I had my face about a foot from the "demonstration." Suddenly Bobby pointed the end of the cow's tit-full-of-warm-milk directly at my face and squeezed real hard. The sudden shock of a face full of warm milk caught me off balance, and I fell backwards, smack-dab into a pile of fresh cow manure. Immediately laughter erupted throughout the large milking barn from the other six milkers, and I realized with embarrassment that I had been "set up" by the jerk. For a moment I just sat there in the warm, mushy, smelly cow manure, the fast-drying milk becoming sticky on my face. The laughter gradually subsided, and activity in the barn returned to normal, the relative quiet broken occasionally by a few residual snickers from the stupid older boys, and a few insulting "stupid new kid" remarks from the quipsters.

"Sorry about that, kid," said Bobby, helping me up from the concrete floor. The sly smile on his face belied the fact that he wasn't really "sorry" at all.

"Come on back and I'll hose off yur pants. They'll dry soon."

He seemed contrite enough. Maybe he was really a nice guy after all.

"Really, Al, when we start milkin' t'morra mornin', I'll teach yu how tu milk."

So I looked forward to the next morning. Nice guy, Bobby. He was just having a little harmless fun. But why was he still smiling, like he knew something I didn't?

Filled with the anticipation all dull-witted new orphan boys seeking approval by the older boys exudes, the following morning I rounded up and fed the cows in record time, eager to get to my first milking lesson and become the first of the "new" boys to learn how to milk.

It was all a part of the desire to be "accepted" as one of the Big Dairy Boys. This meant a lot to me, because even at such a young age, I realized that with "acceptance" by the older dairy boys might come a certain degree of (if ever so slight) "protection" from other older boys on campus. And a large part of being accepted as one of the dairy boys was the ability to take good-naturedly being the butt end of their innovative practical jokes, of which this group seemed to have a limitless supply, and then some.

After completing my morning chores, I found Bobby hunched forward, his head buried into the side of a cow, both hands rhythmically squeezing fresh, warm milk into an open-mouthed stainless steel bucket.

"Here I am," I said expectantly, hoping he had not forgotten his promised milking lesson.

"With yu in a minute," he responded, neither looking up nor breaking his milking rhythm.

The smell of fresh warm milk just as it comes out of a cow is a most pleasant and unique experience. It is a warm, soft, sweet smell.

I marvel at how this wonderful and ever so complicated, docile, trusting monolith can eat grass, bran and alfalfa, then drink gallons of water, and produce milk of exactly the same color, texture, quantity and purity at every milking, twice a day, for ten to fifteen years.

Bobby finished milking the cow, weighed and recorded the weight of the bucket of milk and carried it to the Little Dairy to be processed. When he returned he told me to follow him, and we ended up beside what appeared to me to be the very same cow he had milked the previous morning, the one with the metal-band-thingies on her legs to, as Boney explained, "keep her from falling down." I asked him if this was the same cow, and he responded,

"Yeah, but she's feelin' better this mornin', so's she don't need no shackles."

Sounded logical to me, based on what little I knew about such things. And I had just learned the metal thingies were called "shackles."

"One of thu otha guys a'ready washed 'er bag," explained Bobby.

"Okay," I responded. Nice of his friend to help him out, I thought. For all I knew, Bobby was the official New Boy Milk Instructor. Who knows, perhaps I could some day have that job.

Bobby placed the milk stool to the cow's right side. Remember, mount the mule from its left side, milk the cow from her right side. That's just the way it's done.

"Now, yu sit 'ere." He pointed to the stool. I sat.

"Now, put thu milk bucket 'tween yur laigs." I did as instructed.

"Now, you hafta milk two tits at a time. So jus grab 'er two hin tits." Sounded logical to me. I did as instructed, and reached for the cow's two hind tits.

I don't remember my head hitting the whitewashed dairy barn wall, about six feet from where I first touched the two hind tits while sitting on the stool a split second before. I do recall a dull thud, and when I awakened I saw the milk bucket and stool lying close beside me on the cow manure-splattered concrete floor. I recall thinking that the cow must have crapped at about the same time she kicked.

"You okay, kid?" I looked up into the fuzzy faces of Bobby and two of the other Big Boys kneeling beside me, and they were all looking kinda worried. They were not laughing.

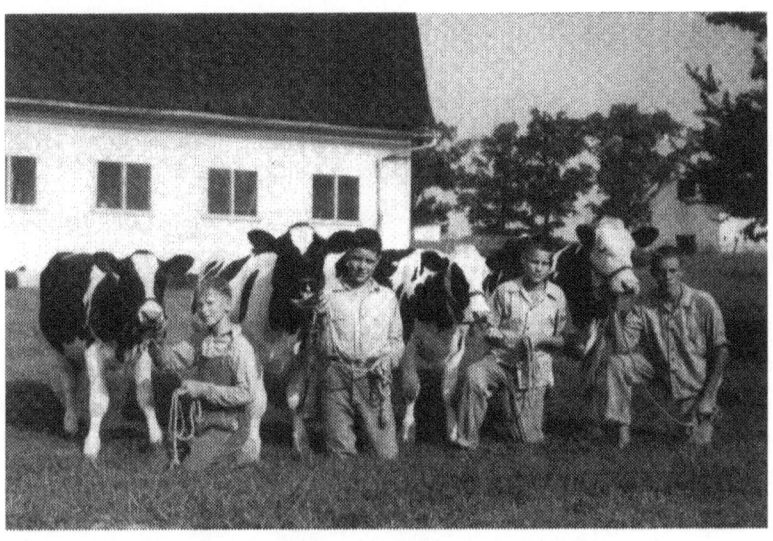

1950. Grooming calves for the state fair. From left: Alton Provost, Frank McMillan, James Strum, Boney Wyatt. Left near background is huge milking barn. Far right background is Long Barn.

"I think so," I said, slowly trying to sit up, and not having much success. So I just sat there against the whitewashed concrete wall where I had just seconds before landed.

"What happened?" No answer. Not from any of them.

Finally the three boys helped me to my feet, and I seemed alright, just couldn't remember what happened from the time I touched the cow's two hind tits until I awoke facing that same cow's swishing tail six feet in front of me. I felt a little woozy and weak in the knees, but continued on with my chores. Bobby said he would teach me to milk on another day. I distinctly remember thanking him.

However, once the Big Boys found out I had actually survived the experience, they began kidding me about milking cows without shackles, especially that mean-son-of-a-bitchin-cow-named-Lucy.

"But I thought the shackles were to keep her from falling down." Stupid. Stupid. Stupid new kid.

No, explained Bill, the shackles were used because she's sensitive to anybody touching her tits, to keep the cow from kicking you halfway to the moon. Then I understood. Good old helpful Bobby. That sorry sonofabitch. Nearly got me killed, dammit to hell. A month later I couldn't recall the actual kick, or flying through the air, or actually hitting the whitewashed concrete wall. But that must have been one really powerful right hind leg. And what *really* hurt was the fact that I had actually *thanked* that bastard Bobby when he picked me up off the concrete floor.

So, what about Bobby? Should I take nearly getting killed as a good-natured practical joke and let it go? Hell no! Bobby's sorry ass was mine. I just had to figure out how he was going to get "his."

An orphan kid eventually will learn to figure his way out of any seemingly impossible situation. This Houdini-like quality is an outgrowth of necessity, and in that vein we had to figure out how to stymie and thwart the wrath of meaner'n hell adults and Big Boys. Except in my case I added to the "stymie" and "thwart" triangle, the balancing hypotenuse-"revenge."

I loved Revenge, and capitalize it out of respect and awe. I'm the original two eyes for an eye guerrilla terrorist engaged in my own private war with anysonofabitchwhodidmedirty. Bobby was all mine. And the most satisfying thought of all was that he didn't even know it.

Laugh at Little Orphan Al? In a pig's eye! Best taste in the world is that of ice-cold milk as soon as it drips from the aerator in the Little Dairy. We used heavy metal cups to drink from, and as we new boys worked in the Little Dairy during the pre-dawn milking, oftentimes the older milkers would "ask" us, no, on second thought, they probably "ordered" us, to fetch them a mug of cold milk fresh from the aerator. Another of those numerous seemingly innocent little things Big Boys do to remind the "new" boys just who was in charge.

So I thought up this ingenious scheme to give measure for measure, and then some. One early morning I took one of the heavy metal drinking cups, walked into the pitch darkness behind the Little Dairy, and calmly pissed in the metal mug. Not a lot. Just a little, for taste-testing purposes.

Then I took the metal cup of about one-fifth urine, stuck it under the aerator spout, and finished filling the cup with ice-cold running milk. The force of the milk created a nice foam on top of the cup, that lo and behold appeared on close scrutiny to take on a slightly yellowish hue. My concoction, I believed, would pass the "color" test.

But now for the all-important "taste" test. We weren't exactly tasting wine, but I didn't want Bobby to kill me for pissing in his milk, either, so I had to be very careful.

About that time Jimmy and Butch walked into the Little Dairy.

"Could one of you guys taste this milk; it may not be cold enough."

"Let me see it," said Butch, reaching for the cup-o-piss. Taking a long swallow, Butch licked his lips and pronounced it cold enough. That's all I needed, an expert's advice, and as I reached for the cup, Jimmy took the cup from Butch and said,

"I'll finish it for you. You can get yourself another cup."

"Okay, thanks, you guys," I said, pulling back my tentatively outstretched hand.

Back to the shadows of night went Little Orphan Al, returning with another one-fifth cup-o-pee. Back to the aerator to complete my Formula of Revenge. Waiting in the Little Dairy for my quarry. Standing there, acting as though I were drinking from the metal cup, careful not to let my lips touch the rim. Here comes Bobby, my very best friend.

"No hard feelings, kid."

"No, it's alright. I'm okay now, just a little ringing in my ears. I'll be fine. I'll get my balance back soon, I'm sure. And my vision is certain to clear up in a week or so. Gotcha a cup of cold milk, if you want it."

"Thanks, kid, yur a'right."

Putting down his bucket full of milk, Bobby took the piss cocktail from me and stood drinking the entire cup full of one-fifth, four fifths.

"Thanks, kid." He handed the empty cup to me.

"I'll get you another cup tomorrow morning."

"Thanks, kid, yur okay."

And you're full o' pee, I said (under my breath) as he walked away. And so you have it-the true story of the Revenge of the Pisser. Don't ever mess with Little Orphan Al-not ever. And tomorrow morning I'd press my luck, and try for two-fifths, three-fifths. At age eleven I was already living "on the edge." If Bobby's milk tasted a wee bit salty, then perhaps the cows had spent too much time at the blue blocks of salt lick interspersed throughout the pasture. But then again, perhaps they hadn't.

CHAPTER 31

Heat, Birthing, and the Mummy

A female calf, or heifer, first comes in "heat," that is, its first ovulation occurs, when the animal is more than a year old. So how do we determine when the "heat" occurs?

Actually, about the only certain way to tell when the young heifer comes in heat is to observe when the other heifers start "hopping" her. If at that time you tie her to the manure wagon and lead old Ace or Vic up behind her for her first "servicing," and it "takes," she has started on the road to becoming a milk cow.

So how do we tell whether the breeding attempt is unsuccessful? Simply observe her. A cow will ovulate about once each month. If this time period elapses and the other young calves start "jumping" her again, then you know for certain this breeding attempt did not take, and you must subject the poor animal once again to the ravages of a bull about twice her size. But such is reality in the domestic animal kingdom.

Let's assume that the bull finally hits the spot, and the heifer is now pregnant. So, when do we get a baby calf? Cow gestation is approximately the same period of time as that of a woman's, about nine months. And there are additional similarities.

So, if after three or four weeks, none of the other heifers start "jumping" our heifer in question, it is fairly safe to assume she is pregnant. So she has been pregnant for about a month. Add eight months to this date and plan for a calf to be born at about that time.

Conception triggers the young female's milk-producing tissue, but the actual secretion of milk remains inhibited until after birthing. At that time the cow is about two years old.

About eight weeks after birthing, the baby calf is weaned, and the mother cow becomes just another walking milk factory. But she continues to ovulate each month. So you find her a boyfriend again, and the process repeats itself. That "process" being that the poor cow is tied by a rope around her neck to the manure wagon, having a half-ton unfriendly bull put all his weight on her hind legs for about ten minutes, while he takes his sweet time poking his red hose at the air playing Russian roulette with her female parts. If for some reason a milk-producing cow will not re-breed, she eventually will "run dry" (stop producing milk) permanently, and at that time she becomes a "beef" cow, and it's selling time for her.

Now, a mature cow pregnant with her second calf did not "run dry" overnight, but gradually over a period of a few weeks would produce less and less milk. She stayed with the herd until about two weeks before birthing, so as not to interfere with her daily feeding routine. But Mr. Davis simply took her off the herd's milking list.

A week or two before birthing, the cow would begin discharging mucous, at which time we separated her from the herd, confining her in a large stall in the Green Barn until her calf was born.

Following birthing, a newborn calf was kept with its mother, usually in the Green Barn, for a period of about eight weeks. At this time the mother was returned to the herd, and the newly orphaned calf was taken to the Calf Barn, really a set of five wooden enclosed and roofed stalls located just across the dirt Farm Road from the Long Barn.

During the first eight weeks, the new mother was taken to the Dairy Barn for the twice daily milkings, and at night the mother was returned to her calf. That is, if the stupid "new boy" could remember to perform this necessary task.

Though certainly not of my own choosing, most of the scutwork at the dairy fell squarely on my skinny shoulders. So it naturally came about that, at age eleven, I was charged with weaning the baby calves. Early in the darkness of each morning, after bringing in the herd of forty-six cows, and feeding each cow silage and bran, I took one or two (depending on the number of calves being weaned) open-top pails of fresh warm milk, and traversed the wide dale between the Dairy Barn and the Calf Barn, to feed the newborns. I referred to this valley as the "Valley of the Shadow of the Mummy."

By instinct the baby calf has been nursing its mother for about eight weeks, and placing my three middle fingers in the baby calf's mouth elicited its sucking response. Keeping my fingers in the calf's mouth, I then placed the pail of warm milk before it, and with the heel of the same hand, slowly pushed the little one's still-sucking mouth down into the warm milk.

The animal has no use for an epiglottis, so it's not going to choke on the milk. The newness of the procedure is disconcerting for a few days, but eventually I could take my hand out of the calf's mouth after a few seconds, and it would continue drinking from the pail of milk. And within two weeks the baby is on its own, weaned except for the solid dairy feed, that we called "bran." A few weeks after beginning with the milk, I started putting bran in my hand, the calf would try to suck on the bran, and in no time it's eating from the feed pail.

The mechanics of this early morning weaning procedure would have progressed smoothly, except for one minor little itty-bitty problem. Even as a child at home I was spooked by the dark. At age eleven I was terrified. The older dairy boys teased me unmercifully because in their experience I was the only boy who had ever carried a Louisville Slugger along when he went into the pasture at 4:00 a.m. to bring in the cows.

However, any slight creaking of a wooden stall door, and I didn't want anything to do with the baby calves or whoever was hiding in the Calf Barn waiting, I am certain, to murder me. When I was four years old, my brothers had taken me to the Paramount on Queen Street to see The Mummy's Tomb, and The Mummy's Curse two years later, and I was terrifyingly convinced that Lon Chaney, Jr. resided (at night, anyway) in the Calf Barn, third stall from the left, on the farm at Oxford Orphanage. Absolutely. No doubt in my scared little mind at all.

Jack walked me through the procedure of weaning the calf-once. Then he told me that this was to be another of my jobs each morning, and that beginning the next morning I was going to be "on my own."

What do you mean "on my own," I stupidly asked the older dairy boy. Just what it says, he replied, and walked away, undoubtedly to find some other job that nobody else wanted, so I could do that job "on my own" also. Jack Barger was a smartass, but we became good friends.

So that first morning at about 4:30, while it was still pitch dark, Onmyown Al took a pail full of fresh warm milk and (reluctantly) set out across the pasture, that broad valley about a hundred yards across. At the bottom of the valley was a square metal drain that carried rainwater underground and downhill. Scared out of my wits by what I perceived to be the bandaged Mummy peering through the broken slats in the Calf Barn, third stall from the left, and determined not to be the Mummy's next victim, I paused by the concrete drain, surreptitiously peered all around me in the darkness to ensure nobody else but the Mummy was watching, and quickly poured the entire pail of milk into the drain, then scampered back up the hill to the Dairy Barn, the chill running up and down my "yellow" spine not going away until I was safely inside the well-lighted milking barn.

Routinely, after the morning milking was finished, we went along the center aisle, unlocked the stanchions securing the cows, and let them back into the pasture during the warm months, but drove them back to the Long Barn during the Winter months, because there was no grass in the pasture for the cows to eat anyway.

So each morning after breakfast, we had to return to the Dairy Barn to collect our flat shovels and wheelbarrow. We scooped up the manure, sloshed it into the wheelbarrow, ran the wheelbarrow up the wooden ramp and dumped the manure into the wagon. About once every other day we would hitch Bell to the wagon, she would pull the wagon through one of the plowed fields, and we would spread the still-wet cow manure as fertilizer. Each morning after collecting the manure, we would use the water hose and push-brooms to scrub and wash down the concrete barn floor. It was a lot of work.

Anyway, while we were cleaning the barn after breakfast the first day I poured the poor calves' milk down the drain, I promised myself I would feed them double at the afternoon milking. Anyway, the hungry little devils started bellowing and making all kinds of racket, and just wouldn't stop. At first I didn't make the connection, but the older dairy boys sure did. One of them inquired of Mr. Davis as to why the calves were complaining, and Mr. Davis turned to me.

"Did you feed the baby calves this morning, Al?" He really didn't say that, but translated into regular normal person English, it came out close.

"Yes, sir," I lied shamelessly. I had become quite adept at lying shamelessly, so long as it could never be proved I had lied.

But suddenly I felt a juvenile twinge of guilt, so I kinda sorta owned up a little bit, adding,

"This was my first time feeding them the milk. Maybe I didn't give them enough. I'll give them more milk this afternoon."

Mr. Davis seemed to be satisfied with my limp explanation. But what was I going to do the next dark morning? I just knew that pesky Mummy would still be lying in wait to ambush me. A terrifying prospect. Deadly.

Feeling quite guilty about pouring the poor calves' milk down the drain, and realizing that Mr. Davis would eventually discover my duplicity, out of desperation I sheepishly confided to Robert that I was "skeered" of going up to the Calf Barn because I swore I'd seen a human moving about in the barn area.

To my astonishment, Robert said he understood, and told me just to put the pails of milk in the shade at the corner of the dairy barn, and take care of the chore as soon as I returned from breakfast. He assured me the milk would not spoil in such a short time. This arrangement accomplished two goals. It took care of my fear of the Mummy (because my brother Bill had told me the Mummy slept during the daytime) and it took me away from most of the after-breakfast manure cleanup. Little (Fast-thinking) Orphan Al had "landed on his feet" yet again.

The Telephone Number

One day when I was well into my third year at the dairy, finally having made that much-awaited transformation from a naïve and quite expendable "new" dairy boy into a feared (and despised) "big" dairy boy, my young buddy Robert Batchelor, of the former category, just happened (quite unfortunately) to be standing in the Little Dairy as Mr. Davis was speaking to the telephone operator, asking her to dial a number for him.

Now here was an auditory comprehension disaster just waiting for an opportunity. As poor Robert recalled, the telephone number Mr. Davis was requesting the innocent telephone operator to connect him with was 333-6333; even for a "normal" person a tongue-twister, but for Bob Davis a veritable speech-impediment nightmare, an insurmountable hurdle.

Bob Davis: "Oheraor, ih ee ree-ree-ree-ih-ree-ree-ree, re."

Now in Normalspeak this simple request would be "Operator, give me three-three-three-six-three-three-three, please."

The confused young operator, who undoubtedly following this verbal exchange wished she had called in to work sick that morning, politely asked Mr. Davis if he could please repeat his request.

Which our dairy manager did, as young Robert recalled, at least four or five times, becoming increasingly more exasperated, his face changing chameleon-like shades of pink-to-red-to-redder each time the confused operator asked him to repeat his tongue-tied request.

Thus in a span of about sixty seconds young Robert had heard the Davisspeak rendition of 333-6333 come out "ree-ree-ree-ih-ree-ree-ree" a half dozen times, to where it had become a permanent and unwelcomed part of the slow-witted boy's somewhat limited, monosyllable-filled word bank.

Having arrived quickly at the end of his very short fuse with the frustrated telephone operator, Bob Davis abruptly thrust the telephone at the unsuspecting lad, instructing him "Ere, ae ee oheraor or ree-ree-ree-ih-ree-ree-ree."

Completely taken aback by the quite unexpected (and unwanted) instruction, young (dumbass) Robert obliged by taking the telephone from Mr. Davis' grasp, and without hesitation (or logical thought) asked the operator, "Operator, give me ree-ree-ree-ih-ree-ree-ree, please," thereby instantly earning Mr. Davis' "gratitude" in the form of a hard slap up against the side of his head from the very put-out, very insulted and equally frustrated dairy manager.

Working at the dairy was rarely ever fun, but it certainly was interesting, at least from a phonetically-challenging point of view. And to the best of my knowledge, no dairy boy who survived to enter Grownupland ever even considered speech therapy or audiology as a life's work. Ree-ree-ree-ih-ree-ree-ree. Damn.

Coley Lee, Bell and Bob Davis

It wasn't so much that Bob Davis had a problem with consonants, or rather with the lack thereof; no, the problem instead lay with us addle-brained preteen dairy boys. Case in point:

One morning while Mr. Davis was standing in front of the dairy barn at the bottom of the long concrete driveway, giving the usual confusing, contradictory and quite unintelligible instructions to a collection of dumb, dumbfounded and quite disinterested dairy boys, Coley Lee appeared at the top of the driveway about fifty yards away, just moseying along toward the dairy.

I say moseying along, or ambling along because, not being exactly the sharpest knife in the kitchen drawer, at times Coley Lee would just wander off, and show up an hour or so later, without explanation. So his instant reappearance that morning was not really all that noteworthy.

Apparently wanting Coley Lee to return to the Mule Barn to bridle Bell, Mr. Davis cupped his hands in an attempt to megaphone his gibberish, and yelled loud enough to contact the unfortunate boy half a football field away, grunting "O'we, oh eh ell," that was the best the verbally-handicapped dairy manager could manage when intending to say "Coley, go get Bell."

Because of Coley Lee's inability to comprehend the dairy manager's consonant-depleted instructions, however, the lad's inner ears received the clear message, "Coley, go to hell," with the somewhat less than luminous boy's brain filling in the requisite consonants where it (quite erroneously) believed they should lie.

And thinking that Mr. Davis was making a joke, Coley Lee replied, without hesitation or rational thought, "Go to hell yourself!" a consonant-filled instruction that was duly received at the dairy manager's inner ears exactly as it was intended by the confused boy, and at the same time landing Coley Lee in a manure wagonload of trouble.

CHAPTER 32

The Balloon Boys

We called it simply the "farm road." From its point of origin at the group of barns and sheds at the edge of the main campus, this decades-old one-lane artery, its red clay surface hardened by the elements of several lifetimes and by just as many years of wagon wheels transporting farm produce, hay, and farm boys, meandered its timeless way through gently waving and seemingly boundless acres of alfalfa, meadows of grazing Holsteins, rich fields of corn and beans, cabbage patches and okra stands, before reaching its terminus at the Farmers Barn more than a mile away.

At approximately its mid-point, the farm road crossed the railroad tracks that traversed the entire expansive farm, and if one followed these tracks eastward, about a mile on, the orphanage property ended, and presently one reached a macadam county road whose purpose was to connect the town of Oxford with its nearest neighbor, Henderson, about fifteen miles distance.

In June 1950, we five or six eleven-year-old former Walker Building boys wasted no time in testing the limits of our new-found freedom. But until we became more familiar with the social hierarchy (read that "pecking order") of our new home, 1-B, found our niche therein, and expanded our network of friends, we "new" boys stuck together in the interest of self-preservation.

Thus on a sunny Saturday afternoon in mid-June, our little group took its first absolutely and totally unsupervised off-campus excursion, exploratory in nature, and soon found ourselves following the railroad tracks to parts unknown, a la Lewis and Clark and John Fremont fame.

The American Heritage Dictionary, Third Edition, defines fantasy as "an imagined event or sequence of mental images, such as a daydream, usually fulfilling a wish or psychological need." The one major fantasy that sustained me throughout my early years at Oxford was the indelible mental picture of my smiling mother approaching me on the steps of the Main Building on a sunny Fall day, bending down, hugging me tightly as she whispered "Come on, Al, let's go home." We boys in the Walker Building spoke openly among ourselves of this shared unlikelihood, which was stoked to a raging flame by the known fact that occasionally word circulated among the children that such-and-such a boy or girl actually had been taken back home by his or her parent. My last thought before falling asleep each night was of my mama and when she would come to rescue me from the physical abuse and psychological deprivation.

Far into the woods we observed, through the dense Southern pines, sudden movement of vehicles off to our right, and in true explorer fashion, decided to investigate this unexpected perceived intrusiveness into our sheltered world. Following a meandering, well-worn path formed by automobile tire tracks leading away from the railroad tracks toward the highway, we began to notice a lot of balloons lying about. Some appeared well-worn, others newer and only recently discarded, and a few that were still in their single packs. Apparently someone had used the area for picnics or parties, but we did not observe any picnic tables.

William picked up one of the balloons, a well-worn one as I recall, rubbed it against his shirt to shake off the dirt, and began blowing it up. As we boys, even at that early age, had great respect for William's wisdom in such matters, presently the five of us followed suit, and right soon six eleven-year-old orphan kids were busily engaged in blowing up balloons on a well-worn automobile path leading to where we had no idea.

It wasn't easy to do, however. The balloons were all the same size, about four to five inches long, none of them was round, and they were of the same light tan color. With a great concentration of lung power, however, we eventually overcame the troublesome inelasticity of our new-found toys. After successfully blowing up a few of them, we tied off the ends, and began batting them about in the air. I distinctly recall wondering at that moment why, since all the balloons we found were of the same elongated shape, were the same size and color, and were difficult as the dickens to blow up, how could the people at the party have had any fun with them?

Now, even at our young ages, we were smart enough to figure out that, as soon as we returned to 1-B, the other boys would want our balloons, so we gathered up lots of them, stuffed them into our pockets, and headed back down the railroad tracks toward the main campus, blowing up more of the uncooperative zeppelins along the way.

When we reached the corn crib and tool shed that marked the edge of the main campus, we found some twine, that we tied to the ends of the long balloons, and proud as peacocks, we marched triumphantly across the campus to our cottage, pockets stuffed with enough treasure to supply every kid in 1-B with balloons for a year, clutching our pieces of long twine at the end of which bobbed in the air above us some twenty or more elongated, tan balloons.

As we approached 1-B, the supper bell was ringing, so we joined our cottagemates, and began magnanimously passing out free balloons to our best friends, who, in turn, began blowing up our presents. Suddenly we heard a swell of loud, derisive laughter from the older 3-B and 4-B boys, and one of the Big Boys grabbed the twine out of my hand, at the end of which bobbed in the air three balloons, and demanded scornfully,

"Boy, what the hell you doing with these rubbers? Did you blow these damn things up?"

"Rubbers?" I asked quizzically. By now a small crowd had gathered around us, the older boys laughing and snatching our balloons from one another, the 1-B and 2-B boys subdued in innocent amazement at the goings-on. Our proud and triumphant balloon excursion had turned abruptly quite sour, and the crowd of taunting older boys began chanting "Balloon boys. Balloon boys. Balloon boys," as they climbed the wooden steps of the dining hall, releasing our precious blown-up balloons into the air as they entered the dining hall.

Fortunately, we 1-B boys took our meals in the smaller basement dining hall with the 1-G girls, and throughout supper we eleven-year-olds asked among ourselves why the Big Boys were laughing at us, why they took our balloons, and why they called our balloons "rubbers." After supper, shocked and embarrassed, the six of us slithered away in the shadows and rushed to the protection of 1-B. One of the better-natured of the Big Boys (if there is such a thing as a good-natured Big Boy) came down into the basement, laughing uncontrollably and looking for the "balloon boys." Finding us, he said in big brother fashion,

"I guess if you don't know, you just don't know. So I'll tell you what you found over on that lovers' lane." And he proceeded to explain to us what a "rubber" was, that rubbers were used by older men and boys so girls would not get pregnant, and that we had been blowing up used rubbers. The thought alone was repugnant to us, even at such an early age. After the Big Boy left, still laughing, the six of us Balloon Boys, along with several other boys no more enlightened than we, immediately grabbed our toothbrushes and tins of Colgate Tooth Powder, and began brushing our teeth and spitting with a vengeance. Not a pretty sight.

Unwittingly, we eleven-year-olds had stumbled into our first lesson in that neverending course known as the "facts of life." I knew that a man and a woman had to do "something" to produce a baby, but not knowing what that "something" was, I could only picture them in my puerile mind's eye, standing close together, fully clothed, looking into each other's eyes. But again, like the Big Boy said, if you don't know, you don't know.

Alone in my bunk that night, my curiosity inflamed by the Big Boy's brief lesson concerning "the birds and the bees," the mental image of the big-titted naked Baby Cottage housegirl flashed before me. But what did her lovely nakedness have to do with "rubbers" and "making babies?" I had looked upon her supple, curvaceous body only as a thing of innocent beauty, affording it no other function save aesthetics. The catastrophic "balloon" fiasco had served only to create confusion on my unfledged mind. By the end of that Summer two events and an unfettered curiosity would aid in completing my understanding of the relationship between "rubbers" and the sexes.

CHAPTER 33

Ace's Show

The only things missing were a Chattanooga Moon Pie and an RC Cola. Ace the Bull was a monstrous, mean-to-the-core bull, and he always drew a crowd of dairy boys, and any farm boys who just happened to notice the mid-morning audience forming were drawn to witness the curious spectacle. This sunny morning in late July 1950 was to be my first "show," though I was unaware of what event merited the sudden work stoppage.

The world of cows and bulls was new to me, and I had just been on the dairy long enough to know what really hurts. What really hurts is to have a goddamn Holstein that weighs about as much as a pickup truck step on your foot. That hurts. But I had learned my lesson. What do you call a new dairy boy who has just had this happen to him? Unfortunate. What do you call a dairy boy who lets that happen to him twice? Stupid.

And what really made me feel like a fool was that when the heavy-hooved black-and-white stepped on my skinny foot, I was in the process of picking my nose. I've never picked my nose again. Not ever.

The "bullpen" was a miniature Long Barn located at the end of an arcing dirt road about two hundred yards from the milking barn. The small wooden structure, its pale paint fading from the elements of endless seasons, had a hay loft above and room for two huge bulls, separated by a sturdy wooden wall.

An enclosed Cyclone-fenced area was attached to the back of the barn; it also being divided into two fenced areas by a double Cyclone fence. Each side of the barn was equipped with its own water trough, and we fed the two bulls twice each day.

The two bulls, Ace and Vic, were enormous, but Ace was by far the largest bull I have ever seen. Mr. Davis had numerous times warned us new boys not to ever enter the barn stalls or large fenced pens.

One of my many daily assigned duties was feeding the two bulls. I performed this task after we had finished milking, distributed the milk to the hospital kitchen, main dining hall kitchen, and Baby Cottage, and had returned to the dairy after breakfast.

I had been working at the dairy for only a few weeks when I observed two quite unusual phenomena, that appeared to my puerile mind definitely out of place. The fence that enclosed the expansive grazing area for the milking herd stood about eighty yards from the Cyclone-fenced enclosure housing the two bulls. The bellowing bulls were ignored completely by the majority of the cows entering and leaving the dairy barn at milking time. However, I noticed that two of the younger cows were trotting back and forth along the fence, making what I could best describe as a "bellowing moan," in response to the call from the bulls. And when these two antsy bovines were forced to join the rest of the herd, the other cows proceeded to "mount" the two young cows-that is, to try to climb on their backs.

Noticing my interest in these seemingly odd goings-on, Bill explained that this behavior indicated Sara and Betsy were "coming in heat."

"And what does that mean?" I asked Bill, having never heard the term.

"Well, there are only certain days the cow can get pregnant, and the cow does these odd things to let us know that she can get pregnant. So we just say the cow is 'in heat.' I don't know why they call it that, but that's what they call it."

"But how does the cow get pregnant just by running up and down along that fence, and having the other cows try to climb up on her back like that?" I asked the question like the dumbass kid I was.

Looking down at me and slowly shaking his head, Bill asked,

"Where you from, boy?"

"Kinston," I answered, not knowing what "The World's Foremost Tobacco Center" had to do with cows "in heat." And with my basic intelligence being called into question.

"Well, better to show you than tell you. Let's let Mr. Davis know who's getting humped. Come on." Humped? What's "humped" mean, anyway? I'd better look it up.

When we caught up with Mr. Davis, Bill told him,

"Betsy and Sara must be coming in heat, Mr. Davis. Both of 'em are chasing the bulls and the herd's humping 'em."

"Okay," said Mr. Davis. "We'll get Sara to Ace in the morning."

I spent the next little while pondering what would be accomplished by "getting Sara to Ace." But not any "deep" pondering, mind you. After all, I'm the fool who got his foot crushed by the cow while picking his nose.

The next morning Mr. Davis told me to keep Sara's stanchion locked, so as to keep her in the barn after milking. After breakfast, Mr. Davis fastened a leather halter around the cow's head, then led her to the manure wagon behind the dairy barn, and tied the halter to the wooden frame of the manure wagon. Then he walked down to the bullpen, returning awhile later "leading" old Ace. And all of a sudden I discovered why each of the two gargantuan bulls had a brass ring in his nose. Mr. Davis had the metal hook at the end of a five-foot-long metal pole hooked through old Ace's nosering, and you could tell that Mr. Davis was in charge. Twist that metal pole just right, and Mr. Davis could have had that sumbitchin bull jumping through hoops. All of a sudden I pictured in my mind's eye all the stupid Big Boys walking around campus with huge brass rings in their noses, and Little Orphan Al chasing them with the metal pole and hook thingy.

Anyway, with the metal hook and rod, Mr. Davis led the huge bull to the south end of the north-pointing cow, and you could see the terror in the poor cow's eyes.

Immediately Ace began licking his lips. But then again, old Ace also licked his lips when he peed or as he was scarfing down his daily diet of bran and silage. Bulls sure do pee a lot. Cows too.

Suddenly Mr. Davis started repeating "Uh, oy. Uh, oy. Uh, oy," by which I believed he was meaning to say "Up, boy. Up boy. Up, boy." I knew that Mr. Davis wasn't too keen on his "p's" and "b's," and I thought for a brief moment I would translate the dairy manager's consonant-less exhortations to Ace into something more meaningful, if not to the bull, to the boys gathered for the occasion. But then I thought of my safety, and kept my big mouth shut.

Anyway, Mr. Davis kept repeating his gibberish as though he were throwing a bone for a dog to chase, while at the same time jerking Ace's nose ring above the cow's behind.

Suddenly, without notice, as if on some magical animal kingdom cue, old Ace jumped up on the comparatively frail young cow's backside, pinning her body between his front legs, and simultaneously this really long red thingy appeared from under Ace's belly. Looked just like an oversized red garden hose, and was about three feet long. Ace started grunting and poking the red hose at the poor cow, who buckled under the tremendous weight of the huge bull.

Anyway, it seemed to me that old Ace was not accomplishing whatever it was that I certainly didn't know he intended to accomplish. The large animal just kept poking the red hose at the rear end of the poor cow, and more often than not he missed the cow and just poked at the air around the cow, and some of the older dairy boys in our audience started giggling at Ace's apparent ineptitude at whatever it was he was suppose to accomplish.

Mr. Davis, showing the frustration that the conductor of the New York Philharmonic might tend to exhibit while conducting a middle school band, quickly admonished them, saying,

"You boys shut up, or he'll take all day." "He" was poor Ace, who really appeared to be doing the best he could under the circumstances.

Standing there with the ten other (now silent) dairy boys, Boney whispered to me "Know how to tell when ole Ace hits the spot, kid?"

"No, I don't." (What does "hits the spot" mean, anyway?)

"Well, when he gets her good, you'll see her smile."

I didn't answer, because I didn't know anything about what was going on. (What does "gets her good" mean, anyway?)

Anyway, ole Ace kept jumping up on the cow's back, her hind legs kept buckling, Mr. Davis kept imploring "Uh, oy. Uh, oy," the poor bull kept poking his red hose at the tired cow, the dairy boys kept quietly giggling at the seeming failure of Mr. Davis, the frightened cow and old Ace to get done what it was they were supposed to get done, and I looked on in utter amazement at the Comedy in One Part playing out before me.

Finally, after poking the air about forty-two times, Ace's red hose disappeared inside the poor cow, and ole Ace started agrunting and ahumping. Anyway, ole Ace's "show" didn't last but about six seconds. Then the big bull grunted and slid off the backside of the tired cow, and his red hose slowly disappeared back into his belly.

"Well, kid, did you see her smile?" asked Boney.

I didn't answer. But I had looked, and I had not seen the unfortunate cow smile. Maybe I had missed something? I'd watch more closely next time. And I still didn't know what had occurred. My neophyte mind could not bridge the wide chasm between "getting Sara to Ace" and the advancement of the domestic bovine population.

You see, there's a really outside chance that I wasn't a very bright child. Many people in our neighborhood in Kinston referred to me as "harmless," whatever that meant. Thinking back on my pre-incarceration childhood, my parents smiled benignly at me and patted my head a lot.

And then one day my cat got really sick, and mama smiled benignly at the cat and patted its head. Was there some sort of connection between me and my sick cat? I wonder . . . Who knows, maybe my lot would improve as I got older. By the time I began growing hair in my armpits, I had been bamboozled so often by older boys I thought I actually lived in Garden Path, North Carolina.

CHAPTER 34

Whipping and Old Ace

I had been working at the dairy about a month, trying my best to avoid the world's most devious, cunning and original practical jokers, expectantly glancing over my shoulder every time I pushed a wheelbarrow full of cow manure up the ramp behind the dairy, computing and analyzing every word of instruction given to me by the nettlesome older dairy boys, wondering what embarrassing situation I was being sucked into this time. I still could not understand what Mr. Davis was saying, avoiding him at all costs, yet listening to him intently and slowly gleaning the meaning of his gibberish from the context in which the conversation was being played out.

Aside from the troublesome language barrier, actually I got along fairly well with Mr. Davis. As noted earlier, prior to the time I began weaning a calf from its mother, it was my responsibility to cull out the new mothers from the herd, and walk them to their offspring in the Green Barn after the morning and afternoon milkings.

So at age eleven I had the responsibility of remembering which cows were to be returned to the whining calves each day.

One morning I had just driven the herd into the milking barn, when Mr. Davis accosted me as I walked up the steep stairs to the feed room, blocking my way at the top of the stairs. Uh-oh. The old "block-the-path" confrontation thingy portended trouble, especially if the "blocker" outweighed the "blockee" by let's say, around two hundred pounds, and had that look on his face as though somebody had peed in his milk mug.

No, didn't look like he was in such a good mood. In fact, the reddened, scowling look and the piercing stare told me Mr. Davis was really quite upset.

"Al, just what is Molly (Omigod, Molly!) doing with the herd? Why didn't you take her to her calf after yesterday's afternoon milking?"

The Orphans' Rulebook of Lies, Number 27, states that you can't get away with a lie if the liee can easily prove you lied. I was trapped! Fast-forward to Rule Number 28, "If you can't lie, grovel." We small, frail, frightened orphan preteens were the world's most experienced grovelers. And liars.

But what *really* gave away Mr. Davis' really, really foul mood was that Mr. Davis was standing, blocking my path, with one balled-up fist resting on his hip, just like Mad Dog Minnie Warwick when she was giving me the one-two in front of all those other frightened kids in the Baby Cottage dining room.

"I'm sorry, Mr. Davis," I stammered, a lump rapidly forming in my throat. Where did that goddamn "throat lump" spring from in these cases? Sensing his rising anger, I figured maybe apologizing would assuage the savage dairyman beast.

"I won't forget anymore. I'm sorry."

Maybe apologizing *twice* would make certain he would go away?

"Well, young man," Mr. Davis said, his voice rising, "This will make sure you don't forget."

And without preamble he unbuckled his big brown leather belt, slipping it through the belt loops and quickly folding it double.

Mr. Davis' actions shocked my senses more than frightened me (did that too), because in the short few weeks I had known him, he seemed for the most part a kind and understanding person.

But just as with Mrs. Tomblin (twice) and Miss Warwick (once), Mr. Davis prefaced his whipping me with "young man." I was not a "young man" when Mrs. Tomblin slapped me hard across my face (ages seven and ten), nor when Miss Warwick (mean old bat) threatened to whip me (age seven). And here I was at age eleven, about to get it again, and here was my assailant du jour berating me with this "young man" horseshit.

Grownups use the expression "young man" when whaling the snot out of young defenseless children, because use of the term seems to provide the much needed justification for their brutality and ease their guilt. Ever hear a six-foot-tall, two hundred fifty pound grownup about to give a vulnerable seven-year-old child an unwarranted thrashing say "Okay, you skinny little seven-year-old defenseless child, I'm going to beat you senseless?"

"Bend over those feedbags," Mr. Davis ordered angrily.

Frightened out of my wits, I did as ordered, and abruptly he brought his leather belt down hard across my skinny eleven-year-old butt, a total of eight times. The boys downstairs in the milking barn counted them.

Out of breath from the exertion of the beating, Mr. Davis told me to get up and I did so, trembling with sobs. I was the first boy Mr. Davis ever strapped. But I believe that as soon as he whipped me, Mr. Davis was ashamed at having lost his temper.

His shaking voice immediately took on a conciliatory tone. He placed his hand on my shoulder, looked into my watery eyes, and said,

"Now, Alton, if you leave the mother out, the baby calf won't get fed that night. So just make sure you take all the mothers to the Green Barn at night. Do you understand?"

His was a voice of apology, and even at that young age, I recognized it as such. And he didn't call me "young man" again, so I felt I was out of the infamous Z.I.D. (Zone of Immediate Danger). In fact, I believe for the decade I was a prisoner at Oxford, I lived on the fringes of the Z.I.D.

"Yes, sir," I said, my bony chest still heaving from hurt and embarrassment.

"I won't forget again."

During the next few days Mr. Davis went out of his way to talk to me, to encourage me in my work. But his shame just would not allow him to apologize for losing his temper. However, I understood his unstated apology, silently accepted it as such, and Mr. Davis became the only person in my life whom I never despised for whipping me. He became my best friend among the orphanage staff members, up there with Maurice Parham, the orphanage controller and main money man. Even after I left the dairy I visited Mr. Davis often and sought his advice and guidance.

But at that moment I was hurt, physically and emotionally, having once again received an unwarranted thrashing.

The day after my belting by Mr. Davis, Butch Mitchell and I had to make the daily trek to the bullpen to feed Vic and Ace. I was still smarting, physically and emotionally, from the surprise assault, and wasn't exactly in a sociable mood. Having my backside soundly whipped within earshot of ten of my peers was humiliating and degrading.

I was royally upset. And I was learning to hold a grudge. After feeding Vic and Ace, Butch and I climbed onto the slats that formed the front wall of Ace's enclosed and roofed wooden "barn," and were just shootin' the breeze and spittin' hawkers on Ace's head, when suddenly and without preamble or comment, I climbed over the top of the slats and eased myself slowly down onto the ground where this big old half-ton or more animal was hard at work feeding his face.

The disparity in our sizes was such that Ace's head alone weighed more than I did. In fact, as huge as he was, Ace's testicles probably weighed more than I did. Perhaps overnight I had developed some sort of weird pubescent death wish. Perhaps it was in defiance of Mr. Davis, who had told us repeatedly never to go into the bulls' pens. Fuck Mr. Davis! Didn't scare me in the least. Scared hell out of Butch, though. Quickly climbing to the top of the slats, he frantically reached for me, thinking I had fallen.

"Al, get the hell out of there. If ole Ace don't kill you, Mr. Davis sure will."

"Fuck Mr. Davis! And fuck Ace, too!" I said, in determined defiance, waving my hand dismissively at the dehorned monster standing patiently beside me. Noticing the wave of my hand in his periphery (bulls also had finely-tuned side glance vision, apparently), Ace looked my way. I didn't flinch. But just to be safe, I didn't do any more stupid dismissive hand waving either.

Old Ace took one look at me, quickly computed that I was no threat to him, grunted, snorted, and farted (in that order) and just kept on eating. With a temerity born of a mixture of stupidity, youth and frustration, I reached over and tentatively began rubbing the huge monster's head, being careful to navigate my hand around mine and Butch's gobs of spit.

Ace shook his head, and I jerked back reflexively. He kept on eating. I decided not to rub his head anymore. Butch just stood on the slats all bug-eyed, shaking his head in silent awe at this stupid-assed friend of his.

"Come on in, Butch," I said. "He's not gonna hurt you. You didn't hurt him, and we're the ones who feed him."

"We'd better leave, Al," Butch replied, still shaking his head in disbelief, apparently not fathoming my dumbass dirt-clod "logic."

"You go on, Butch," I replied with confidence, all the time not taking my eyes off my mammoth new-found "friend."

But Butch stayed with me, whether from morbid curiosity or friendship I did not know. After Ace finished foundering himself on his feed, I cautiously walked alongside him (though not exactly touching) as he moved to the outside Cyclone-fenced area. Ace continued to ignore me, so I finally mustered up the courage to touch his side. He still ignored me, so finally I gently patted his side.

Finally it came time to return to the dairy. As I walked away I said to Ace, "Sorry we spit on your head, Ace. We won't do it again. You're a good bull."

I'm certain I really meant to say good "friend," so much was I in need of another, be it human or animal. On the way back to the dairy, I felt elated. Butch said he thought I was crazy. We agreed never to mention our little adventure to anyone.

What causes a skinny-assed eleven-year-old kid to climb into an enclosed area with a huge bull and risk being trampled to death? My only explanation is that it was an act of defiance growing out of the previous day's thrashing by yet another callous and unbridled grownup.

I've never regretted my act of stupidity, or bravery, or whatever word one might choose to describe my foolish actions. However, I firmly believe the entire episode of Mr. Davis and Ace became a solid rung on my ladder leading to maturity. And Butch and I agreed that we never would again spit on Ace's head. The lesson learned is that one does not spit on the head of one's friends, be they animal or human.

An event occurred about six months after the above-related incident that caused me to pause and reconsider what I had done. Vic was the younger of the two bulls, and he still had his horns. Ace, the older bull, had been dehorned. A double Cyclone fence separated the two outside pens, one bull in each pen. Apparently one night or early morning Ace got mad at Vic, tore through the bottom of the Cyclone fences, and trampled young Vic. I decided after that day never to enter Ace's pen again. But I still looked upon the ferocious monster as my friend.

CHAPTER 35

Cornsilk Fags

On a late afternoon in August 1950, after the milking was completed, the cows had been let out to pasture for the night, and we were busy shoveling cow manure and hosing down the concrete floor of the dairy, Jack asked us "new" boys if we had ever smoked a "fag," which was what a cigarette was called in Great Britain and in our confined little world. Almost in unison, Arnold, Butch and I shook our heads.

"Okay, may as well show you how," said Jack. "You guys go down to the cornfield beside the bullpen, and grab a handful of cornsilk off five or six ears of corn. Make sure it's brown, not green."

"Cornsilk" is the bunch of styles and stigmas that appears as a tuft or tassel sticking out of the unattached ear of corn that has not yet been shucked, and is often used as a diuretic in herbal medicine. It is the pollen-bearing influorescence of the corn plant. At first colored light green, as the weeks pass it dries up and turns light brown in color.

Eagerly and quickly the three of us did as instructed, and shortly three pairs of skinny legs were racing back to the dairy, carrying our precious cornsilk, while three tiny hearts raced with anticipation of smoking our first fag. Another small step, we figured, on our way to becoming "Big Boys."

Jack then tore a page from a funny book, and when we placed the dried cornsilk on the table in the milkroom, he tore the sheet of paper widthwise into three equal strips.

"This is how you do it," Jack calmly instructed, picking up a portion of the dry brown cornsilk. He proceeded to expertly and gently twist the cornsilk, then when it had a somewhat cylindrical shape, rolled it between his open palms several times to better shape and compact it.

Next he placed the cylinder of cornsilk onto the paper, and rolled the paper around the cornsilk twice. Licking the length of the paper as he would an envelope, he pressed the wet edge against the paper. It stuck like glue. Then, pinching off the end of the roll that contained no cornsilk, he proudly handed it to me.

"Okay, kid, I'll light it for you. All you got to do is drag on it with your breath. Now take a big pull."

Not a problem. Sounded simple enough. As Jack struck the large kitchen match and held the flame under the end of the fag, I exhaled quickly, then with all the lung power I could muster, sucked in what must have been the then orphans' all-time record volume of cornsilk smoke.

Immediately my lungs filled with the hot smoke, the shock of what had occurred literally knocking me flat on my back, and I couldn't breathe. In panic, I kept trying to inhale, flailing my arms about as I began writhing in panic on the ground behind the dairy.

Sensing what had happened, Jack quickly jerked me off the ground and began hitting me on the back with the heel of his open hand.

"Breathe out! Breathe out! Breathe out!" he shouted, holding me up while he continued pounding me on my back, with Arnold and Butch looking on in helpless terror.

Trembling with fright and shock, I finally caught my breath and sat down on the ground, dazed, light-headed, my lungs on fire.

"Dammit, kid, you ain't supposed to drag on it *that* hard," said Jack, squatting beside me, visibly relieved that I had not died from the experience.

Well, I had just smoked my very first fag, got the daylights scared out of me for my troubles, and swore then and there I would never smoke another. And for the rest of that day, I didn't. Did smoke another two days later, and like most orphan boys, became a connoisseur of cornsilk fags. And in 1950, the best smoke an orphan kid could get for the money. Of course, we didn't know at that time the diuretic effect of cornsilk, but looking back, we boys sure did pee a lot after smoking one of them there fags.

CHAPTER 36

Dabs

You could play "dabs" on any sized spot of ground that was bare and hard, and that had fairly good drainage. The favorite central location was what a few of us termed the "battleground" (after reading accounts of the Korean War in the Raleigh *News and Observer* and the Durham *Morning Herald*), a widened-out area along the dirt pathway leading from 3-B and 4-B to the school.

The basic games of dabs were "triangles" and "circles," and much like the game of horseshoes, a game we played with real well-worn horseshoes, dabs was a game of skill, certainly not for the lighthearted. However, unlike the game of horseshoes, that was enjoyed by boys from 1-B through 4-B, dabs was played mainly among the younger boys ages ten through twelve, who lived in 1-B and 2-B.

We didn't have to mark a triangle or circle in the hardened, well-worn ground-several of each shape had been grooved for us permanently into the red clay years before I ever first mustered the courage to match my "skill," so it was, against a taunting older playmate in my first game of "keepsies."

"Triangles. Tens up. Keepsies," the ten-year-old sixth-grader challenged, massaging a large steelie about the size of a regular glass dab between his left thumb and first two fingers, all the time eyeing the bulge that at my young age could only have been a goodly number of dabs in the left pocket of those stupid-assed knickers we were still forced to wear.

But the dabs "sharks" could always spot the "first-timers." It was late Summer of 1950, and in June I had moved from the Walker Building to 1-B with five other kids who had also just completed the sadistic Baby Elephant's fifth grade. The previous Saturday afternoon I had braved heat and thorns, toiling alone for three hours in an area of the expansive pasture we called the "thicket," where the ground was low and overgrown with thorny shrubs, and chock full of delicious, plump blackberries. Resisting the overpowering urge to eat up all my profits, a malady to which many orphan boys before my time had succumbed, I had filled five medium-sized paper lunch bags with the precious harvest, and, cautiously circling the main campus in order to avoid the stupid and equally ruthless "raiders" from 3-B and 4-B, who might take by force my five bags of "gold," I sold them to an elderly lady who lived about two blocks from the main gate of the campus. The blue-rinsed lady and her equally snow-topped husband did not have any children, and I was seriously considering asking them if they could be my parents.

The kind old lady had paid me a quarter for each bag of blackberries, and I had scampered as fast as my skinny white thorn-scarred and bleeding legs could carry me, to the small mom-and-pop candy store (that we now call "convenience" stores) that was located on Alexander Avenue a block from the main gate, clutching my dollar bill and quarter, where I purchased my first ever two cloth-mesh bags of multi-colored regular dabs, each containing about twenty of the treasured spheres, and had duly celebrated my ingenuity and newly-acquired status as a dabs owner, with an orphan's greatest reward save a peanut butter and molasses sandwich, that being a Moon Pie and an RC Cola.

So here at last I stood, alone on the famed "battleground," eagerly anticipating my first ever game of "keepsies," which, as the name implies, what you were skillful enough to knock out of the triangle or circle, you got to keep. At last I had graduated from the neophyte world of "funsies," where the timid players got their marbles back after each game, to the "big time." It was euphoria. Little did I know I was about to "lose my ass."

"Funsies," a child's game (of which I swore I had never taken part), was played with dabs borrowed from friends, but I had soon tired of the lack of challenge, feeling somewhat akin to the only horse running in the Kentucky Derby, and I was determined to make my move up the social ladder, to gain the admiration and respect a dabs champion enjoyed among his peers. A nagging concern at that critical moment, however, as I stood on the cusp of certain (that is, certain in my own mind) fame and (quite literally) fortune, was the fact that I did not yet own a coveted "steelie," which is a steel ballbearing used as a "shooter" for the quite obvious reason that a steel ballbearing will hit a glass dab much harder than will another glass dab. You know, physics and all that.

"Tens is good," I responded, mustering all the confidence I could.

"Keepsies is good," I added, then hesitated momentarily.

"Circles, not triangles," I added with a note of intractable protest in my raspy voice.

"Why not triangles?"

"'Cause you got a steelie, and I don't got one. You'll stomp me in triangles with a steelie." The big kid weren't talking to no sucker. I had observed the older boys playing dabs for about a month. By historical convention, circles were much larger than triangles and, I might add, a heckuva lot rounder.

To determine the order of shooting, each boy stood about four feet from a long groove that had been cut into the dirt long before, and tossed a dab, trying to get as close as possible to the line. The order of proximity to the line determined the order of shooting. Then, if you were playing triangles, each kid's dabs were bunched in the center of the triangle with those of the other players. The initial shot for each player was not made from the perimeter of the triangle (as was the case with "circles") but from a grooved line outside the triangle.

The game of dabs was similar in some respects to billiards, or "pool," as everyone called the game. If the player shot his shooter into the triangle or circle, and he knocked a dab out of the enclosure, he got to "keep" that dab; thus the obvious name "keepsies." In addition, if he knocked a dab out of the enclosure, and his shooter remained inside the perimeter of the triangle or circle, he was allowed to continue shooting as long as his shooter remained in the enclosure after each shot.

The unwritten rule was that each player had his choice of what he wanted to use as a shooter, a regular-sized glass dab, a steelie, or a "gollywhopper" (that we called a "golly" for short). A gollywhopper is just what the word implies; it is a glass marble, or dab as we called it, about three times larger than a regular dab. However, gollies were rarely used as shooters, because the size makes it too cumbersome for nine- and ten-year-olds to grasp and shoot straight. The most desirable shooter was the steelie, and an experienced dabs combatant knew just how to spin the steelie so that, when it struck a glass dab, the struck dab would be propelled out of the circle or triangle, leaving the steelie spinning in its vacated space. This we called "sticking" the shooter, or "hit and stick" the shooter.

Because I have never seen the word "dab" in any dictionary, and have never heard the word used in the context of the game of marbles outside the orphanage, I believe the word "dab" to be a nonce word, that is, a word that is invented or used just for a particular occasion.

Anyway, my challenger figured that since he was more experienced than I, and his shooter a commanding steelie and mine a mere glass dab, that in just a few minutes he would render me dabless anyway. However, apparently impressed with my tough bargaining stance, and my determination not to meet him on an uneven playing field (glass dab versus steelie), the older boy said,

"Tell yu whut I'm gonna do, kid. I got another steelie. How many dabs yu got?"

"Two bags full," I said, pulling the unopened mesh bags from my pocket and holding them out in an orphan's tentative "see-but-don't-even-think-about-touching" stance.

"Okay," he said. "That's twenty dabs in each bag. Tell yu whut I'm gonna do. Put one bag back in yu knickers." Older kids have all sorts of ways to belittle younger kids. He specified that I put my dabs back in my "knickers," when he could just as easily have said "pocket." The "knickers" comment was to let me know that he was older than I, and that he did not have to wear the stupid knickers anymore. Don't play with my mind, you stupid prick. But this was a thought, not a spoken comment.

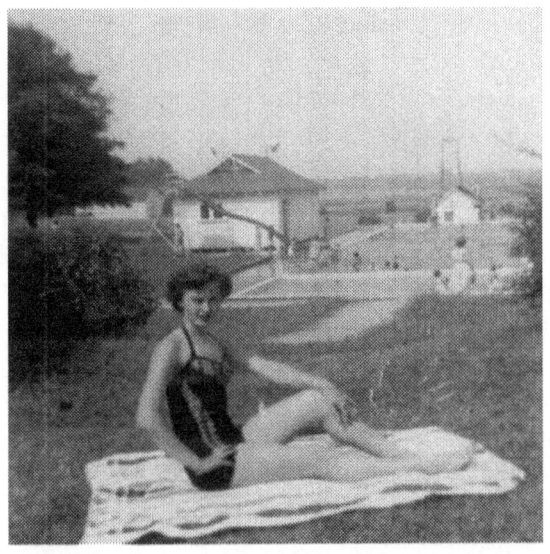

Swimming pool and shower house. Pool is divided into "baby pool" and "big pool."

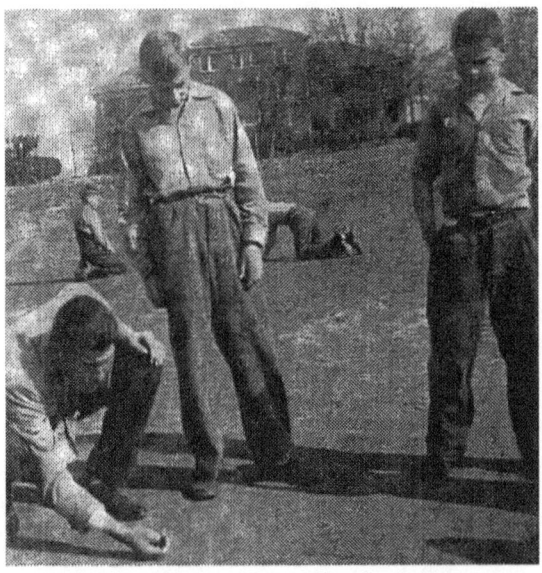

1950. Playing "dabs" on "battleground" beside school. "Big Boy" Paul Davidson is "knuckling" a shooter. The author, age eleven, is in near background, far left (in overalls).

I did as instructed, feeling a mild sense of relief.

"Now, I'll give yu one of mu steelies fur ten of yur dabs. This way, yu'll allus have a steelie. Then we ken quit footlin' 'round an' play dabs."

We made the trade, and with great pride I realized I had reached a milestone along my arduous path to maturity-any kid who can at such an early age come into possession of a "steelie" was definitely a cut above his peers. I was really proud. Since we had agreed on keepsies, circles and tens, I gave the older boy my remaining ten marbles from the opened mesh bag, and he counted ten marbles from the bulge inside his front pants (not knickers, mind you) pocket. Placing the twenty dabs in the center of the circle, he expertly corralled the dabs between his thumbs and index fingers.

"Justa be fair," he said, "We won't throw 'tsee who goes first. Yu go on an break 'um."

My "time" had arrived. This was my big chance. I was going to get an opportunity to prove myself. I wasn't going to fail. Nosireebob. Nervously I placed my new steelie between thumb and first two fingers, took careful aim at the twenty spheres of gold amassed in the center of the circle, and with all the force I could muster, thrust my right thumb forward, propelling my precious steelie against the mass of glass.

My steelie bounced harmlessly off the concentrated dabs and out of the large circle. I knew then that I had a lot to learn. Then, without expression or comment, as though this were routine stuff with him, my teenage opponent "broke" the mass of dabs, knocking three of the dabs out of the ring, and I watched in silent awe and dejection as the expert nearly "ran" the circle of dabs, half of which had just a moment before belonged to me. I had made a colossal blunder, a lesson learned. It was back to the blackberry patch for me.

More out of pity than not, I ended up with three dabs out of the twenty we had put up for the match. Then the kid who had solidly trounced me said,

"That's okay, kid, yu did good." Then he silently counted out seven dabs from his winnings, said "Hold out yur hand, kid," and put the seven dabs in my open hand.

"What's this for?" I asked. "You won 'em fair and square."

"You're okay, kid," replied the boy, and I knew I had found a lifelong friend.

The expression "playing dabs," when done among young orphan boys on the "battleground" located beside John Nichols School in the 1940's, was undoubtedly a glaring misnomer. To us kids the "game" was as serious as cold snot, as real almost as death. I never saw a smile or heard laughter-you could at times cut the tension with the blade of a trusty Barlow knife. Those were *my* five dabs bunched together with the ten from my two opponents. I had picked a lot of blackberries, or stolen a lot of strawberries, in order to earn the money to purchase those precious multi-colored gems, and I didn't want to lose them. So my unannounced goal was to recover my five spheres of gold, then take as many of the others as possible. Unfortunately, this was also the unstated goal of the kids playing against me. Almost seemed unfair. To me.

If a kid had to say something, he did so between shots or between games. And he damn well better not decide to rip a loud fart while some other kid was shooting. Such conduct was unacceptable, to put it mildly. That is, unless you were a Big Boy. A Big Boy was by definition allowed to fart as often and as loud as he wished anytime he wanted to. I just couldn't wait to grow up to be a Big Boy. Lots of prestige and meaningful perks.

To shoot, the player would get on his knees, brace his non-shooting hand (or forearm) on the ground for better support, and "knuckle" the shooter in his shooting hand. "Knuckle" is the act of shooting a dab when the thumb is placed over the bent forefinger. The shooter hunches his shoulders, tensing his entire body, then puts all the energy he can in his shooting hand, and lets go. This great concentration of bodily energy when knuckling a dab is the origin of the term "knuckle down" as used in its secondary meaning "to work energetically or seriously." This term means to really apply oneself to a task, which is exactly what you had to do in order to win at dabs.

Coley Lee Hackett was one of the better dabs players. Shooting with his (evil) left hand, Coley Lee could make a steelie spin in place of the glass dab it had propelled about five feet away. And he rarely ever missed. Javon Frye was really good, and Van Edwards wasn't far behind.

The game of dabs taught me one lesson in life, of which I am forever grateful-that is, you don't have to be an expert at something in order to enjoy it. Dabs was just such a game for me. A chipped, battle-scarred shooter was a source of pride, and some kids were not averse to hitting their shooter against a concrete sidewalk in order to attain this false self-esteem.

I was proud of myself at age ten for entering the realm of "keepsies" in playing dabs. I was so proud of the town I was from, Kinston, but must admit I was ashamed that those other two of my peers from Kinston, Red Albertson and Ersul Sowers, were still playing "funsies" when they were in tenth grade. No guts, no glory.

CHAPTER 37

The Blue Flame

One cold and rainy Sunday afternoon in late Fall of 1950, after I had been in 1-B for several months, some of us kids were playing various board games or listening to the radio in the first floor study hall. The heavy afternoon rains had kept us indoors, and after an hour or so, boredom, that instigator of youthful mischief, had descended like a black cloud over our little group.

The favorite inclement weather indoor sport among 1-B and 2-B boys was what we called "knee football." The first floor study hall in every cottage consisted of a large room with a hardwood floor, that was kept waxed and polished as one of the daily duties of several boys in each cottage. On rainy weekends we read funny books, played pick-up sticks with wooden popsicle sticks and played jack-rocks with real pebbles, and checkers. When we tired of these games, somebody would say the magic words "knee football" and we would begin moving the chairs and wooden study hall tables against the side walls, quickly converting the first floor study hall into a shiny slippery football field. Miniature rubber footballs had just become popular, and if we did not have one of those handy, several thick socks were rolled up and tied with string and this became our football du jour. Two boys elected themselves to choose players for their teams.

One of the most striking sociological phenomenon that surfaces among thirty preteen boys living together is how quickly they establish the "pecking order." Rarely did the proverbial "bully" last that long at the orphanage. The Big Boys, i.e., the older boys in tenth, eleventh and twelfth grades, usually had younger brothers, and, if not, had established a friendship with some younger boys because such friendship gave the older boy access to the younger boy's older sister. These things just seemed to sort themselves out. It was an unwritten but very real rule among the older orphanage boys that the way to a girl's heart was through friendship (read that "protection") with the girl's younger brother. The best example I have of this is my sister Eoline, who was two years older than I, and was blessed with natural good looks and a bulky blouse.

Of course, at the age of eleven I was not quite certain why Bobby Boyette and Javon Frye had suddenly become my "friends," but they sure did talk a lot about my sister and what good friends of hers they were. But that was good enough for me.

Thus as ten- and eleven-year-olds in 1-B and 2-B, the Big Boys protected us as best they could from the stupid dork banditos in 4-B, a few of whom we younger boys became firmly convinced had years before been fathered by our collective nemesis, the Reverend A. DeLeon Gray himself.

The pecking order referred to above concerns the balance of strengths and weaknesses that became established in the Walker Building and remained with us throughout the years. I could run faster than the other boys. When I made the varsity football team in the ninth grade, I could outrun any boy on the team. Three years later, as a senior, I could still outrun everyone.

Beginning with our days in the Walker Building, nobody ever "messed" with Newton Wilder or Blockhead Johnson. If a boy was dumb enough to challenge either of them, he was fortunate to escape the encounter with minor bruises. Yet I never saw Newton or Blockhead pick on any younger boys. The other kids were certainly not afraid of these two classmates-let's just call it a "healthy respect."

Bill Herrington and Van Edwards were the most dependable. Even as youngsters they reminded me of a pair of bulldogs. Both were nearly as fast on their feet as I . . . but not quite. Red Albertson was tall even as a ten-year-old, and could jump a lot higher than any of us.

Frank McMillan was a few years older than our gang, but was in the same grade as we were. I always felt safe with Frank on my team. He was kinda slow on his feet, but always carried his weight on the football field. You could depend on his friendship and loyalty, and no opposing running back got past his side of the line.

Anyway, when we chose up sides to play knee football on a rainy weekend afternoon, one "captain" chose a player, then the other "captain" chose one, just as when we played on the outside ball fields. Since we were aware of each other's strengths and weaknesses, the teams were always evenly matched.

So on that particular rainy Sunday afternoon we chose up sides. The following rules were observed in knee football. You had to stay on your hands and knees. You could not raise one or both knees off the floor to propel yourself forward. This was called cheating, and some opposing player would demand that any touchdown that occurred on that play be called back.

Likewise, you couldn't raise your hands off the floor to block an opponent. So you blocked by using your head and shoulders. There were no out of bounds markers except for the walls. You tackled the ball carrier by knocking his knees from beneath him, thereby flattening his body. If an opponent by "mistake" hit you in the mouth with his head or shoulder, you committed the same "mistake" a little later. Rarely did we play a game of knee football in which no blood was spilled on the shiny hardwood floor, or at least one kid did not receive a black eye from an errant elbow.

We were a competitive, rowdy, mouthy bunch of boys, and all of us were "poor" losers. Likewise, there were no graceful winners; suffering defeat in a game of knee football meant to lose face, and we played until we were exhausted, or until Witch Robinson forced us to quit for fear we would really hurt one another, or the supper bell rang.

Anyway, on that particular bleak, cold and rainy afternoon, we had just started to choose up sides for our knee football game, when I noticed the absence of some of the older boys, simultaneously being drawn to bursts of uproarious giggling and laughter emanating from the cottage basement.

Presently we heard shouts of "Let me try it," "My turn," and "Gimme dem matches." More preteen raucous laughter. Then quiet. Then spontaneous howling.

Our curiosity definitely aroused, we crept out into the hallway and down the stairs leading to the basement. Halfway down the flight of stairs, I peered between the balusters into the basement.

In the center of a circle of giggling older boys, Bobby was on his hands and knees, his trousers and undershorts down around his ankles, his skinny bare white ass pointed skyward. About two feet to one side of Bobby's bare ass crouched Butch, a large kitchen match in one hand and the closed box of matches in the other.

"Ready!" said Bobby. This apparently was Butch's cue, and quickly striking the large matchhead against the matchbox, Butch held the lighted match about a foot from Bobby's bare ass.

Upon hearing the matchhead strike against the side of the matchbox, we heard Bobby grunt and strain, his face reddening. We next heard a loud fart, then watched in utter amazement the blue flame shooting about two feet behind Bobby's ass. Looked like a human rocket, he did, straight out of a Flash Gordon funny book.

This dramatic spectacle was followed immediately by howls of laughter and cries of "I'm next. I'm next!" I sat speechless on the stairwell, having just observed my very first session of the orphans' *real* favorite rainy day sport, burning farts, and I'll never forget the experience. And I discovered that, in the atmosphere of competitiveness that was just as much a part of our lives as playing dabs, running footraces and lifting weights, the kid who could burn the longest blue fart was on par with the kid who, standing in two-foot deep snow on a freezing January day, could pee the farthest on a full bladder.

From 1950, flash forward half a century, to the Fall of 2002, so that you may become convinced of the wartime and postwar sport of burning farts. Anyway, I took my wife to see the latest picture show entitled *Hart's War*, starring Bruce Willis. The picture show concerned captured American soldiers being held in a German POW camp during World War II.

After lights-out one night, we observed one G.I. flick a cigarette lighter in the darkness, whereupon a blue flame shot out of the darkness of the barracks, and appropriate boasts were made by the "flamer." My wife asked what the cigarette lighter had to do with the resultant blue flame. So I explained it to her. She refused to believe me.

CHAPTER 38

The Return of the Balloon Boys

Tip-toeing quietly through the stand of scrub pines, interspersed like midgets beneath the tall oaks, we were dead certain of one thing-somebody was hurting somebody, real bad. Had to be. No doubt about it. The labored grunting like an old root hog, emanating though muffled from the back seat of a large shiny black sedan, definitely came from a man. No doubt about it. And the high-pitched squealing like a stuck pig was frantic and panicky, imploring it seemed to us, to stop the old root hog from hurting what could only have been a teenage girl. No doubt about that, either.

This bouncy duet was being played out before our unflinching gazes and furrowed brows in the Fall of 1950, in the back seat of a 1948 Ford sedan, a heavy vehicle that took a lot of energy to make it move back and forth like that. And it was really beating a two-step.

Butch Mitchell and I had been just moseying along through the woods on a brisk Saturday afternoon. The dying, multi-colored Fall leaves blanketing the ground crackled beneath our well-worn brogues as we approached innocently the edge of what we had come to call the "lovers' lane" at the far edge of the orphanage farm.

Because we tended to focus on the ground before us as we trekked the expansive farm and woods, you know, snakes and other slithering creatures, the initial sounds of the car's occupants startled us, and we stopped short about twenty yards shy of the ruckus. The big vehicle wasn't moving, but then again, it *was* moving. It wasn't going straight ahead, but swaying left and right, like it couldn't make up its mind whether to make a right or left turn, or was building momentum for a forward thrust.

From our vantage point, Butch and I could see that the windows were all fogged up. And all that godawful grunting and squealing going on inside the big car. Orphan kids are if nothing else curious little devils, what with leading such a structured existence and all. So we orphan boys sought out the unusual, the surprise, the extraordinary, as a welcome diversion. Butch and I just had to see what was going on inside that steamed-up automobile. Apparently whatever the mean sonofagun was doing to the little girl, she was begging him to stop, and we had to do something to help her.

We crept closer, as silently as our brogues would allow through the sound of stiff leather crushing dead Fall oak leaves. Butch reached the car first, and, cupping his opened palms over his eyes to keep out the glare, peered inside. Ole Butch may have seemed a little nutso at times, but he sure possessed an enviable degree of moxie. Butch Mitchell and Coley Lee Hackett. I learned a lot about courage from these two little hell-raisers.

About that time I heard the muffled pleas of the young female squealer emanating from inside the vehicle become more distinct.

"No! Don't! Stop!"

"No! Don't! Stop!"

Her cries were interspersed with the mean old grunter's steady grunts, indicating that he had no intention of stopping whatever it was he was doing to the little girl. After a few seconds, Butch turned and motioned me with a wave of his arm to the other side of the vehicle. Copying Butch's glare-reducing technique, I got real close to the rear window, cupped my hands over my eyes a la Butch, and peered into the seemingly perpetual motion machine. Through the light fog on the window, I saw cupped-hands Butch's face pressed against the window, peering back at me in wonderment. Omigod! I had never before seen anything like this! Between our two amazed pairs of bulging eyes lay a tangled mass of naked arms and legs, some large of both body parts, with a lot of ugly hair, some slim, smooth pretty body parts. Seemed like the large ugly mean man was trying to crush the fair-skinned young girl, whose long blond hair cascaded across her face and spread out on the back seat. And amid cries of fear, both Hairy and Pretty were doing a lot of grunting and squealing and moving. And she was still pleading with her attacker.

"No! Don't! Stop!"

"No! Don't! Stop!"

Judging by the round bald spot at the back of his gray head, he (the "grunter") appeared old enough to be her (the "squealer") daddy, which, in rural North Carolina in the Fall of 1950, might well have been the case. In a panic I wondered how best to make the mean old bastard stop hurting the beautiful teenager.

Suddenly, the young girl's hair parted, and two beautiful blue eyes stared up at me over the grunter's shoulder. She blinked a few times, as if trying to clear a picture. Then she let out a terrified shriek, and apparently sensing Butch and I were there to save her, shouted "Goddamn you, you sonofabitch!" and pushed at the old man hurting her.

Drawn into their little melodrama, I stood frozen, peering in through the car window, wide-eyed and hands cupped, when suddenly the grunter turned, which in itself was quite an accomplishment, given that the two of them were interlocked seemingly permanently.

"You little sonofabitch, you!" he screamed, trying desperately to extricate himself from his contortionist's predicament. As I turned to escape I heard the rear car door on my side open, followed quickly by the rustle of leaves beneath pounding bare feet, and then there the grunter was, bounding after me like a naked hairy demon from hell, and I was shocked to see that his peepee seemed to be covered by one of the "balloons" we had discovered at an earlier time, and the "balloon" was flopping to and fro before him. I ran for my little ole Peeping Tom life. Butch was nowhere in sight. Seeing the grunter chasing after me, Butch had lit out in the opposite direction. Sometimes old Butch was about half smart. And sometimes I wasn't.

Sprinting through the trees and certainly not looking back anymore, I heard over my shoulder,

"Come back here, you little bastard! I'll break your goddamn neck! I'll kill you!" And then he called me what must have been some really awful names, because I didn't understand much of what he shouted. Sounded like he was really, really upset, though.

Finally, the sound of bare feet pounding dry oak leaves subsided, and I cautiously slowed to a brisk walk, panting and out of breath. Pointing my (best hearing) left ear in the direction of my escape, presently I heard the welcome roar of an automobile engine, that I hoped belonged to a shiny black 1948 Ford sedan, followed by the screech and slide of blackwall tires across a blanket of dead leaves, and soon the sounds faded into the distance.

Still frightened out of our wits, Butch and I used the orphan's favorite proven means of communication to locate one another.

"Butch!"

"Al!"

"Butch!"

"Al!"

"Here I am. Is the old bastard gone?"

"Yeah, I think so. He must have been really hurting that little girl."

"You know, I didn't really see her crying."

"Come to think of it, neither did I."

And not yet understanding the meaning of such goings-on, we continued our trek through the beautiful, multi-colored Fall orphanage Saturday afternoon, feeling somewhat proud of ourselves that we had saved the beautiful blond teenage squealer from further harm, but at the same time wondering in the backs of our naïve, unsophisticated minds why she had not been crying. She must have been a brave young girl, to scream like that, yet not cry. She certainly would be an inspiration to other young girls under the same or similar circumstances. Or so I reasoned.

On the way back to the campus, Butch got very quiet, and I realized he was in deep thought. After a long while he said,

"She sure was pretty. Maybe we could come back next Saturday. She might be here again."

"Butch, you're crazier'n heck. That guy could of killed us."

He was off his bean if he thought I was going anywhere near any more big black Fords moving left and right while standing still in the desolate "balloon" area. Nosireebob. Little Al was gonna mind his own business from now on. Weren't gonna save any more big-titted blond-haired fifteen-year-old country girls what might not have wanted to be saved. Not ever again. Damn. I could of been killed. For nothing.

CHAPTER 39

Mr. Walker's Firewater

At a point about three years into my open-ended prison sentence, I came to equate Trouble (always capitalized, of course), with quicksand-I was forever falling into it, and it sucked me under every time.

The lovers' lane way over yonder aways past the railroad trestle near the road to Henderson had early on produced two events of unflagging interest, 1) an overabundance of "balloons," a continuing embarrassment among my peers, and 2) an unexpected encounter with a terrified(?) teenage girl and her hairy-assed, mad-as-a-hornet "attacker."

Now, that first event I had tried my darndest to expunge forever from my memory, being constantly thwarted in this attempt by callous and dimwitted 4-B yahoos. But the latter, that glorious image of the ample-bosomed blond teenage beauty, apparently had been painted indelibly onto my puerile, innocent mind's highly-impressionable and receptive canvas.

And most assuredly on the mind and imagination of my friend Butch as well. The end result of this downy-cheeked sexual arousal (although I'm certain neither of us recognized it as such at the time) was that periodically my voyeur buddy and I would return on a Saturday or Sunday afternoon to the scene of the "assault," just to see if perchance the object of our infatuation had returned for yet another back seat romp with her uncle/daddy/much older brother. Moths to the flame, and all that naturally follows.

Thus on a cold and damp Saturday afternoon in mid-December 1951, Butch asked me if I wanted to trek to the farm "just to see what we might find." I knew exactly what Butch meant, and because the back seat of the big black Ford sedan had but two windows through which to gawk, unfortunately we could not invite any of our comrades along on our fact-finding excursion into the forest. And personally, I did not relish having to fight Blockhead Johnson or Mad Dog Wilder for a window position.

As we cautiously approached the near edge of the large clearing that apparently served as the centerpiece of the area's "balloon" rituals, that certain slant of light on that particularly dreary Winter's afternoon glinted off what at first blush appeared to be a cylinder of glass propped against the base of a half-century-old oak tree. In the midst of the gloom and drabness that Winter seems to inflict on everything it touches, Butch and I momentarily forgot about the purpose of our mission, and approached the source of the reflected light, that as we drew closer, seemed to take on the color of golden honey. The glass cylinder appeared to be propped up against the trunk of the large oak, waiting for its owner to return and claim it.

Which is exactly what Butch did, without hesitation, invitation or comment. Turning the large bottle pensively in his hands, Butch and I quickly deduced from the evidence before us that 1) the bottle never had been opened, 2) was filled halfway up the neck, and 3) appeared to contain, oh, if pressed to give an estimate, about one-fifth of a gallon, or possibly four-fifths of a quart, of the rich-looking yellowish-orange liquid.

The large label on the heavy bottle advised that apparently its contents at one time had been owned by a gentleman named "Johnnie Walker," and even showed a likeness of Mr. Walker, who appeared costumed as an eighteenth-century member of British aristocracy. Could even have been the Prime Minister or Mayor of London, for all I knew.

I was about to ask "I wonder who left this bottle here?" when Butch deftly popped the cap from the neck of the bottle, thereby breaking the very official-looking paper seal that had covered the upper neck and cap, and took a really big whiff of the contents.

Reminded me of when the previous year I had first taken a big drag off Jack Barger's cornsilk fag out behind the dairy barn. The powerful ninety-proof aroma galloped unchecked through pristine, uninitiated, suddenly flared nostrils, arriving at Butch's tender olfactory apparatus with such acid force that the shocked lad backed up about three giant steps, all the while not releasing his death grip on the neck of the bottle. A lasting memory indeed for a young orphan boy.

My perceptive and insightful friend must have figured that, if the contents of that bottle *smelled* that powerful, certainly the *taste* must be out of this world. I stood in that open "balloon" arena transfixed, as my stupid but curious twelve-year-old buddy threw back his head, tilted the large bottle about forty-two degrees north of horizontal, and took a really grownup-sized pull on the contents of what theretofore had been *Mr. Walker's* golden liquid. And right then and there I realized why in my pre-incarceration Saturday afternoon matinees at the Paramount on Queen Street, them pesky Injuns had referred to what flowed over the cusp of long-necked glass bottles as "firewater." Indeed!

Whatever it was in the dapper Englishman's bottle of spirits completely stole Butch's breath away. My startled friend immediately dropped the bottle, clutching at his throat with both hands as he fell backwards onto the bed of dried oak leaves and "balloons."

Rushing to my light-minded cottagemate's side, I knelt down on one knee beside him and, looking up into my awe-struck, terrified eyes, Butch gasped "Put the top back on that bottle." Not "I'm about to die, please help me," or "What in the world was that?" but "Put the top back on that bottle," was his urgent, breathless, strange yet barely whispered request.

In a fit of panic, I sat Butch up and slapped his back (a la Jack Barger and the cornsilk fag), and when my friend's breathing had gradually returned to about two-thirds normal, he looked up into my pained eyes and in a deadly serious, suddenly soprano Godfather-like half-whisper, said "Al, you just gotta try that stuff."

Which I did. On my first (quite tentative) pull, the stone-cold serious effects of that ninety-proof bounced right off my stomach lining and shot like a 155-millimeter Howitzer shell straight north, simultaneously sharpening my sense of smell and blurring my vision on its way to attacking my (very) small and (quite) uninitiated brain.

Pretty soon two reasonably calmed preteen orphans were sitting in the cold, damp air, on the cold, damp ground, at the base of that big old oak tree, passing Mr. Walker's firewater back and forth between us, taking small sips until, after we had consumed about half of the bottle's exotic-tasting contents, we began to slur our speech somewhat, seemingly at nothing in particular.

Suddenly the "balloons" surrounding us were funny, all our teachers, work supervisors and cottage counselors were stupid, and a lot of our cottagemates had developed theretofore unknown faults and idiosyncrasies.

We were amazed at how the "firewater" had made us more intelligent, brave and insightful, and had encouraged us to feel like stepping lightly and giggling as we danced among the "balloons" and dried oak leaves on that fading Winter's afternoon.

And as I sat propped up against that big oak tree, sipping the magic elixir, gradually a really strange warmth spread its way through my body, the golden liquid continuing to burn its way down my esophagus and radiate in a warm glow in my stomach. Suddenly I became consciously aware that I really didn't need my heavy woolen coat anymore, and my shivering from the effects of the December cold definitely subsided. I felt . . . , I felt . . . , well, really warm all over. And peaceful. I recalled wondering if this is what people meant when they spoke of "finding happiness."

Apparently fearing that a genie would surely escape from the treasured bottle should we consume its entire contents, Butch suggested that we might save the last third of the magic liquid for another day. Because in my tipsy, fully inebriated state I would have volunteered to walk to the Business Office and tell Old Man Gray to kiss my drunken little ass, I readily agreed with my friend.

So two happy, boisterous preteen orphans took a couple of sharp tree limbs, dug a shallow hole near the base of that huge oak tree, and buried our treasured bottle. We agreed that the first one of us to receive a whipping after that day would inform the other, and we would return to our hideout and finish what we had started.

Recovering (somewhat) our sense of balance, we made our way back across the Winter woods toward the campus and 1-B. Although we were walking side-by-side, we kept bumping into each other, so finally I decided to just follow along behind Butch, and I noticed that my intoxicated buddy was "weaving" moreso than walking. I had to hold him firmly by the shoulders so's he didn't misstep and fall off the railroad trestle.

Not a week passed before Mr. Davis strapped old smart-mouthed Butch out behind the dairy, for some real or imagined serious infraction of dairyhouse rules, and that Saturday afternoon we kept our pact. Butch Mitchell was probably the first dairy boy to actually try to get a whipping. And I was probably the first dairy boy to be happy that he did.

That Saturday afternoon we two eager (alcoholic) beavers couldn't wait to dig up our precious "firewater," and none of our cottagemates seemed to notice that we appeared much happier returning from the woods than starting out.

Every month or so Butch and I would revisit the condom patch, scour the ground like we were huntin' Easter eggs or something, and occasionally we got lucky. One day we found a nearly-full bottle of Jack Daniel's Tennessee Whiskey, and we were fascinated by the fact that the shape of the bottle was square.

And there were other "finds" containing lesser amounts of the precious "firewater," and two orphan preteens searching for the extraordinary in our Oliver Twist existence, were happy for any diversion from our humdrum lives, especially if it flowed from a long-necked glass bottle and sported the likeness of our dapper English aristocrat, or came all the way from Tennessee, wherever that was.

CHAPTER 40

Hog Killing

Holding the menacing, blood-soaked butcher knife down by his side with his right hand (he was right-handed) and reaching toward me with his left hand (that being his only remaining free hand), the killer instructed me in his most serious and commanding tone of voice.

"Gi me dur ri-ul, ow-un."

Having somehow by now mastered the Language of Bob Davis, the "ri-ul" was the .22-cal. rifle he had numerous times that same gray December morning handed to me after touching gently the business end of the slim metal barrel to a point just behind an unsuspecting 200-pound porker's left ear and calmly pulling the trigger, instantly paralyzing the animal with a small bullet to its brain, freeze-framing the theretofore mobile bacon factory's final moment.

For what seemed like the umpteenth time that cold morning we traded bloody knife for shiny rifle, and as I held the knife the dairy manager almost nonchalantly took aim behind the ear of his next victim, and pulled gently on the trigger. As though celebrating its last hurrah, the oinker remained perfectly calm, as if willingly accommodating Mr. Davis, who numerous times that same gray morning had just as calmly reached for the bloody blade I was holding outstretched in my left hand, and, bending at the knee for added momentum, plunged the blade nearly up to its hilt at a point just beneath the chin of the no-neck walking lard bucket.

This early December 1950 morning surrealistic slaughter of which the central figures appeared to be Mr. Davis, the collectively doomed grunters and I, was to remain forever an indelible part of memory.

I was at the time eleven years old, and why Mr. Davis chose me to play the role of Death's Assistant in this bizarre phantasmagoria I'll never know. But here I was once again, caught smack-dab in the middle of the action. The Creator in all His infinite wisdom apparently had selected Little Orphan Al to be an active participant in this continuing tragicomedy called "Oxford Orphanage," and not merely a spectator. I gladly would have opted for the latter, and would not have jockeyed for a front-row seat.

It took about twenty minutes to kill the hogs, and by the sound of the last report of the rifle Mr. Davis and I had perfected our timing of the transfer of blood-drenched butcher knife for the heavy-framed .22-cal rifle. And each time I heard the sound of the rifle fire I winced and closed my eyes tightly, reliving that cold Winter afternoon of my daddy's death, but a few years before, and by the day's end had firmly resolved never again to take part in this bloody nightmare-evoking ritual. And I never did. The traumatic memory of that day lasted for months afterward, and it was several years before I could bring myself to discuss the incident with Mr. Davis.

The gestation period of a sow is about 114 days, or close to four months. The average litter consists of seven of the cute little buggers, each weighing about two and a half pounds. You can call a pig a pig until all at once the animal gets so big you feel it's more respectful to call it a hog. Let's say, then, for point of reference, that a pig weighs less than 180 pounds. We slaughtered "hogs" at between 200-300 pounds.

Pigs, and the "Big Boys" of the swine family, the hogs, are excellent feed-to-food domestic animals, who quite literally eat about anything you slop before them. A hog will eat a dead human; however, the domestic hog will not attack a human, even if it believes the human is going to castrate it. So even as eleven- and twelve-year-olds, we kids were not afraid of even the largest hogs.

It has been said by more than one Southern country sage that the purpose of hog killing is to use every part of the hog but the squeal. And this is just about a fact. The larger parts of the hogs were cured with salt for bacon and ham. The small intestines of the butchered hogs were carried from the meat house to the vegetable house behind the kitchen. These small intestines were slit lengthwise, cleansed of food content, then cut into small sections. These pieces were then boiled or parboiled and then dried in the open air. And Presto, you have just made yourself a wash basin full of "chitlins."

Many common-usage words change their spellings and pronunciations over time. Say "North Carolina" twenty times quickly and it starts coming out "Nathcalina." Same with "chitlins." Say the proper word "chitterlings" twenty times quickly and you get "chitlins." Anyway, chitlins, the end product of this process, was a tasty, grease-filled delicacy on which we boys quickly foundered ourselves.

Then there is my daddy's favorite, pickled pigs' feet, or "souse." "Pickle" is the name given to a solution of brine or vinegar used to preserve and flavor foods. Thus a "pickle" is much tastier than the plain old cucumber from which it is transformed. "Souse," then, is any food steeped in pickle, more particularly pigs' feet.

"Foundered" is another of those "Southernisms," as I like to call them. The word "founder" means "to become sick from overeating," and originally was used in reference to farm animals, such as a cow or mule. However, we orphan kids used the term when we wished to express the idea that if we ate any more ice cream, or Musky Dines or (stolen) strawberries, we would become sick at our stomach.

In the Winter of 1947, the year I arrived at the orphanage, the farm and dairy boys slaughtered and dressed sixty-eight hogs to supply meat and lard for the children and staff. I specify "Winter" because as there was no freezer locker available with the capacity to store such an enormous quantity of meat, "hog killing" was not conducted during the warm months. The hams and other meats were cured with salt.

In 1948, forty-nine hogs were killed, furnishing nearly seven thousand pounds of dressed meat. The following year sixty-one hogs were slaughtered, and in 1950, my first year on the dairy, we killed fifty-one hogs that December. In 1951, the orphanage constructed a modern, all-brick freezer locker building behind the vegetable house, at a cost of $15,279.07 for the building and equipment. This expanded freezer storage facility served two purposes. First, it enabled the farm to slaughter hogs year round, even

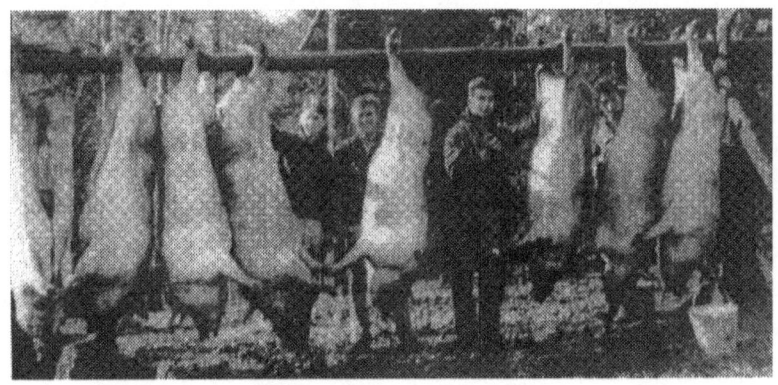

Hog killing time. "Bleeding" the hogs by suspending the carcasses head-down.

during the heat of Summer. Secondly, it allowed for an expansion of the capacity of the hog farm.

To this end, on April 1, 1951 twelve gilts (a young sow that has not yet "farrowed"-not yet given birth to a litter of piglets) were purchased from North Carolina State College in Raleigh. These gilts were added to the eleven sows and ninety-three hogs on hand. These hogs were slaughtered between April and September of that year. Thus construction of the freezer locker allowed the orphanage to nearly double (from fifty-one to ninety-three) the number of hogs slaughtered each year. Pork consumption at the orphanage totaled more than thirty-two thousand pounds, compared to seventeen thousand pounds in 1948.

There came a time about three or four months after a litter was born, that the poor males had to be relieved of any urges that might interfere with their eating. So Mr. Adams or Mr. Davis would round up about ten of us "lucky" boys, select a sharp (or dull, if no sharp one was readily available) knife, pick up a few metal containers of tar, and off we would go to the hog farm, to harvest "mountain oysters," as pig testicles are referred to in mixed company down South.

"Mountain oyster" harvesting was one of the most genteel, refined and solemn events at the orphanage. Not really. Never be fooled by a pig's passive nature-the males seemed to sense when their routine has been interrupted. The procedure goes somewhat as follows:

First, a couple of preteen boys chase down a young pig, tackle the squealing, writhing, slippery thing, and throw it on its back. Next, four boys, one holding down each kicking, pig-manure coated leg, pin the creature to the equally pig-manure covered concrete slab of the pig pen.

Next the two boys holding down the pig's hind legs pull the legs forward, causing a tightening up of the scrotum, the covering of the testicles. Mr. Davis (or Mr. Adams) then makes a long incision over each of the two testicles, reaches into the scrotal sac, pulls out the testicle, and with the reasonably sharp (or reasonably dull) knife, severs the spermatic cord holding the testicle (at times taking two or three swipes at the ever moving spermatic cord to complete the job) and drops the testicle into the "balls bucket." Ditto for the remaining testicle.

Then Mr. Davis puts down the knife, picks up the container of tar and, like an old Southern grandma dipping snuff, pours an ample amount of the black tar into both jagged holes of the scrotal sac. Young boys are possessed with overactive imaginations anyway, and every cut made by Mr. Davis elicited spontaneous wincings from the four young holders-downers. Truly the stuff of which nightmares were made.

For the duration of this non-delicate, certainly non-sterile surgical procedure, the poor porker has been screaming bloody murder, and you can't shut him up because no kid has the nerve to try to clamp his snout shut. Definitely no job for the faint of heart. To Mr. Davis it was just a job. As far as Mr. Adams goes, I believe the sadistic sonofabitch enjoyed it, as he always smiled throughout the procedure.

And then we had to repeat the routine for the remaining dozen or so young male pigs. Afterwards we kids had to go hose off all the pig manure. We smelled awful, and none of the other farm or dairy boys would get anywhere near us for the rest of the day.

The dairy supervisor, Mr. Davis, and the farm supervisor, Mr. Adams, possessed equal authority. One did not work for the other. Some tasks, however, called for additional hands, for example, cutting the fields of stripped-barren cornstalks in order to fill the two huge seventy-five ton capacity dairy silos for Winter storage of silage, and both farm and dairy boys pitched in to complete this unavoidable major task.

Another of these special endeavors was "hog-killing" day, that occurred several times each year, and farm and dairy boys alike were shanghaied for this most distasteful event. When compared to purchasing ham, bacon and other wholesome meats supplied by the domesticated hog, raising hogs on the orphanage farm was indeed a bargain. Space certainly was not a problem, as there was an abundance of that on the 350-acre farm.

The decades-old long, winding, quite picturesque dirt road leading from the barns and dairy proper, to the Farmer's Barn nearly a mile away, had no name. When we were instructed to go to a certain location, such as the Beef Cattle Barn or the forty-acre field, the speaker simply referred to the specified location; one never had cause to say "go down the such-and-such road to the bridge over the creek, etc", because our beloved farm road led to every location of interest on the farm, and it was the *only* road one could take to reach these destinations.

To get to the "pig pen," as it was commonly called (though Mr. Davis referred to it as the "hog farm"), one went down the road away from the farm buildings about a third of a mile, then turned right onto a narrower dirt road, and followed this road for about a hundred yards, and there it was. The pig pen could accommodate literally hundreds of hogs. The intervals between the slaughter of the hogs for food, and the number of hogs killed on each slaughter date, easily could be determined, because the population of orphans and staff to be fed remained a constant at approximately three hundred eighty students and staff.

The pigpen consisted of a wide, roughly square-shaped fenced area, with enclosed wooden stall-like structures to protect the swine from the oftentimes bitterly cold Winters. A portion of the penned-in area, alongside the fence paralleling the dirt road, contained a wide rectangular concrete slab. Food and water troughs had been constructed along this concrete slab, adjacent to the fence. The leftover food from three hundred persons eating three meals each day quite easily filled several fifty-five gallon garbage cans. Daily these large containers of "hogwash," or as we usually referred to it, "slop," were transported by mule and wagon, and in later years by pickup truck, to the pigpen, where they were emptied into the long, open concrete troughs. All pigs grunt while eating.

The word "hogwash" has two meanings, 1) kitchen waste, or "slop," and 2) useless or insincere talk or writing. The farm boys fed hogwash to the pigs daily; old man Gray fed hogwash to all us kids at Vespers every Sunday night. We youngsters envied the pigs.

Construction of the modern, all-brick freezer locker building in 1951 made a laborious and distasteful task a little easier. "Sticking" the hog is the act of Mr. Davis or Mr. Adams severing the carotid artery and jugular vein of the doomed porcine, and the dying animal almost immediately fell on its side. We boys then lifted the heavy hog off the concrete slab by its hind legs, to facilitate bleeding, after which the animal was loaded onto the truck and transported to the "meat house," the aforementioned new brick structure located behind the vegetable house.

The driver of the truck backed the truck (or wagon) up to a small loading ramp, and the hog was dragged off the vehicle bed and into a metal vat filled with scalding water, heated by a gas heater underneath to 135-145 degrees Fahrenheit. This process was called "scurfing" the hog. The scalding water loosened the hog's course hair and removed dirt and other impurities from the skin.

After about five minutes in the scalding water, the carcass was pulled onto a roller bearing bed, where we used flat metal scrapers to scrape off the hog's hair. After this was completed, the hog was suspended by hooks through the gambrel tendons on the hind legs. The head was severed, and one of the older boys opened the carcass by a straight cut in the center of the belly of the hog. This caused the hog's digestive system and other body organs to drop into a large metal tub placed beneath the carcass, along with the associated fat, that we called "leaf" fat. Everything that fell into the tub we referred to as the "innards" of the hog. The boys then used hacksaws to split the center of the backbone into two sides, and later the boys cut the carcass into side, shoulder, leg and loin. From a small child spectator's view, it was quite interesting. From an older boy's view, because he had to perform the arduous task, no fun at all.

Chapter 41

The Disappearance of Wun Hung Lo

Because hogs were raised to put on the supper table, and so as we kids wouldn't have to cry into our already salty plates of bacon every morning at breakfast, we never gave them names. Except one. The Chinese hog. It's an interesting story. Not exactly Joe Pulitzer-class prose, yet thought-provoking in an uncultivated sort of way.

It was an especially sweltering mid-morning in August 1951. I had turned twelve a few months earlier, and was into my second year as a "dairy boy," chronologically only a year older, but certainly wiser by half. Although still a mite slow on the uptake, I was definitely making progress, though still getting picked on by the scumbag Big Boys.

As explained above in lurid detail, most of the male pigs were eunuchized three or four months after birth. We youngsters never figured out how the godawful huge monster of a male hog managed to retain his testicles for so long, unless it was Mr. Adams' intent to use him as a stud in the pigpen, or possibly because nobody was brave enough to try to separate his "hoghood" from him.

Anyway, on that muggy Summer morning the Prince of Darkness' mangy mongrel, Tom Adams in the flesh, had shanghaied four of us dairy boys, and off we rode in the bed of his pickup truck down to the pigpen.

As soon as we alighted from the truck bed we saw him. *Saw* him? Hell, you couldn't *miss* him, that's for sure. Damn biggest, meanest-looking hog I ever saw, ever. And the first time I heard him grunt, I felt like snapping to attention and answering "Yes, Sir," and swearing to him that never before in my miserable young life had I ever even thought about eating bacon, or pork chops, or even the lowly chitlins.

Naturally assuming that we had been brought along to perform some menial, non intelligence-provoking, unimportant, make-work task, certainly not one that would likely place our collective lives in immediate jeopardy, once we had recovered from our initial shock at the enormity of this behemoth, we four totally clueless young dairy boys quickly reverted to our normal adolescent mindlessness, and began staring at this huge hog, giggling and pointing at the cob-roller's massive scrotal sac. It looked like somebody had strapped a huge hairy knapsack onto his rear end.

"C'mere, Provost!"

I turned from the impressive porcine spectacle to see Tom Adams holding out to me what appeared to be a large can of black tar in his left hand, and an equally large and threatening rusty-looking butcher knife in his right hand, his body language unmistakenly indicating that he expected me to take the articles from his grasp.

But I just stood there before him, momentarily dumbfounded and speechless, my theretofore unimaginative young mind certainly not wanting to make the obvious, staring-in-my-own-face connection.

Let's see here now. Surely I could figure this one out rationally. Four reasonably dull-witted preteen dairy boys. Biggest goddamn uncastrated hog on the Maker's green ground. One very large, unopened can of black tar. Ugliest-looking terror-invoking unsharpened butcher knife this side of Jim Bowie's eleven acres. Four legs on the Masterhog. Therefore one (very large) hog shank for each (very small, frightened) dairy boy. Methought, if Tom Adams had in mind what I believed he did, no way in hell were we gonna survive this. I was destined to die at an early age trampled into pig shit by a monster hog that outweighed the four of us no-hips preteen orphans put together.

My saliva-drooling stupor was interrupted by a caustic, demanding "Dammit, Provost, put these over on top of that shed!" "These" were the aforementioned very large can of black tar and rusty blade of terror half the length of a sixteenth-century Samurai's sword. I timidly took the large can of black tar and the rusty mini-sword from Mr. Adams' grasp and placed them where he had indicated. Now what, I thought. But I thought I knew. And after about five years in this flippin place I was certain of the actions of these dumbass grownups about one hundred percent of the time.

Waving his stupid hand in the direction of "Mr. Big," Adams instructed us, "Now you boys catch 'im and throw 'im on his back." Now, you've no doubt heard that tripe about the devil and the deep blue sea?

Well, that worthless bastard Tom Adams was the former, and the "deep blue" in this case weighed about three hundred eighty pounds. But alas, we were dumbshit orphan kids, doubtless more expendable than .50-cal. shell casings scattered at the base of Mount Suribachi, so we did as we were ordered, and after the longest ten minutes ever put on a clock, managed to wrestle Big Balls to the concrete slab of the pig pen.

"Now each of you boys grab a leg," Adams ordered, and like a flash the smallest among us, the one some called Little Orphan Al, but others referred to as "that stupid kid from Kinston," jumped on a flailing, slightly (but only) less than deadly front leg. I wanted no part of that monster's back shank.

But as was ever the case with my yellow-bellied buddy Butch Mitchell, the little bastard started whining, so that was Tom Adams' cue to make me trade shanks with Butch, and I ended up with my skinny arms wrapped around the monster's deadly left hind leg anyway.

"Now just sit on 'im," ordered Adams, "And you boys pull 'is hind legs up toward 'is front legs."

We did as instructed, and Adams picked up the rusty butcher knife, and with a long, slicing motion, split the thick scrotal sac on my side.

The huge hog shrieked and bucked, but by some miracle we managed to hold on. Then the Butcher of Oxford reached into the gaping scrotal sac, pulled out the biggest nut ever seen on a hog, and took three quick slices at the moving spermatic cord.

That damned hog shrieked and squealed so loud and long you'd of thought Adams was trying to cut off the poor cob-roller's balls. Which he was. Trying to, that is. But the three slices of the dull blade still hadn't done the trick, and the frightened monster porker started bucking like a West Texas bronco.

"Hold down 'is legs, dammit!" Tom Adams screamed at me, drawing the dull knife back out of the danger zone.

"I'm tryin'," I responded, my pig shit-coated hands grappling for the left hind leg that had slipped from my grasp and was waving frantically, trying in vain to get purchase in the open air. My fear of incurring further the wrath of Lowlife Adams finally overcame my fear of having my arms gashed by the enraged hog's razor-sharp toe, so I quickly wiped each crap-coated hand on my pantsleg and grabbed cautiously at the big animal's flailing errant hind leg.

Once firmly (firmly?) in control, I hoped to hear a "Good boy," or a "That's the way to do it," from Adams, but got instead the idiot's expected "And don't let it go again, dammit!"

About that time, Big Guy screamed an awful scream, jerking his entire body back and forth, and we four boys lost our already slippery grip and sprawled back into the slimy pig manure that coated the concrete slab. Sensing his chance to escape, Bigun raced like a terrified three hundred eighty pound hog for the opened gate, his razor-sharp toes scraping haphazardly across the manure-coated concrete slab, making like he was the featured favorite at Pimlico.

"Go get 'im, dammit!" screamed Tom Adams, frantically waving his dull half-Samurai in the direction of the "hogscapee" who was now galloping into the woods toward the edge of the orphanage property, the edge that contained no fence.

It was as though somebody had drawn the porker a map. We kids chased after him, but he was much too fast for us, and the last we ever saw of Big Balls was his massive backside, sporting a long red cord attached to an enormous oval-shaped blood-red mountain oyster, bouncing wildly in the air with each short but determined stride of the huge animal.

We never recaptured the monster hog with the one dangling testicle, and eventually Tom Adams also gave up and, cussing and berating us four preteens, drove us back to the dairy in his pickup.

It took us four quipsters only a moment to recount to the older dairy boys our suddenly and now hilariously comic tale, and it took these comedians about half that moment to tag the errant hog with the moniker "One Hung Low" that sounded enough like a Chinese name that we would spell it "Wun Hung Lo." Just another day in the life of never a dull moment called the orphanage dairy.

CHAPTER 42

Sick Call and the Dreaded Polio

"Sick call" was held in the hospital basement infirmary each morning immediately following breakfast. Any child who felt ill or who had sustained cuts, abrasions or bruises, simply reported to the infirmary and took a seat in line on white-painted, well-worn benches situated along the wall. A well-represented number of crybabies, whiners, goldbricks and hypochondriacs were interspersed among the ill.

Temperatures were routinely recorded, aspirin, or a good dose of Epsom salts or soda were dispensed liberally by The Great White Witch, for headaches and assorted pains and injuries, and any child clutching at his or her throat and speaking in a low, raspy voice automatically received a throat swabbing with Mercurochrome. Same treatment for abrasions, small cuts, and skinned shins, knees and elbows.

If a child came in clutching at his stomach or intestinal area, his or her temperature was taken immediately. A high temperature might possibly indicate appendicitis. A normal temperature brought on the next question: "When is the last time you did No. 2?" Better have a quick answer for that one; vacillation in responding got you an enema or a good dose of Epsom salts or Castor Oil.

Mercurochrome is an antiseptic that first used mercury to obtain an antibacterial effect. Its purpose was to prevent infection, and it stained the skin tissue surrounding the cut or abrasion bright red tinged with a yellow-green fluorescence.

It was nearly impossible for a child to skip school and not get caught. Being admitted to the hospital was the only excuse. Roll was called each morning in class. Absences were reported to Mr. Regan's office, and Mr. Regan's secretary telephoned the hospital. If the child were not in school, and not in the hospital, in all probability he had run away under the cover of darkness. And it happened a lot.

The omnipresent Mercurochrome was in widespread use during the 1940's, even though it was really a weak antibiotic. It was not until 1938 that researchers at Oxford University in England succeeded in isolating a fairly pure form of penicillin, and not until 1944 that commercial production was great enough in the United States to be used in wartime. Thus Mercurochrome remained in widespread use well into the 1950's and beyond.

The angst-producing polio epidemic was at its most alarming stage during the late '40's and early '50's, and the dread of contracting the deadly virus blanketed the orphanage campus like a rolling morning fog scene from *The Mummy's Curse*. In fact, the only thing more real and equally as frightening to me than The Bandaged Guy was the fear of having to spend my claustrophobic young life trapped in a shiny metal cylinder, unable to pee or poo or even scratch my nose when it itched. Painfully I discovered that possessing an overactive imagination is indeed a dual-edged broadsword.

Thus seated quietly each morning after breakfast on the well-worn wooden benches along the wall in the basement of Hicks Memorial Hospital were a representative number of paranoid youngsters who suspected they had overnight surely been ambushed by the dreaded "Fever" associated with the symptoms of the ghastly "Unspeakable." And it was easy to spot these children; it appeared that their hands were permanently glued to their forehead, checking their temperature. And Little (Frightened) Orphan Al was often right there in the middle of the pack, hand attached to my forehead.

After picking himself up off the ground one too many times, a bruised and battered Job complained to God that it appeared to him (Job) that nobody else ever got "dumped on."

God assured Job he was not alone in his misery. Job did not doubt The Word of God, but being just a wee bit curious, Job raised his hand, like he was in the third grade or something.

God acknowledged Job. Job asked God if he could but ask one small question.

"Just one, Job. But make it snappy. You are already on Mr. Gray's List for this coming Saturday."

What else is new, thought Job, wincing in the anticipation of spending this coming Saturday bent at the waist grabbing his ankles. But Job asked his question just the same.

"Who is this other poor unfortunate soul?"

"People will know of him as 'Little Orphan Al.'"

"That's a funny name," replied Job.

"Look who's talking," came The Almighty's quick retort.

And as if I didn't have the continuing (bad) luck of my soulmate Job to deal with daily, my generation was cursed by the tail-end third of the dreaded POLIO epidemic. That's an all-capper for sure. (Insert Giant Prolonged Drum Roll Here.) And it scared the living daylights out of us kids, for years.

Poliomyelitis, that everybody just called "polio," is a virus that causes the disease "infantile paralysis." This lightning-fast crippling condition results in deformation of the bodies of mainly children and young adults.

The virus polio is transmitted via water contaminated with fecal material. The virus enters the body through the mouth, multiplies in the intestines, and then migrates to the central nervous system. The virus results in inflamed nerves in the brain and spinal cord, causing paralysis of the muscles of the chest, legs and arms. Because of the manner in which the virus is transmitted, contaminated feces or oral secretions, children are most vulnerable.

The dreaded polio could cripple a small child overnight, leaving his limbs limp and useless. As terrible as is the AIDS virus in the latter part of the twentieth century, it pales in comparison to the deadly fear that polio engendered throughout the United States, and the epidemic years were filled with a widespread and quite intense paranoia among the young orphanage inmates. Just one case in a town could lead to the immediate closing of municipal swimming pools and school playgrounds.

Poster children were used widely to concentrate the public's attention on the plight of those crippled by the disease, and many a night I fell asleep picturing in my all too vivid mind Little Al as a poster child, my pitiful face and racked-in-pain body draped in what resembled shackles like those we dairy boys used to subdue ornery milk cows. I discovered what real fear was. The fear of polio was as real a fear as you got.

The polio epidemic in the United States lasted from 1916 to 1961, the year I graduated college. And the disease attacked adults as well. Franklin D. Roosevelt, who became President of the United States in 1933, contracted polio in 1921, although he hid his infirmity from the public for many years.

It was not until 1943, when I was four years old, that a vaccine, consisting of killed-virus influenza and developed by Dr. Jonas Salk and Thomas Francis, proved successful in clinical trials. And it was not until I was in first grade, in 1946, that Herald Cox and Hillary Kaprowski began research on a live-virus polio vaccine.

However, the end was a long time coming. In 1950, when I was eleven years old and therefore smack-dab in the middle of the high-risk group, 33,300 new cases of polio were reported in the United States. Scary stuff, that; such statistics sure made believers of us preteen orphans. At the beginning of the twenty-first century, there were 1.63 million polio survivors in the United States. And those are the "survivors."

Those unfortunates suffering chest paralysis were confined to a Drinker respirator, the seemingly ever-present "iron lung." This frightful metal cylinder, that resembled the heavy-duty clothes dryers in the orphanage laundry, encased the entire body save the head, exerting a push-pull motion on the patient's chest to aid in breathing. And yes, many a night I dreamed about being confined to a Drinker respirator, fighting to breathe, and, something I have never been able to explain, being worried that I could not scratch my nose if it itched. And every time my face itched, I would immediately scratch it, for fear I would one day not be able to enjoy that freedom.

Because in the late '40's there existed no specific cure (or really effective treatment) for infantile paralysis, and because twenty-five percent of those afflicted with the disease sustained permanent disability, including muscle atrophy, we youngsters in Walker Building, 1-B and 2-B lived in perpetual fear of contracting the dreaded disease. I was still only sixteen years old when the much-heralded "Salk vaccine" came into widespread use in 1956.

To us kids, then, the fear of contracting infantile paralysis was as real as death. Because the highly infectious "Kiss of Death" was caused by a virus and transmitted via water contaminated with fecal material, the cottage counselors, including Miss Hobson, Witch Robinson and Mrs. Dye, routinely cautioned us youngsters to wash our hands after going to the bathroom, and I spent many pre-poo and post-poo hours at the sink, hands immersed in hot soapy water. And before wiping my skinny ass I literally encased my hand in toilet paper. It was akin to cleaning myself with a miniature mummy. And my fear put an immediate halt to biting my fingernails and picking my nose, two of the three main pleasures of preteens.

And fear of contracting the dreaded infantile paralysis sure put the quietus on some of us kids re the indiscriminate claiming of "Leffuns!" every time we heard the crinkling of a candy wrapper.

During my decade-long incarceration at Oxford, the stigma attached to even the word "polio" was so great that in only one of the Annual Reports of the Oxford Orphanage does the dreaded word itself appear. The Annual Report of the Oxford Orphanage for the year ending December 31, 1948, the year I moved from the Baby Cottage to "Firetrap Towers" (the Walker Building), states in the "Health" report on page 23:

> We feel especially fortunate since none of our children were afflicted
> with Poliomyelitis during the recent epidemic in North Carolina.

The Annual Report for the year ending December 31, 1947, my first year at the orphanage, deftly sidestepped *the* word, by stating, on page 22:

> The health of the children has been exceptionally good during the
> past year since we have not experienced any serious epidemic on
> the campus.

Similar statements were made in the Annual Reports for the years 1949 through 1954. And without giving even the reason for the newly-discovered polio preventive measure, the "Health" sections of the Annual

Reports for 1955, 1956 and 1957 state ". . . and our children received the Salk vaccine."

In 1948 the polio epidemic was so great that the entire campus was quarantined, and all vacations were canceled for the Summer. And on page 33 of the Seventy-sixth Annual Reports, dated December 31, 1948, Mr. Talton, the Scoutmaster, reported,

> We were disappointed that we were not able to attend the opening of Camp Durant this year, but due to the polio ban we had to spend the Summer on the campus.

We boys never did figure out whether our hapless classmate William Thomas ("W.T.") Bass had contracted polio. The muscles in our friend's left arm and left leg had atrophied, and he shuffled along, putting as little weight as possible on his left leg, his left arm seemingly bent permanently at the elbow, and the fingers of his left hand curled loosely into a flabby half-fist. He was a piteous sight.

Whatever the actual cause of W.T.'s infirmity, word quickly spread around the boys' side of the campus that the poor lad had been stricken with the dreaded infantile paralysis, whereupon we youngsters began to question among ourselves as to who had recently drunk from the same water ladle, glass, Nehi grape or RC Cola bottle as had W.T., or who had stupidly claimed "Leffuns!" off a candy bar, apple or orange after W.T. had taken a few bites.

And because one of the initial complaints of a person who had contracted polio was a high fever, it was not uncommon to observe, in the classroom, at the dining table, or during study hall at night, boys inadvertently reach up and press their palms against their forehead, or a child holding both hands against his forehead, and at the same time his breath, in deadly fear of that "Kiss of Death," the unspeakable "Fever."

Youngsters often tend to equate the word "prayer" with a hope or a wish (is there really a difference?), and we Walker Building, 1-B and 2-B boys "prayed" our hearts out, that the Almighty would be merciful and spare us from our friend W.T.'s horrendous fate. At lights-out every night I would lie still under my covers, murmuring softly what became rather quickly a nightly paternoster, that if the Merciful would but spare me from the dreaded "infantile paralysis," I would faithfully do my morning "duty" and rake *all* the fallen leaves on my side of the yard, that I would never rake my leaves onto my "friend" Bill Herrington's duty area again, that I would never, never ever utter another cuss word, even promising to trade in the commanding "hell" and "damn" for the anemic, sissified "heck" and "darn," and that I would help W.T. Bass in any way possible . . . so long as I didn't have to touch the poor sod.

And just before falling asleep each night, I would rest my palm on my forehead . . . just checking. Years later we boys admitted to this instantaneous and quite sincere, need to be closer to the Maker. And I vowed to myself that whatever scrumptious goodies W.T. might come to possess, I would never ever claim "Leffuns!" from him again.

Somewhere along my arduous path to young adulthood, I developed a capacity to empathize with those less fortunate than I, such as "road kill" for example; to imagine myself as that other person, to put myself, so to speak, "in his shoes." I feel quite certain this positive outlook on those less fortunate all started with W.T. Bass.

To all us healthy youngsters, W.T. was a piteous sight, and instantly upon seeing our once-robust and happy classmate in his permanently wilted condition, my heart went out to him. Ostensibly the doctors had prepared a certain "physical therapy" regimen for W.T., straight out of the parchment pages of "Stone Age Medical Science." Apparently in an attempt to force the crippled youngster to use the atrophied muscles in his shriveled up left arm and hand, the unfortunate lad was required to carry around the campus in his left hand a pail, filled to varying degrees with sometimes rocks and at other times dirt. As explained to us youngsters, the "physical therapy" goal was to gradually increase the weight of the rocks and dirt in the pail, as the muscles in W.T.'s hand and arm regained their strength.

Didn't work. After several months of suffering juvenile mockery and teasing from some of the 1-B and 2-B boys, and much harsher ridicule from those callous nitwits in 4-B, out of humiliation, embarrassment and eventual disappointment at the lack of a desperately hoped-for quick cure, W.T. simply gave up. He flatly and defiantly refused to ever again pick up the stupid bucket of rocks and dirt, and eventually we boys forgot our friend's physical limitations, and just accepted him as one of us 1-B boys. Worked out better for everyone.

CHAPTER 43

Why We Talk Funny

Oxford Orphanage is the oldest orphanage in North Carolina. For a hundred and thirty years, since its founding in 1872, the orphanage has been a close-knit community, a small town unto itself. And, I might add, a really spooky place to spend ten years of a young boy's life.

Because children past the age of about ten (more or less, give or take a few special cases not fitting the rule) were not admitted to the orphanage, the average "big house" sentence, if the child remained to graduate high school, was approximately eight to ten very long years.

It logically follows then, that the majority of children entering the orphanage did so between the ages of five and eight, and that during their early years at Oxford, any connatural speech patterns, localisms and slang developed at home, became diffused almost immediately by the constant daily interaction with more than three hundred other children from various regions of the state. Accents and even personal identities were expunged from the "new" boy or girl with blinding celerity.

The logical outgrowth of this constant replacement of incoming accents with those of a population of nearly four hundred students and staff, was the unique phenomenon of a Southern community without a Southern accent, or, perhaps more precisely, one with its own unique accent.

Speech patterns in the region of North Carolina that encompasses Kinston and Oxford fall into the specific Southern dialect some linguists once called Hill Southern, but now refer to as the South Midland dialect. We called fireflies "lightnin' bugs," a burlap sack we knew only as a "tow" sack, that if we'd been forced to spell it would have come out "toe," soot from a chimney was called "smut," a harmonica was simply a "harp," and a wishbone or breastbone from a chicken was a "pulleybone," all one word.

In our closed orphanage society of the late 1940's and early 1950's, children and staff alike used certain words, expressions and terminology not to be found outside the confines of our little "city." And though not an orphan's invention, every boy, by the time he moved up to 1-B at about age ten, learned and commonly spoke to his buddies in "Pig Latin."

Pig Latin is a jargon formed by transposing the initial consonant of a word to the end of that word, and suffixing an additional syllable. Words usually end in "ay." The sentence

"The boys are going to play a joke on John after supper tonight," in Pig Latin would be,

> "Ethay oysbay areay oingay ootay aplay aay okjay onay Onjay afay ertay uppersay ootay ightnay."

We (stupid) preteen boys thought we "had it over" the young girls, that certainly being inferior females they would be old-and-eighty before they could ever hope to decipher our "secret" boys' language, so at the supper table we spoke in Pig Latin, and in a short time I became quite fluent, able to speak the language as fast as I could regular English. The fun ended abruptly, however, when one morning at breakfast Betty Jean interrupted our aimless juvenile jabber with the scornful quip, "Iwhay ontday ooyay upidstay izegay utshay upay." Sure ended it for me. Abruptly.

During the first half of the twentieth century, Southerners seem to have elevated aphesis, which is the dropping of a weakly-stressed syllable at the beginning of a word, to an art form, thereby greatly expanding the American English language horizon. As in 'sylum dog.

In my pre-captivity life we kids used to smack skeeters at my granddaddy's cabin in Swansboro during the hot Summer months. At the orphanage we chased possums, picked and ate taters, "got a whuppin" if any of the staff caught us with a chawtabaccer.

"Coastal Southern" speech originated along the mid-New England states, being carried south by migration into first Virginia and then North Carolina. These accents and dialects were then eventually transported from the colonial settlements in these Eastern Seaboard states, southwestward into Georgia, Alabama and Mississippi.

"Lower Southern" idiomatic regionalism is a mainly North Carolina patois, a further refinement of "Coastal Southern" speech. Oxford lies smack-dab in the middle of this subregion. Examples of the centuries-old refinement of this dialect abound in Southern literature and everyday social intercourse.

Late seventeenth and early eighteenth century settlers moving into Granville County and eastward to the Outer Banks of North Carolina were of mainly English descent and had transmigrated from Tidewater Virginia, their farm animals, personal belongings and Tidewater brogue in tow. And this brogue has remained to this day in Granville County. We orphans called it the "Oxford brogue," some of which over the years had become infused into orphanage life. The word "brogue" means both a strong dialectal accent and a heavy shoe of untanned leather, and this Irish word became part of Southern culture a century or two before I arrived at the orphanage.

Out of necessity and circumstances, we boys used the word "gyp," past tense "gypped," instead of the word "cheat," past tense "cheated," for example, "He gypped me out of my dabs." One heard the word "gypped" quite a bit at the orphanage.

"None of your business" means "Mind your own business." But to us kids, the term for "butt out" was "None of your beeswax, cornbread and shoetacks." And a threat to punish a child for certain infractions of the (grownups') rules, real or contrived, might come out as "I'm going to fix your little red wagon!"

"Chaw" is a uniquely Southern word. It is a variant of the word "chew." It is both a noun and a verb. A "chawtabacca" is a twist of chewing tobacco. The expression "He really chawed him out," means he scolded him. "Lightwood" is a word used mainly in the South. It is dry, resinous pine wood that burns readily with a bright light. Lightwood is used as a "starter" for wood or coal fires in stoves, and is made from the heart of the Southern pine. Any kid who grew up on a farm in North Carolina in the first half of the twentieth century can locate for you the "heart" of the Southern pine.

The word "lighterd" is what finally evolves when you say "lighter" very fast twenty-five times in succession. This word is used in that region of North Carolina moreso than "kindling."

The words "window shades" are also more apt to be used than "curtains," even though the speaker is referring to curtains. And Southerners sometimes use the expression "them there" to provide greater specificity about the location of persons or things, moreso than just indicating "them" or "those" in the same setting educated non-Southerners might use "those."

The term "carrying-on" was widely used at Oxford. In scolding us boys for engaging in too much horseplay or boisterous laughter, the cottage mothers or teachers were apt to use the expression "You boys stop that carrying-on." Food was loosely referred to as "grub," and a description of what a boy was doing at the supper table might be that he was "scarfing down his grub," meaning that the boy was greedily consuming his food.

My mother's sister was my "aunt," pronounced as the insect, rather than "ahnt." Some of the Southern Virginia accent found its way to Oxford, located fifteen miles south of the Virginia state line. For example, some folks around Oxford called a house just that, a house; others, however, called a house a "hoose," rhyming with "goose." That same person would be apt to say "aboot" instead of "about."

The "picture show" had two meanings; the theatre itself was called the "picture show," and the movie, or film, being shown also was called the "picture show." In reality then, we kids used to go to the picture show to see the picture show. If you are old enough, you can recall the picture show "leader," "An RKO Radio Picture" in the 1930's and 1940's.

A "funny book" was what today is called a "comic book," and the "funny papers" were the newspaper comic strips.

Double-modal and multiple-modal constructions were quite common in the South and at Oxford Orphanage during the forties and fifties. The words "counta" and "onacounta" were used a lot, and meant "on account of" or "because of." "Might coulda" meant "might be able to."

If a boy was "fixin' to" do something, it meant he intended to perform the act in question. "Oughta" meant "ought to" or "should." "Should oughta" and "shouldn't oughta" were also commonly used, with the latter expression carrying with it the admonition of unpleasant consequences should the person continue with said conduct.

As a term to indicate a long distance from the speaker, the words "over yonder" were used mostly, by the orphanage staff as well as by the children. The term "over yonder" referred to the location of a thing, person or event farther from the speaker than simply "over there," that was used to indicate the location of closer things that could be seen readily by the speaker. An object or person that was within sight "over there," most likely could not been seen if located "over yonder."

In describing a boy running fast, especially in a non-direct route, we used the colloquial expression "He lit out across the pasture after the cows." And the word "summers" had nothing to do with the seasons; it meant "somewhere." "Where's Bill?" "Iono, he's around here summers."

The word "aways" (always in the plural) was used in "our neck of the woods" (the region in which we lived) to denote a longer distance (possibly in terms of miles) from the speaker, and was by conventional usage understood to be a distance farther than "over yonder." However, it was not altogether uncommon to hear the expression "over yonder aways" used in the forties and fifties by elderly folk. At times this expression was used when the speaker was not inclined to give you directions, or possibly not seeking for looking, and couldn't explain how to get from here to "over yonder aways," even if his life depended on it.

The expression "a spell," as used in the sentence "Let's go back a spell," could mean, depending on the context in which it was spoken, an unstated distance, or an undetermined or unstated period of time.

The word "amite" and the words "a mite" were in common usage in that region of Nauthcalana to mean a degree of temperature or a span of time, that could mean a few minutes or a few hours, depending on the situation in which it was used. Thus, "It was amite (a mite) cold last night," carried with it the connotation that it was colder than expected.

Also, "He got there amite (a mite) late," signified that the person arrived later than expected.

Folks in that region of the state are more likely to say "a quarter to eight" rather than "a quarter til eight," and when I was growing up during the postwar South, that same person never would use the expression 7:45 in giving the above stated time on the clock, no more than he would say it was 6:25; rather he would say it was "twenty five after six."

Any North Carolina tobacco farmer can tell you than an "armload" or "armful" is actually a scientific unit of measurement of any bulky object, even though that object is not being carried in one's arm. The "local yokels" as we orphans sometimes referred to Oxford townspeople, used the term "corn husks" where others might say "corn shucks," though to the indigenous, the act of removing the "husks" was called "shucking the corn."

If anyone asked where I was from, I answered "Kinston, Nauthcalana." And my hometown, Kinston, was a "baccer" center, but it was also a "t'baccer" town. And any fool could tell you that if you drove nauth from Nauthcalana you'd soon come to "Aginya" (Virginia).

A "perfective" is a word that expresses the completion of an action, and perfectives abounded in everyday Southern speech. The perfective "done" is commonly used for emphasis, as in "I've done told him to wash up for supper." The expression "liked to" means "almost," as in the sentence "I liked to of killed him," or "I liked to have killed him."

And it is an established (Southern) fact that "you all" or, the beat-to-death-and-then-some contraction "y'all" is a proper second person plural pronoun. Use of "y'all" avoids any likely confusion when a speaker is addressing a group of two or more persons. If the speaker uses the word "you" in that instance, each Southerner wonders whom among the group the speaker is addressing.

I know it's difficult for educated Southerners to believe, but even the somewhat less than luminous Yankees have come up with their own confusion-avoidance word, "youse," that in reality is a "nonce" word, that is, a word either invented, or just used for a particular occasion.

"Youse" is used "up North" in exactly the same situation as a Southerner would use "You all" or "Y'all." Appalachian hill country dwellers, and their cousins who have escaped the coal mines and made it to Pennsylvania and Ohio, use the expression "you-uns" for the same purpose, and some Yankees and especially Californians use "you guys" in similar situations. Limited education sure plays havoc with vocabularies.

The contraction "ain't" is in widespread use throughout the English-speaking world, and I have several English friends who use "ain't" in everyday social intercourse. Charles Dickens and other nineteenth and twentieth century English writers used "ain't" liberally in their works.

Not to use ain't in appropriate circumstances means you often must "talk around it." And ain't is a versatile expression; it can be used in the first, second or third person, singular or plural. The use of "aren't I" is quite stilted in everyday use, and who among us feels comfortable asking "Am I not," when forming first person questions in everyday conversations? Thus there were a lot of "ain'ts" in common use at the orphanage, among all ages.

Following are a few expressions used by the orphanage students and staff that, while found in more in-depth dictionaries, I have rarely heard used since leaving the orphanage in 1957.

"Studin'" is the shortened form of the word "studying" and was used a lot among the orphanage boys. This word was used only as part of the expression "I ain't studin' it," its actual meaning being that the boy making the statement refused further to argue the issue at hand, and the expression signified there would be no more discussion on the matter. Period.

More likely than not, the boy making the statement in actuality had already lost the argument, and the expression of finality was uttered as a means of saving face without conceding he was wrong.

To "take up" for someone meant to protect that boy from physical harm from older boys. Protection from older boys was generally not necessary in the Walker Building, because the boys in that cottage were not free to move about the campus, and never ventured onto the farm except under supervision. Literally then, we Walker Building boys were kept out of "harm's way."

The ideal person to "take up" for you would be an older brother. My brother Pete, four years my junior, arrived at Oxford Orphanage in 1952, and by then I was well able to protect him from any older boys. A 1-B or 2-B boy of age ten or eleven could best find someone to "take up" for him, if he did not have an older brother, by befriending a boy in his cottage who had an older brother.

"Duty" was a word used to indicate a task involving the expenditure of energy for the common good, performed during the forty minutes between the "first" bell at 6:00 a.m. and the "twenty-minute bell" at 6:40 a.m. The proper completion of the "duty" was inspected by the cottage counselor between the twenty-minute bell and the "five-minute bell." Every child, regardless of sex, size or age, was assigned a "duty," that might involve any task from sweeping the room to raking leaves to cleaning toilets.

Duties were assigned by the cottage counselor, and for reasons made obvious by the preceding sentence, duties were rotated periodically, in order to prevent a mutiny among the toilet cleaners. How in heaven's name I was blessed in that regard, but for the entire decade I was at Oxford, I never once was burdened with the duty of cleaning toilets.

"Ros'neers." We grew acres and acres of corn on the orphanage farm. The "red" corn was used as feed for the livestock, that is, the pigs and mules, and after harvesting, the red corn was shucked and stored in the "corn crib," a low, square-shaped, screened-in building constructed solely for the storage of corn, located adjacent to the "tool shed" and in front of the mule barn.

Farm tools and small implements were stored in what through common usage was referred to as the tool "shed." The word "shed" generally implies an open-sided shelter. Our tool "shed" was actually a large one-room, one-story structure, enclosed on all sides, with a door that was locked when not in use. However, everyone referred to the tool "room" as the tool "shed."

Corn used as food was referred to as "ros'neers" and throughout my youth I never knew that the word was a shortened form of "roasting ears" of corn. We kids ate a lot of "ros'neers."

"Founder." The word "founder" was in common use among boys and girls at Oxford during my ten-year stay. Loosely translated, the statement "I got foundered on that watermelon," meant "I'm so full I just can't eat another slice," or "I'm so full I'll get sick if I eat another slice."

Possibly the word found its way over time into the orphanage's extensive word inventory from the fact that occasionally a cow would eat so much rich pasture grass it would just lay down on its side and die. I've seen it happen just like that. The common dictionary definition of the word "founder" is used in the context of livestock becoming ill from overeating. Anyway, we dairy boys foundered on strawberries many a morning, on the way to milk the cows at 4:00 a.m.

As one might expect to occur in a self-contained little "city" such as Oxford Orphanage, "nonce" words were quite common, especially among the orphanage boys. A nonce word is a word invented, or used for a particular occasion, and many of the words contained in this book are indeed nonce words, and although in common and widespread use among the orphanage children and staff, will not be found in any dictionary. A few nonce words are as follows.

The word "dab" or "dabs" was orphanage slang for the word "marble," "marbles" or the game of "marbles." A boy would not ask his friends "Let's play a game of marbles." Instead, he would state "Let's play some dabs." The game of dabs was a serious game of skill, and was considered to be the unspoken great leveler among boys of all ages.

The general classification of "dabs," used in the context of the physical marble and not the game, included the small glass marble, called just a "dab," the large glass marble, called a "gollywhopper," or just a "golly," and the small steel marble, called a "steelie," that was in reality nothing more than a steel ball bearing. Any one of these, the glass "dab," the "golly," or the "steelie," could be used as the "shooter." Thus in 1949 a game of dabs being played among a group of 1-B and 2-B boys on the red clay infield outside the fifth and sixth grade classrooms likely would amount to a colloquy deemed quite foreign to a visitor from outside the hedges.

A great dabs player was held in the same revered esteem as the boy who could burn the longest blue flame fart, or who could pee the farthest in a snowbank on a full bladder, feats or attainments normal persons might find socially repulsive, but in our confined little postwar world were accomplishments to be sought after.

The word "mud" was in constant use at the orphanage, among boys and girls of all ages. The word was used only in the context of the expression "to mud for" and it meant to stand lookout for any adult who might come upon and discover the wrongdoing being committed by one's partners in crime. The term "to mud for" was well understood and used by orphanage supervisory personnel as well as orphans, and upon either catching the perpetrator red-handed, or determining his identity after the fact, the first demand by the supervisor was "Okay, now who was muddin' for you, young man?"

The punishment meted out to the mudder was generally the same as that given to the actual doer of the crime, except in those instances wherein by the great disparity between the ages of the actual culprit and the mudder, the supervisor was convinced the mudder had been coerced (read as "threatened) into aiding the older criminal.

"Mountain oysters" was the common term given for the testicles of hogs or pigs. At each "hog killing" any testicles yet attached to the unfortunate porcine were separated therefrom, placed in pails, and distributed among the five colored farm workers.

The lasting beauty of the South is its traditions of expanding outward to its meaningful limits, our rich and diverse English language. Thank God for the South. If it had not been for the South, the North and Abraham Lincoln wouldn't have had anybody to beat up on during the War of Yankee Aggression, that scholars north of the Mason-Dixon Line still refer to as the U.S. Civil War.

CHAPTER 44

Mountain Oyster Hunting With Red Ryder

I moved up to 2-B in June 1951, just after finishing the sixth grade. Mrs. Ethel Dye was our cottage counselor, and for the most part the somewhat frail, silver-haired lady was harmless. "Harmless" is really a "good" description. The word was reserved for any cottage counselor who either did not physically abuse us, or cause Mr. Regan or Mr. Gray to do the deed, or in my case, the plural form of the word.

If we didn't do our morning duty to her satisfaction, Mrs. Dye punished us in one of two ways. You either spent Saturday afternoon picking weeds from her large flower garden located behind the cottage, or if you (like me) couldn't tell the difference between a weed and a flower (from my unrefined perspective, most of the "weeds" were prettier than the "flowers") you were put to work building what we kids called "Mount 2-B." Smart kids that we were, we even caught the play on words, Mount 2-B and Mount To Be.

Those poor British sods who were forced to help my friend William Holden construct The Bridge on the River Kwai had nothing on us. The building of Mount 2-B (or To Be) entailed taking one of the many metal buckets Mrs. Dye used to store her flowers, walking way the hell over yonder across the expansive football practice field beside the school to a field where in the Fall we planted turnips and rutabagas, filling the large bucket with rocks, carrying that heavy-as-a-bucketful-of-rocks bucket of rocks all the way back across that expansive football practice field to the cottage, and dumping the rocks onto a pile.

And then you got to repeat the procedure again. And again. And again. For about three hours. In the Winter, not terribly bad. In the "dog days of Summer" almost unbearable. Ever see these stupid Georgia chain gang prison movies, where they show the dumbass prisoners cracking jokes. Sure weren't no joke-cracking going on during the construction of Mount 2-B. Nosireebob. Lotta goddamn work, that's what it was. Only things missing were the chains and the whip, and we felt certain that had Ethel Dye asked, Regan or Gray would have supplied those also. And she wouldn't have had to ask them twice.

I had long desired to own a Red Ryder B-B gun, and on vacation in July of that year Doc asked me if there was anything special I wanted. I thought he was serious. So I got serious. What I *really* wanted was a brand-spanking new Thompson submachine gun, just like the one my friend the picture show actor James Cagney had.

Doc ignored my request. Okay, next on my wish list would be the above-mentioned Red Ryder, I explained, trying my best not to show my disappointment at my brother ignoring my original request. Doc said no problem. I had already found a place to hide my air rifle.

Let me tell you something about the policy of the orphanage administrators concerning the ownership of air rifles by the orphan boys. Plainly put, I knew without asking, that if Regan or Gray discovered I owned a Red Ryder, they would beat me to within an inch of my sorry life, confiscate the gun, and probably pack me off to the notorious Jackson Training School.

The boys' cottages were heated during the Winter by metal radiators or heat forced up through vents in the floors. Steam was supplied to these radiators by heating the basement boiler by means of a coal-burning furnace. A boy in each cottage was paid extra cash each month to stoke the furnace. For a year while I was in 4-B, I had this job. It paid five dollars per month. Might not sound like much, but it was five dollars more than anyone else had.

I had located the perfect hiding place for my B-B gun, beneath the massive pile of coal in the 2-B basement coal bin. So Doc purchased the Red Ryder and enough B-B's to hold off the Germans at the Siege of

Stalingrad for about three years, and before we drove through the main gate, I ran the barrel of the Red Ryder down my pantsleg, tucked the butt of the rifle under my right arm, and ambled along stiff-legged toward the cottage, around to the basement and into the furnace room. Doc had covered the rifle with a heavy oil paper, and I pushed back the coal and hid the gun alongside the near right wall of the large coal bin.

I was willing to share my new gift with a few close-mouthed friends, so I told Bill, Van, Newton, Marvin and Red. On Saturday and Sunday afternoons, those of us who had not been (unjustly) sentenced to hard labor on Mount 2-B or in Mrs. Dye's flower garden, would bunch together in a tight group, with stiff-legged Little Orphan Al in the center, pockets full of packs of B-B's, and off we would hike to the far woods to target practice for the afternoon.

We were the original "Wild Bunch," a bloodthirsty, transgressive, lawless group. Each of my friends knew that if discovered, he would suffer the same fate as would I, but their attitude was the same as mine. We really didn't give two hoots to hell. Had to catch us first.

We shot everything, moving or stationary, big or small, weak or strong. We took turns shooting cows in the hindquarters with B-B's. we made the small male pigs jump by popping their "mountain oysters" (testicles) with B-B's. The poor pigs were easy pickings, because their testicles are not located underneath their bodies, but attached to their rear, so they made perfect targets.

We shot at big barn walls, glass soda bottles, squirrels, snakes and every other living animal. We all became pretty good shots, got better with practice, and even held competitions. We were just a bunch of kids having fun, and nobody ever found out about the "Ryder" as we referred to it.

Half the fun was just knowing we were having a good time with a B-B gun that was definitely forbidden on campus. We knew that once off the main campus and down the farm road aways, there was no cause for concern. Never once during my entire time at the orphanage did I ever see Mr. Regan off the farm road.

We boys enjoyed the B-B gun for nearly a year, and nobody ever knew we had it. One night it rained buckets, a real frog-strangler, and a few weeks later when I went to collect the rifle, I discovered the coal at the bottom of the bin was soaked, and when I unwrapped the rifle it was covered with rust and ruined. I took it to the woods and threw it in the deep part of the creek that traversed the farm. But the Red Ryder had supplied us boys with many months of clandestine distraction from our daily routine. And none of us got his eye shot out. Nary a one. Honest.

CHAPTER 45

Birthdays and Friendship

I turned twelve on April 30, 1951, "celebrating" it alone as usual. Adolescents crave sympathy and recognition, that support their fragile, emerging egos and give them a sense of much-needed positive self-worth. However, each downy-cheeked 1-B and 2-B boy was too naïve and self-centered to fathom that his peers also sought this much-needed attention.

Almost universally then, beginning about two weeks before the boy's birthday each year, he would start hinting to the other kids that his birthday was on such-and-such a date and day of the week. These initially subtle and fairly wide-spaced in time "reminders" increased in frequency and decreased in subtlety as the special day drew nigh.

The number of "Happy Birthday" greetings received on that child's special day determined just how homesick the boy would be at day's end, and in the days that immediately followed.

In many respects our microcosm mirrored that of any similar small town; cliques were formed by the age of twelve or thirteen. At times Bill Herrington, Van Edwards, Newton Wilder and I were as though one person. We trusted and "stood up" for one another, and discovered that a mean-spirited big boy was less likely to harass a group of us. And, sometimes not.

I learned that if I remembered the birthdays of my closest friends, and wished them "Happy Birthday" on that hallowed day, they would be more inclined to return the favor as my birthday approached.

It was in this and similar settings that I learned the most valuable lesson in advancement through life, which is, go out of your way, I mean *really* out of your way, to help people and show them that you are genuinely interested in their welfare, and you will be rewarded in like kind.

This attitude has served me well throughout life. I left the orphanage on February 15, 1957, with two twenty dollar bills given to me by my friend Mr. Maurice Parham, the orphanage comptroller and business manager, and a large suitcase full of clothes "lifted" the night before from the Industrial Building by a few of my friends.

Six months later, in my first semester at Berry College in Rome, Georgia, I was elected President of the Freshman Class. I was a student government officer the entire four years at Berry College, ending up in my Senior year as President of the Men's Student Government. As a Junior I was awarded the Jessie Pritchett Parish Student Leadership Award, that honored each year the one student in the entire student body for his or her leadership abilities on campus.

These leadership qualities were not born overnight. They were developed as a snot-faced orphan kid of eleven and twelve in 1-B and 2-B, where I learned that if I helped my friends, they in turn would not let me down. I realized even before I left Oxford at age seventeen, that I had been an inspiration to my peers and the younger boys, for standing up to the abuses of Regan and his twin Hound from Hell, Pig Talton. In turn I had learned a lot from my peers and a few of the Big Boys who and befriended me. My story could never be finished without mention of some of them, to whom I owe a neverending debt of gratitude.

Van Edwards taught me to help others, out of the goodness of my heart, expecting nothing in return. From my first day in the Baby Cottage until I left Oxford in 1957, and beyond, I sought Van's opinion and guidance.

Coley Lee Hackett and Butch Mitchell taught me, by example, to question abuse and authority, and I learned the defiant "Fuck you!" (spoken very loudly under my breath) from these two hell-raising nonconformists.

Newton Wilder taught me not to fear physical abuse from older boys. Newton was not afraid of anything or anybody. And the older boys knew it, and left him alone. Newton was the role model for my rebellion against physical abuse from grownups.

Javon Frye and Bobby Boyette, both several years older than I, were the Big Boys who befriended and protected me from any potential physical harm. They started out as good friends of my sister, and they remained loyal during their stay at Oxford and beyond. Each of them told me on several occasions that if any older boy ever picked on me, just to let him know. On the night of my altercation with Mr. Regan at age thirteen, both boys came to the basement of 4-B to try to talk me out of leaving the orphanage that night. When they failed to convince me to remain, Bobby gave me ten dollars and the two friends wished me well.

Maurice Parham, the orphanage comptroller, took an interest in me at an early age, and gave me advice and encouragement, being cognizant at all times of my hate-hate relationship with Mr. Gray and Mr. Regan. Not once did Maurice Parham conceal his friendship with me from any member of the administration.

CHAPTER 46

The Bell

Life at the orphanage, as well as the lives of hundreds of townsfolk living within hearing distance, for better or worse, was regulated daily by "The Bell."

Certain tasks performed on campus warranted monthly cash payments; for example, the boy who turned on the campus lights at night and turned them off in the morning, the boys who cut hair, and the boys who maintained the coal furnaces that supplied hot water and forced heat to the cottages.

The "bellringer" was likewise a paid position. The upside of this job was the extra money, always a big plus for us orphans; the downside of the job was undoubtedly early hearing loss.

Regulation of life on campus went somewhat as follows. The "Six-o'clock Bell" brought the orphanage abruptly to life each day. This was the longest ringing of the Bell each day, and lasted for several minutes. The simple message sent by the Six-o'clock Bell was a well-punctuated "Get up!" Every child sleeping at the sound of this Bell had forty minutes to get out of bed, do his "duty," wash his face and hands, and get ready for the cottage counselor's inspection of the performance of his duty.

At 6:40 a.m., the Twenty-minute Bell sounded, at which time the cottage counselor inspected the performance (or non-performance, as was often the case) of the duty, and if the child's performance was found lacking, he did the duty again to the satisfaction of the cottage counselor. Orphan kids thus learn at an early age to "get it right the first time."

At 6:55 the "five minute bell" sounded, and the children knew they could enter the dining rooms at the next bell, that rang at 7:00 a.m. This bell was called the "seven o'clock bell" or the "breakfast bell." No child was allowed to enter the dining room until the seven o'clock bell sounded, regardless of the weather.

During rainy weather, the girls usually waited on the large covered porch of the massive dining hall, and the boys crowded together on the covered porch on the ground floor of the Main Building. This grouping had been set in stone by custom, and never changed while I was at the orphanage.

Ringing the large bell properly was an art; it had to be learned, and one experienced bellringer taught his replacement. If a boy desired to ring the bell, he had to "butter up" the bellringer. Mary Jane candy or Bazooka bubble gum usually got the bellringer's attention and cooperation. Just one of the perks of the job.

Concerning the art of bellringing. A neophyte was the one who jerked the large hemp rope, causing an erratic, rapid "clang-clang" followed by silence. The experienced bellringer pulled on the thick rope with a practiced rhythm, and after the first slow, measured pull on the rope to get the process started, only helped continue the bell at its own pace. This was evidenced by a "clang-pause-clang-pause-clang" pleasant to the ears. And an awful lot of responsibility went with the job, because more than three hundred children relied on the bellringer being accurate. Couldn't ring the 6:00 o'clock bell at 6:10 a.m. Try that trick and the bellringer would lose his job.

The endearing peal of the bell carried with it a certain reassurance, that life at Oxford went on at a fixed, predetermined, steady pace, that whatever your troubles might be, the Bell signified a sense of, well, let's call it stability, in our lives. Or, at least we sought to view it in that light.

The Bell became my friend, because I knew I could rely on its consistency and faithfulness. It never demanded anything of me, rather, it informed me, or reminded me, if you will, of what time it was and where I was supposed to be at any given moment. Other than as a status symbol, as in "look what my mama brought me . . . and yours didn't," we kids had no practical use for timepieces, either clock or watch. And respect for the Bell was universal. During my ten years of incarceration at Oxford Orphanage, I never once heard a child curse the ringing of the Bell, or speak in any derogatory manner about it.

The normal sound of our Bell was a commanding CLANG . . . CLANG . . . CLANG. However, when the weather was damp and the temperature outside fell below thirty-two degrees Fahrenheit, ice quickly coated the poor Bell, resulting in an anemic ting-a-ling, like a muted timpani of thunder many miles distant.

"Can I ring the Bell?" I asked my question rather timidly, fully expecting to be soundly rebuffed in my attempt to control *something* in my eleven-year-old world.

"Why would a skinny little fart like you want to ring the Bell?" the Big Boy replied, somewhat amused at my request. But before I could form a feeble reply, he added "Yu got any candy?"

"No, but I can get some," I blurted out, not knowing if or when I could obtain the bribe.

"Okay, get me a Mary Jane and I'll let you ring it."

"Thanks a lot." And I scurried away.

I had exacted a promise from the Big Boy. For a measly little Mary Jane candy I could control the lives, even if for an instant, of more than three hundred kids. What a rush! And what's more, I had never seen any of my peers ring the Bell. Poor, jealous sods!

On the first day of the following month, no sooner had Josephine pressed the shiny quarter into my sweaty palm, and I was at the door of the business office, down the steps, across to the Candy Corner in the Main Building, and demanding from Betty Evans (gosh, she sure was pretty, and she looked great from behind, too) a whole quarter's worth of Mary Janes.

But would the Big Boy remember me? What if he had changed his mind? Would I know how to ring the huge Bell? And just how many rings did I get for a quarter's worth of Mary Janes? My thoughts were jumbled as I approached the Big Boy. I wanted to ring the Twelve O'clock

Bell, that told several hundred hungry kids that I, Little Orphan Al, was going to give them permission to enter the dining rooms. What a sense of power!

I watched the Big Boy chatting with his friends while keeping a close watch on his watch. It was drawing nigh onto noon, so I had to make my move. At a pause in the conversation, I tugged at the Big Boy's shirt sleeve. Opening my palm to reveal a goodly number of pieces of the coveted Mary Janes, a right good-sized fistful of the goodies, I said,

"Got your Mary Janes."

"For me?"

"Yeah, you said you'd let me ring the Bell if I got you some Mary Janes. Can I ring it now?"

"Sure, but I don't need all your candy." And he took two large pieces from my outstretched palm. I recall thinking at that moment, that usually I would be hiding my candy from the Big Boys, and here I was actually extending my hand to give one of them some candy. Sure hope none of my buddies saw me seem to capitulate in this manner, it would have destroyed my image for good. They probably would have painted a yellow line down my back, and banished me from the Seventh Cavalry outright.

"How many times can I ring it?"

"Okay, since you're so eager to ring the Bell, you can do the Twelve O'clock Bell and the Six O'clock Bell. And it's about time. Get ready."

My tiny palms began to sweat, and I started having the same heart palpitations as though standing in front of Old Man Gray on a Saturday afternoon. However, these were happy sweaty palms and joyful heart palpitations, and were signs that I was about to experience something wonderful and exciting.

"Okay, grab the rope one hand over the other."

I did as instructed.

"I'll pull with you the first few strokes, then you're on your own." And he placed his large hands over mine.

"How many times do I pull on it?"

"Don't worry, I'll tell you when to stop."

"Okay."

We pulled the thick rope together, the Big Boy's hands clasped firmly over mine. The pulls were slow and measured. Now Little Orphan Al was in charge. What a thrill!

Suddenly the Big Boy released his grip on my hands, saying,

"Keep it going just like that. I'll tell you when to stop."

And I kept it going, using slow, measured pulls, with the same rhythm we had just used together, more helping the Bell ring itself, maintaining the established cadence.

Finally the Big Boy said "Okay, just let it go."

I did, and the Bell made two more fading peals, then fell silent.

"You did good, kid."

"Thanks."

"See you back here before six o'clock. Don't be late."

"I won't be late."

"And by the way, here's your Mary Janes," he said, handing back my candy.

"Thanks." I had just found another friend.

The Big Boy let me ring the Twelve O'clock Bell each day for several days, then periodically thereafter. It was the high point in my young life during that time. And the Big Boy remained my friend long after he graduated and left the orphanage. He called me "Bellringer," and I wore the nickname with pride.

I seldom hear bells ringing anymore. Many churches today tend not to use them. But whenever I hear the peal of a distant bell, memories flood my mind. If only they were all good ones . . .

CHAPTER 47

Orphans' All-Time Favorites Peanut Butter and Ice Cream

The orphanage purchased large quantities of peanut butter and molasses, and massive amounts were also donated, as was butter, by the U.S. government. We used to go with Mr. Adams and Mr. Davis down to the railway depot, Camp Butner, located about fifteen miles from Oxford toward Durham, and pick up loads of these foodstuffs that were government surplus, the result of subsidized farming and dairying in the United States. We were grateful.

We kids usually had peanut butter and molasses for Wednesday and Sunday supper. Because everyone was required to attend Vespers on Sunday evening (old man Gray's weekly moment of glory) rarely was any cooking done for Sunday supper, even in the Baby Cottage. That was fine with 300-plus orphan kids, as we all enjoyed the simple menu of peanut butter, molasses, deviled eggs and pimento cheese.

Half a century later my favorite foods remain peanut butter and Grandma's Molasses, the love of which must have found its way into my gene pool. Early on my four children developed an orphan's craving for peanut butter, and even my wife, who rarely tasted the delicacy before we married, keeps her special jar of "reduced fat" peanut butter on the dining room table, that we still call the "supper" table.

In October 1997 I attended my fortieth high school class reunion during Homecoming. After church services on Sunday, I stood in line with more than a thousand former orphans for the traditional Homecoming Southern Barbeque Dinner. When I approached the last server in line, my plate already piled high with delicious greasy pork barbeque, cole slaw and baked beans, I looked down and there before me sat a huge plastic tub, big enough to bathe a St. Bernard in, filled with already-stirred peanut butter and molasses, beside which lay several large stacks of bread.

Instantly the nostalgic shock of the moment formed a lump in my throat and brought an embarrassment of tears to my eyes. Without giving it a second thought, I placed my (suddenly unwanted) plate of barbeque on a table to my left, said "Lots, please," to the orphan server, who, giving me a smile of perfect understanding, filled my plate half full with the delicious mixture, plopped about eight slices of white bread on the other side of the plate, reached back and poured me a large glass of cold milk, and I sat with former classmates and enjoyed the best meal I had that year. Tears of remembrance mix well with peanut butter and molasses. One of a few priceless moments of a lifetime, simple in form but infinitely important in meaning.

At the orphanage we kids ate breakfast, dinner and supper. The word "lunch" never was used. Standard English-language dictionaries define "lunch" as any light meal, "supper" as an evening meal, and "dinner" as the chief meal of the day, whether eaten in the evening or about noon.

Children on the main campus enjoyed peanut butter and molasses every Wednesday and Sunday for supper. The pint-sized prisoners in the Baby Cottage ate deviled eggs and pimento cheese sandwiches on those two nights.

So how do you prepare peanut butter and molasses sandwiches for more than three hundred hungry orphans? Not on any small scale, that's for sure. Peanut butter came packaged in these really oversized glass jars. Molasses came in what looked like a fifty-five gallon oil drum, that when turned on its side a la a cask of aging Chardonnay, Merlot or Burgundy, exposed a kind of faucet, or spigot, that we kids pronounced (and would have spelled) "spicket."

To prepare this twice-weekly Southern Epicurus delight, several huge jars of peanut butter were scooped into a whopping metal basin. The kitchen girls held large milk pitchers under the "spicket," turned on the handle, and filled the pitchers with the rich, black, frothing molasses.

The girls then poured the molasses over the basin of peanut butter, then stirred the ingredients until it produced a blackish-brown homogenous mixture. Bowls filled with the preparation were placed at each end of the dining room tables by the female waitresses, that we called "head girls," and the children scooped out what they wanted, either eating the mixture as it was, or making sandwiches.

Probably the most ignored rule of conduct on the campus was the prohibition against taking any food from the dining rooms, except for the fruit given as dessert (apples, oranges and bananas) nearly every night at supper. This rule presented a grand dilemma for peanut butter and molasses starved orphans, because we ate this delicacy that we considered more of a dessert than a main course, only twice each week.

So every Sunday and Wednesday at supper, we kids would stuff ourselves with peanut butter and molasses, and tuck one (or two or three) peanut butter and molasses sandwiches under our shirts or coats, depending on the weather. During the Winter months a peanut butter and molasses sandwich could last about two weeks before going bad, or so Ersul Sowers told me.

At the time my good friend and dairymate Frank McMillan arrived at the orphanage in 1944, the students were treated to homemade ice cream, and Frank recalls that as a Baby Cottage inmate, he enjoyed cranking the mixture.

At home in Kinston, at about that same time, it was my task to determine the quantity of salt to be sprinkled on the ice at the appropriate time during the process, and to supervise closely my older brothers Bill and Kenny as they cranked the mixer.

By the time I arrived at Oxford three years later, in February 1947, the sacrifices and hardships of wartime had eased somewhat, such that for Sunday dinner dessert, each child was treated to a square-shaped block of ice cream, consisting of equal parts vanilla, chocolate and strawberry, and it seemed to me that chocolate was always the center flavor.

These blocks of ice cream, that we kids called "bricks," were called "Neapolitan Squares." The bricks came individually wrapped in a sort of waxed paper, to keep them separated. The Neapolitan Squares were purchased from Pine State Dairies, and we all looked forward to this weekly treat.

In the early 1950's Mr. Pruitt and the bakery boys began making our own ice cream, and a storage room off the downstairs dining room was converted to an ice cream room, complete with ice cream machines and storage freezers. Using us children as testers, Mr. Pruitt experimented with the ice cream machines. At first the ice cream came out slushy and tasteless; you either could not taste the chocolate, or it was so filled with chocolate you never wanted to taste chocolate ice cream again.

Braving an onslaught of ridicule and taunts from dissatisfied, unforgiving and demanding children, however, Mr. Pruitt and his boys persevered with their experiments, eventually producing ice cream that was both palatable and toothsome. Strawberry and peach ice creams were chock full of fresh strawberries and peaches from the orphanage farm, and the chocolate and vanilla ice creams were rich in flavor. And because ice cream's main ingredient, milk, was produced in abundance by the orphanage's fifty-cow herd, rich, creamy and delicious ice cream of many flavors instantly became the dessert of choice for children and staff alike. The brand of ice cream mixer was called a "Kool King," and the ice cream was stored in one and a half gallon metal containers. Pine State Dairies made the blend, and Mr. Pruitt and the bakery boys added the milk and when in season, the peaches and strawberries.

When we started high school, our old dairy buddy Frank McMillan gave us boys a key to unlock the padlock on the large metal bar that secured the metal ice cream containers. At night we would unlock the main kitchen door, go into the basement and feast on delicious just-baked bread and other food. Periodically we would swipe a few gallons of ice cream and some large tablespoons, and take our contraband down to the skating rink near the Baby Cottage, soon founder ourselves on the delicious ice cream, then leave the empty containers in the drainage grating that was located in the grassed center of the skating rink. Crafty little bastards we were. Eventually some younger kids would notice the containers shining up from under the grating, and eventually the containers would be returned to the bakery.

One night at supper, just after we had said the blessing, Mr. Pruitt called for quiet, and announced if whoever had been stealing the ice cream would please return the metal containers. While he was making his request, he was staring directly at me. After supper Van Edwards, Bill Herrington and Newton Wilder swore that Mr. Pruitt was staring directly at them.

We boys gave it some serious thought, then decided if we didn't return the five empty ice cream containers, Mr. Pruitt might get mad and just quit making ice cream altogether. And this just wouldn't do. So we retrieved the metal containers from the drain and the bushes, and just left them lying on the ground. And sure as hell, next night at supper, Mr. Pruitt made an announcement thanking the thieves for returning his containers. We were all offended that Mr. Pruitt referred to us as thieves, but we decided to let it slide. We were thieves, yes, but we also were magnanimous thieves.

And just where did we boys get all these keys? Simple. At the end of our Junior year in high school, just prior to graduation, one of the graduating Seniors extracted from his private locker a large key ring, on which hung about twenty keys of various sizes and shapes, and handed the keys to one of our group.

"You'll have to figure them out," said the departing Senior, then added,

"But they'll fit any building and room you need to break into." The boys in 3-B and 4-B would have turned Ali Baba green with envy.

CHAPTER 48

Snow, Snow Cream, Sledding and Frozen Tits

Kids love snow because it's soft and fluffy, there's a lot of it, they can eat it and it can't hurt them. And to us orphans the three or four quite generous snowfalls that quietly blanketed our section of northern North Carolina each Winter lifted our homesick spirits, if only for awhile. To this day I have discovered no Winter scene that equals in grandeur the four hundred acres of Oxford Orphanage covered by a few feet of white powder in January. Truly the stuff of which Christmas cards are made.

But times sure have changed. Any kid who grew up in North Carolina during the forties and fifties knows well what "snow cream" is. Alas, however, I could not find the term in any of my favorite unabridged dictionaries.

We enterprising orphan children needed five things to make snow cream, 1) a large metal pan, 2) milk, 3) a bottle of vanilla extract, 4) sugar, and, of course, 5) snow. Numbers 1,2 and 4 we could get anytime. All you needed to acquire Number 3 was a girl friend or sister who worked in the kitchen. For Number 5, we just had to wait and hope we got lucky.

So, along toward the middle of December the kids in 1-B through 4-B eagerly awaited the first snowfall of Winter, that was usually fairly heavy. After it had snowed for a few hours, we boys would grab our large metal pan, look for the largest wind-swept snowdrift we could find, gently rake the top layer of snow away, fill the pan with loose snow, then gently, very gently, pack it down to give it some consistency, but not packed too hard.

Next we poured in the milk, added generous amounts of vanilla extract and sugar, and stirred the mixture very, very slowly. Snow cream was as tasty as vanilla ice cream; after all, the ingredients are nearly the same.

Topographically, the main campus was relatively flat. So about the best (read that "steepest") snow sledding area at the orphanage was located on the far side of the hilly pasture where the cows rested at night during warm weather. The steep hill overlooks the small creek and railroad track that run the width of the orphanage farm, near the blackberry patch.

Following a snowfall, at the earliest possible moment, we kids grabbed whatever we could find that was flat on at least one side, and headed for the top of the long hill. We kids made sleds out of any metal garbage can lid or sheet of wood that would slide across snow. Snow sleds were of the makeshift variety, limited only by the ingenuity of the owner.

When not making snow cream, sledding or engaging in snowball fights, during snowfalls the normal kids stayed inside hugging the radiators or trying to crowd their buddies off of hot air vents located in the floor. A Winter January wind fifteen miles from the Virginia state line could quickly bite your nose and crawl like a frozen crab beneath the soft woolen flaps of your toboggan.

I'm not certain whether stupidity begets meanness, or vice versa; however, some of those 4-B hoodlums were as mean as they were dumb, so even during heavy snowfalls in the dead of Winter, I learned to negotiate the becalmed, white-powdered campus, head bowed, glancing furtively left, then right, then left again, and so on, because in the orphanage in 1948 and 1949, furtive, surreptitious left and right glances were the order of the day as a basic survival skill among us preteen orphan boys. And we youngsters stayed the hell away from 4-B like everybody who lived in that cottage had the Black Plague or something.

Still and all, it paid to be vigilant, because at times during such awfully cold weather, we younguns would observe one of the stupid-assed 4-B yahoos venture outside in the freezing snow halfway up to his ass, stand there shivering in his T-shirt, pack a few oversized snowballs, sling them aimlessly at a large, six foot diameter oak tree trunk or some other non-moving, non-threatening inanimate object, sniff the still, freezing air like a friggin' bloodhound, then meander on back inside to discuss more ways to harass us 1-B and 2-B preteens.

So, 4-B was not exactly a repository of intellectual advancement. Being at times not too swift on the uptake, some of these mental midgets would be apt to ask a drugstore clerk whether hand lotion came in powdered form, or what time the six o'clock bell rings on Thursday morning. But then again, in their defense, none of them ever mistook a rubber for a goddamn balloon.

When I say I was more intelligent or more perceptive than most of my peers, we're not exactly comparing my intellect to that of any Al Einstein, but to that of my peers, of which the I.Q. of a goodly number of them seemed to hover somewhere in the vicinity of the 1947 North Carolina speed limit for rural roads. One night Coley Lee and I broke into the case worker Miss Broadwell's office and looked at our personnel files, and at the personnel files of three hundred other kids. Coley Lee instantly regretted coming, after looking at his file. But at least Coley Lee would be able to remember his I.Q.; as I recall it was an even ten points lower than the normal body temperature for white Southern boys.

At that same midnight breakin-a breakin is when you just get information, a raid is when you break in and take goods from the Industrial Building or goodies from the kitchen-I learned that my I.Q. was two points higher than my sister Eoline's. That was understandable and to be expected. However, my brother Pete's I.Q. showed on his record to be four points higher than mine. I made a note to have Miss Broadwell correct the obvious typographical error, since the fact that I was four years older than my brother naturally meant that I was more intelligent than he.

I rarely if ever did anything really stupid . . . that I'd admit to, anyway. But ever so often one of the older boys mistakenly thought I had done or said something dumb. And in that case the Big Boy would ask "Where you from, boy?" spitting out the "boy" like it was a cold snot he had got stuck 'tween his teeth, that was likely the case.

I would of course quickly reply "From Kinston," then proudly add, "World's Foremost Tobacco Center." The answer was always "Yeah, you told me that already."

Then one day one of the Big Boys, cocking his head to the right and kinda slanting his eyes to the left in order to compensate and keep me in focus, asked "Ersul Sowers and Red Albertson. They from Kinston, too?"

"Yes," I replied proudly.

"I thought so," came the answer.

I don't know. Perhaps it was something they put in the Kinston Municipal Water Supply.

The first snowfall of the Winter of 1950-1951 turned out to be a small blizzard. A dense shower of white began to hit the ground about the time study hall started, and by the time it ended two hours later, the boys in 3-B and 4-B were already in the midst of a snowball fight. Fearing she would not live through the night if she dared hold us back, Witch Robinson released us, and by then the ground was already covered with a thick blanket of white. As usual once the 1-B and 2-B kids came outside, the dumbass Big Boys quit fighting each other, and we younger boys got the worst of it.

Of course, years later when I was in 3-B and 4-B, we older boys never picked on the 1-B and 2-B boys when it snowed. Well, maybe just a little bit. And then again, maybe more than that. Anyway, getting hit with snowballs was no big deal. But the dumbass Big Boys would chase us down and put handfuls of snow down our shirts, or rub snow in our faces, or both. Usually both. Rarely ever not both.

At the orphanage we could always tell it was snowing or icing simply by listening to the sound of the ubiquitous Bell in the belfry of the Main Building that controlled our lives (and the lives of literally hundreds of persons living on the periphery of the orphanage grounds).

The usual sound of the huge Bell was a commanding "DING! DONG! DING! DONG!" that got everybody's attention. Impossible to sleep through it, or to ignore it. I used to imagine The Maker's day beginning with the command of the Main Building Bell.

However, during snowfalls and ice storms that, being located a mere fifteen miles from the Virginia state line, we had our share of each Winter, the moisture in the air coated the Bell with ice, and the only sounds emanating from the bell tower were the quite anemic "ping. ping. ping. ping." If ever we had sympathy for an inanimate object, it was *our* Bell when the temperature dropped below thirty-two degrees on a damp Winter night.

The orphanage campus was a most beautiful place, and the seasonal snowfalls transformed it further into a Winter Currier and Ives print, both on the forty-acre main campus, and the 350-acre farm and dairy. During the Winter months the milking herd was kept in the Long Barn at night, and even during the day if it turned really cold. Didn't serve any purpose to keep the cows in the pasture-no grass for them to eat anyway.

To secure the cows, I had to drive them through the pasture, up the hill, through two wide wooden gates, right onto the Farm Road for about a hundred yards, then left into the Long Barn. Reverse these directions when going the other way. It puts you back at the dairy barn.

When bringing the herd to the dairy in the morning darkness, if the cows can see the road, they are smart enough to see where the road ends and the gate is located, and so long as I guided the leaders, the rest of the herd would follow. But I still had to roust the old cows and the lazy (yes, there are lazy cows-it's not just a human trait) ones, lest they get left behind.

It snowed so hard throughout the night, and was still snowing when I was awakened at 3:30 the next morning by the big dairy boy. So off I trudged, in snow up to my skinny ass, stumbling, slipping, sliding (and cussing my predicament) all the way to the Long Barn.

The gate to the pasture was left open at night during the Winter (Who was going to get out of an empty pasture?), so I slid open the large wooden front gate of the Long Barn, prodded out the first few lumbering beasts, and headed them down the road toward the gate leading to the pasture. Then I returned to the barn for the rest of the herd of forty-six cows. Trouble was, the snow was so deep the cows couldn't possibly see the road, missed the gate off to their left completely, and just kept walking straight, into the glorious blackness or a moonless night.

As I unknowingly brought up the rear of the herd and got them to the gate, I looked straight ahead and there before me, eerily disappearing into the early morning darkness were forty-six freezing udders, from which dangled 184 freezing tits, spread out from hell to yonder. Totally disoriented because of the deep snow and pitch dark, the entire herd was heading *away* from the dairy barn, toward the hog pens a half mile away. Dammit to hell!

Cows are herd animals-they tend to follow the lead cows . . . that is, if they can see or at least localize the cow's mooing in the dark. However, in three-foot snow drifts, on now unfamiliar ground and a moonless night to boot, scattered cows mooing incessantly because their (184) tits are turning to icicles, you end up with forty-six disoriented cows heading in forty-seven different directions. Try rounding up that herd!

After trying desperately but being unable to turn any of them around, I finally gave up and trudged back through the snow and face-biting cold to the dairy, and told the older boys what had occurred. Apparently they had had the same experience in years past, because nobody kicked my (cold) butt or yelled at me or called me "stupid," and off we all went, the ten of us cow-hunting in the dark. More than an hour later we had rounded up all forty-six of the unhappy, frozen-titted beasts, all of us cold and wet and hungry and tired before the day had even started.

Mr. Davis called Mr. Pruitt at the kitchen, and Mr. Pruitt saved breakfast for the ten of us. When he found out what had happened, he fed us all heaping portions of oatmeal, scrambled eggs and bacon, and finally we warmed up a bit. All of us dairy boys liked Mr. Pruitt, and we appreciated him even more after that morning. Another lesson learned for dumbass little Al, another experience to tuck away in the recesses of my rapidly-expanding mind. The salient lesson learned that memorable snowy night: Never, never, never, ever work on a dairy. Not ever.

CHAPTER 49

Tom Adams

I wasn't in a very good mood. It was the end of June 1951, and I was a few months into my twelfth year on this Earth, and the same period of time into my fourth year on Hell's Four Hundred Acres. Earlier that month Eoline and I had been allowed to go home on vacation for two weeks, one of those glorious weeks of which we spent with Doc, Bill, Kenny, J.B. and their families in Washington, D.C. Good time. Bad move.

By the end of the Shortest Two Weeks of My Miserable Life, when mama brought us back I was already well into the Seventh Stage of Depression, you know, when self-immolation spells relief, and when you begin searching for a really sharp double-edged Gillette, and you aren't supposed to start shaving for another five years or so?

Back at the dairy, Mr. Davis did his level best to stop my bawling, but to no avail.

He became so exasperated that he asked Robert Wyke to try to reason with me, but after several days Robert told Mr. Davis that I was inconsolable and that he didn't want to have anything to do with "that stupid crybaby from Kinston."

I really didn't give a damn. I was homesick, I didn't belong in this stupid, hateful place, I wanted to go home, and "home" sure as hell wasn't Oxford Orphanage. I was not a happy lad, didn't care who knew it, and spent long hours each day in the doldrums.

A week or so after returning to Oxford Prison Farm, I was loitering in front of the dairy barn with Frank and Butch, just idling away our free time, debating the cons and cons of life in "this damn place," placing side bets on which of us was more homesick, when we looked up the concrete driveway leading to the dirt farm road, and observed Tom Adams, who had been farm manager only for about five months, sauntering toward us down the driveway.

Now, in the few short months he had been manager of the orphanage farm, Tom Adams had engendered about as much respect among the boys at the orphanage as a follicle mite on the left testicle of a rabid pit bull. This despicable low-life, who had made a sport of physically threatening and abusing defenseless preteen farm boys since his arrival in January 1951 straight from a training school, appeared to be headed straight for the three of us, though as farm manager he had no real authority over us because we worked for Mr. Davis. But here came the Hound from Hell just the same.

Tom Adams was wearing his patented permanent derisive smirk, that showed us young orphans just how much disdain and contempt he had for us and our lot in life.

As he drew near, we just looked at him without speaking, believing he had come to see Mr. Davis, who was inside the dairy at the time. From an early age at the orphanage, we kids were taught to speak only when spoken to by a grownup, and Mr. Adams had yet to address us with his patented vilifying tone of voice.

As he approached us, he kinda sorta veered more toward me than the other two boys, like he was some sort of human heat-seeking missile and I was the only boy smoking a cornsilk fag. Clearly not expecting it, the lightning blow from his open right hand caught me squarely on the side of my face, knocking me off my feet and bouncing me like a well-worn tennis ball off the whitewashed lower wall of the dairy barn.

Dazed, my left ear ringing weirdly, and experiencing a strange sense of lightheadedness, I looked up as the bastard said,

"I know you didn't say anything, but you were thinking 'dammit.'"

Looking down at me with his patented contemptuous glare, the slick-skinned abuser waited for me to say something.

This sadistic son of a bitch was the *exact* reason I hated "this damn place," and for fear of antagonizing him further, I just sat propped up against the whitewashed dairy wall, buried my face in my hands and began sobbing uncontrollably.

The next thing I recalled was being jerked to my feet by a very large hand holding on to about ninety-nine percent of my hair, the bastard's reddened face pushed about an inch from mine, with him literally screaming in my bruised, tear-filled face,

"Now, if you don't stop your damned crying, you'll get more where that came from!" Visions of The White Bitch Tomblin, Baby Elephant Baldwin and the sadist old man Gray flashed through my terrified mind.

I tried my best to stop crying, fearing the worst, but the bastard only tightened his grip on my hair, shaking my head back and forth like it was a rag doll, and through a blur of tears I saw his free hand coming at my head again.

From sheer terror I twisted loose, leaving his hand clutching a tuft of my hair, and bolted into the dairy. Luckily, Mr. Davis was inside still, giving some work instructions to the other dairy boys, and had not heard the ruckus. I moved quickly along the aisle until I had Mr. Davis between me and Tom Adams, and stood at the rear door of the dairy barn, determined to keep on running if I had to.

Tom Adams poked his still-red face through the front barn door, but when he noticed Mr. Davis standing in the aisle, turned without comment and walked back up the long concrete driveway, undoubtedly to vent his spleen on other unsuspecting preteen farm boys.

I was probably the first frightened orphan boy to run from Mr. Adams and live to tell the tale. At this age in my young life, hatred, scorn and insurgency began to push themselves into and claim a place in my oft-wounded psyche. Following the traumatic incident, I avoided the cruel bastard at all costs, and vowed openly that I would run from the abusive child-beater if ever he approached me again.

Fortunately for me, he never did, and after awhile turned his venomous nature to other poor vulnerable farm boys. I was a fast study. My "list" was growing. Mentally I penned in "Tom Adams" below Baby Elephant Baldwin.

Tom Adams had accumulated all the practice and experience in child cruelty to fit in real well at Oxford Orphanage; prior to becoming farm manager at Oxford, this abuser of orphan boys had held a similar position at an infamous training school in the state.

D.P. "Soapy" Peake had been an employee at Oxford Orphanage for thirty-eight years, most of this time as farm manager, when I began working at the dairy in June 1950. Five months later, on November 5, 1950, Soapy Peake died, and Mr. Davis assumed the farm manager's duties until a new farm manager could be hired.

Thomas R. "Tom" Adams arrived in January 1951 to take over as farm manager. Even then, mechanization was reaching the orphanage farm. The kitchen inventory at the end of 1951 showed more than eight thousand pounds of vegetables and berries in the freezer lockers. During the year several new implements had been purchased for the lone DC-3 tractor that had been purchased a year earlier, and this allowed the orphanage to sell two of its ten mules.

Mr. Adams predicted that if the orphanage purchased another tractor, a hay baler and a forage cutter, he would be able to sell another two mules. Given such progress in farm mechanization, Tom Adams no doubt envisioned a mule-less farm within three years. Didn't happen.

Doubtless from years of practice on the poor unfortunates at the training school, Tom Adams possessed an ingrained proclivity for mental and physical abuse of young boys. He held a position on campus similar to that of Mrs. Tomblin in this regard.

At the beginning of a child's stay at Oxford, the child was under the direct control of the insensitive, uncaring and abusive Mrs. Edith Tomblin for a week or ten days, at a time when no doubt every child who passed through the Main Gate desperately needed love and care and understanding. Didn't get it from that hateful old bitch. What a greeting!

And at one time or another, nearly every adolescent and teenage boy worked at the orphanage farm for a few years, and thus fell under the curse of the abusive predator Tom Adams. If you took Oliver Hardy, shaved off his moustache, and gave him the depravity attributed to Adolf Hitler, you would have a pretty good picture of Tom Adams. Had this beer-gutted, slick-skinned, moon-faced, constantly antacid-munching pornographer left his attitude and cruel disposition at the training school, he would have been an asset to the orphanage. He really knew his farming.

However, as other supervisors before (and after) him, Tom Adams learned quickly that his pattern of ill-temper and physical abuse would not be held in check by those orphanage administrators to whom he answered.

About thirty boys worked on the farm in Winter and about sixty during the Summer, and from the beginning Tom Adams' baseness stuck out like a red flag. Nobody liked Tom Adams; nor did anybody cross him.

I never forgot the humiliation I suffered that warm Summer morning. For weeks I seethed in anger over the crass insult. I had committed no act that would have caused the evil bastard to assault me. Butch, Frank and I were quietly discussing our vacations; and we were not even laughing or joking or talking in loud voices. It was at this point in my young life that indignation began to smolder beneath my veneer of fear of bodily harm.

CHAPTER 50

Colored Farm Workers

Even as an artless youngster of eleven, I could read the hard times chiseled like granite statues into the aging features of the five colored orphanage farm workers. Their bronze faces etched with a patina of lines and wrinkles doubtless from decades of trudging behind plows pulled by Missouri mules in the baking North Carolina sun, these five gentlemen were as kind as saints, as gentle as the mules with which they toiled, as loyal as patriots to The All-Powerful.

In 1950 the colored farm workers included Jesse Montague, Henry Martin, Hubert Laws, Silas Gooch and Claude Satterfield, although during the grass-growing months, Henry's more or less fulltime job was cutting the fast-growing campus grass with his very large, very noisy riding lawn mower. As of that year these five men had worked for Oxford Orphanage an average of twenty-eight years each.

Like so many of my peers, I am a product of my postwar Southern upbringing. Daddy and mama taught us kids to respect the coloreds who lived near us and who were customers in the family "convenience" store that took up the large front room of our house. So as I worked alongside the colored farm workers at the orphanage, I showed them the same respect I afforded the white staff members and teachers. We youngsters answered the colored workers with the Southern honorific "Yes, sir," as we were taught to address any adult, regardless of his or her station in life.

We orphan boys easily could empathize with our colored co-workers, because a disadvantaged child, having become cognizant of his deprived social status (by comparison of his lot with that of those more fortunate) is thereafter able to spot his soulmate in what we Southerners call "a New York minute."

One muggy Summer afternoon in 1951, when I was twelve, I was walking through the warm rain on my way to the dairy, when I passed the corn crib, where alone sat skinny-as-a-rail Claude Satterfield, who later retired in 1957 after thirty-eight years as an orphanage farm worker.

Claude had sought respite from the elements; can't do a whole lot of plowing in a muddy field. So there we paused for awhile, seated on well-worn wooden steps beneath the protection of the corn crib overhang, an unpretentious, innocent preteen white orphan boy, and an aged-beyond-his-years scrub pine bluegum, enjoying an impromptu discussion about the similarities and differences between our lots in life, he reminiscing over a lifetime of toiling alongside literally thousands of similarly-situated displaced orphan kids, I in turn listening in dumbstruck awe, empathy and appreciation to a kind old colored gentleman, whose chances for education and a "good life" in what he labeled, without recrimination or spite, the "white man's world," were nonexistent, and when he surprised me with the self-denigrating observation "We's jus' a bunch o' ole coons," suddenly my problems shrank to the size and consequence of dry spit in the furrow of a just-plowed crooked August cornfield, and I resolved firmly at that seminal moment in my unfledged youth that I never would be poor, that unlike Claude Satterfield, I did have the chance for a good life, and I wasn't going to muck it up. These five colored men were gentlemen in the truest sense of the word, and my friendship with them was genuine and lasting.

And the colored farm workers seemed to sense and understand our predicament, making us as close to "soul brothers" as is possible between mixed races. The negative imagery of blacks about blacks, which runs polluted and unchecked half a century later, did not exist in the 1940's small Southern towns of Kinston and Oxford.

There was one "job" at the orphanage that you didn't have to ask for volunteers to accomplish. Every Christmas, as long as I was at Oxford, the boys in 4-B and 3-B delivered a heaping bushel basket full of candy, fruit and vegetables to the home of each of these five gentlemen, and it was such a joy to see the appreciation and friendship on the faces of them and their families.

CHAPTER 51

The "Bonecrushers"

As a group, I cannot say we kids really dwelt on the fact that we were "orphans." Each of us had his story to tell; that most of us decided not to tell, either from embarrassment or fear that telling the story might cause painfully repressed memories to resurface, only to haunt us over and over again. I did my best to apply my own simplified form of child's logic to the tragic events surrounding my daddy's death, to no avail. Cause and effect just would not mesh. I did not have Doc around to explain why he had killed the one person in my life who had most loved me. Nor could my sister supply the answers. Years later, when I was around Doc for a more extended period, the seminal event was sufficiently faded on the horizon of my distant memory that I deemed it unfair to my brother-turned-father to demand an explanation of the disturbing events of February 9, 1946.

And it's not that I consciously blocked out the trauma. More likely than not, the move from the Walker Building, where not much in the way of responsibility was demanded of us, to 1-B in the Summer of 1950, where my time was absorbed by my dairy "education," more responsibilities in school, sudden increased freedom to roam the vast woodlands on Saturday and Sunday afternoons, and the disquieting wonderment of the onset of puberty. A child's mind can assimilate but a certain volume of new material, and thoughts of my family past were pushed farther and farther into the recesses of my still disconsolate mind, only to be recalled at times of physical or mental abuse at the hands of uncaring adults and bullying Big Boys.

Crowded into this busy schedule of events in my young life was organized sports. What we called "midget" football leagues flourished in eastern North Carolina in the late '40's and early '50's, and any sixth grade boy could try out for Mr. Thomas Currin's midget league team that we called the "Bonecrushers." Mild-mannered and sincere, "Coach" Currin taught Civics at school, and is best remembered for his habit of ending every single spoken sentence with a slight clearing of his throat, followed by ". . . on that." However, the benignness of Tom Currin, Mrs. Ligon and Bonnie Davis could not overcome the malignancies that were Baby Elephant Baldwin, old man Gray, E.T. Regan and Tom Adams.

During the second week of midget football practice in late August of 1951 I was sitting on the grass watching the action of the bigger boys on the team, when Coley Lee Hackett suddenly fell prostrate, clutching his (evil) left arm and complaining that somebody hurt him when they tackled him on the previous play. Damn sissy crybaby, I thought with disgust. Can't even take a little tackling, what with all them shoulder pads, knee pads and hip pads. Disgusting, I thought.

"Who wants to go in for Coley Lee?" asked Mr. Currin, scanning the group of us propped up on one elbow along the sideline. Taking the mere shifting of my weight in order to get more comfortable as an offer to replace Coley Lee, Coach Currin motioned me over to the huddle.

"Now, Van is going to move to quarterback, and you (pointing to me) are going to play fullback . . . (cough) on that. Now you (looking down at me) are going to take the handoff and run off right tackle, on two . . . (cough) on that."

Handoff? Right tackle? On two? On that? On two what? Guiding me by my bulky shoulder pads, Coach Currin positioned me behind Van.

"Okay, let's go. On two . . . (cough) on that," intoned the Coach.

Straight ahead of me, Van hunched over the center, and I followed the other players' cue and bent forward slightly at the waist.

"Hut one, hut two," squeaked Van. Turning with the ball toward me, Van waited. Nothing happened. I didn't move. I just remained in the slightly bent-forward position. Van figured that I didn't want the ball. But he didn't want it either. So he flipped the football underhanded to me. Terry Johnson and Red Albertson hit me about the same time the football hit me, and I felt my head bouncing around inside the flimsy helmet like a glass dab in a walnut shell. My knees buckled from the impact, and I felt like four kids were trying to fold me like a paper airplane. And I couldn't see out of my left eye. Everything was dark. About the time I began to panic, I adjusted my helmet, and recovered binocularity.

Lying still on the ground, I had to think fast. I quickly figured out my escape from this trauma called "football practice." Now, if I got up, Coach Currin would make me do it again. So, in the interest of self-preservation, I grabbed at my left arm a la Coley Lee, and began moaning and rolling on the ground. Out of the corner of my right eye, I glanced up toward Coach Currin, who was for some unknown reason shaking his head. In disgust? In sympathy? In indifference?

Waving in the direction of Coley Lee sitting on the grass (now the fool was clutching his "right" arm) the Coach said "Okay, sit over there with him." There I was again, put in the same class as Coley Lee Hackett. Damn. Football was going to be a tough sport.

CHAPTER 52

The Four Visions and the Famed Middle Distance

Fact. All orphan boys lie. It's a defensive mechanism learned as a seven-year-old frightened "new" boy in the Baby Cottage. Recall the famous "My mama told me I didn't have to eat anything I didn't want" lie? By the age of twelve, orphans have attained the status of "'sylum dogs," an honorary title that they carry with them to the grave proudly. Only accomplished liars are allowed into this brotherhood.

Lying is the ammunition used by orphan boys in their neverending battle with that despicable class of grownups, work supervisors, teachers and cottage counselors, whose sole purpose it seems is to accuse orphan boys of lying. It got to the point with Little Orphan Al that an accusation of some grievous transgression was automatically prefaced by "Now don't lie to me, boy (or young man)," followed by the nearly always fact-based accusation. But I lied anyway. Force of habit.

To determine whether a 'sylum dog is lying, the hated "bigun" has only to look the accused in the eye; the grownup is ahead of the game already because in ninety-nine percent of the cases, it's a given. Orphans who are lying will answer the accusation by either a blank stare, an open-mouthed look of incredulity or a Mona Lisa half-smile.

Orphans who are not lying will answer the accusation by either a Mona Lisa half-smile, an open-mouthed look of incredulity or a blank stare. It's a habit. And we all quickly mastered The Four Visions and the Famed Middle Distance.

Orphan kids, especially smaller boys, quickly master the Art of the Four Visions, namely, Glancing Up Vision, Glancing Down Vision, Side Glance Vision, and that old surreptitious standby, Corner of the Eye Vision. By his tenth birthday every orphan, from a mountain's worth of (bad) experience, has finely tuned these Four Visions to perfection.

Becoming Argus-eyed is one of the many means of self-preservation in an orphanage where a small child's inveterate enemies are those two classes of equally feared and despised predators-an uncaring, abusive staff and an equally piratical group of stupid-assed Big Boys, though I believe firmly that we were forced to call them "Big Boys" just to keep the rest of us in our place. In this regard, I mean "big," as opposed to "little," and all that naturally follows as night follows day.

Glancing Up and Glancing Down visions are quickly mastered in the orphanage hospital and Baby Cottage. These defenses are natural reactions to unwarranted and unprovoked physical abuse and/or threats of same. Glancing Down Vision is the ocular position of gaze utilized when a small (and naturally by definition quite defenseless) child suspects he (or she) has performed some act that will meet with certain displeasure from those two decrepit gargoyles (while keeping in mind that all gargoyles, by convention, are male), Minnie "Mad Dog" Warwick and Edith "Mad Dog II" Tomblin, or one of Miss Warwick's teenage bitchgirl surrogates, such as refusing to eat *all* of that regurgitated quiche on your plate, or harmlessly and forgetfully and innocently crapping in your boxer undershorts. Petrified, defenseless tykes glance down in these situations mainly for two reasons.

First of all, these little ones silently pray that when they glance back up, the mean old tormentoress will have disappeared off the face of the earth. But this rarely, if ever, happened. And it never worked for me, though I kept on trying . . . and praying . . . er, hoping.

In the alternative, the frightened child hopes that as he (or she) glances down, he will find the answers to all of life's problems in his shoes, or shoelaces, or the pattern on the hardwood floor or bathroom tiles, or in some unfixed middle distance between his eyes and the above mentioned thingies. Again, this rarely, if ever, happened. And alas, it never worked for me. However, we small, vulnerable tots had only hope on our side, so we kept doing a lot of glancing down anyway.

Glancing Up vision, or "Expectant" vision, is not exactly the opposite of Glancing Down vision. This ocular gaze is utilized infrequently, when the child's blatant lie is met with silence as if the old bat cottage mother was speaking but you didn't know if you heard her question, "You don't really expect me to believe *that*, do you, young man?" Needless to say, Glancing Up vision is usually followed almost instantly by the aforementioned Glancing Down vision, the latter ocular gaze lasting for either an indeterminate period of time, or for eternity, whichever came later.

The third of the Four Visions, Side Glance vision, is used in those specific situations involving avoidance of eye contact with adults or despised-and-just-as-feared Big Boys. This position of ocular gaze is called for when the young child must determine the source of the physical threat, but doesn't dare turn his head in that direction to let the aggressor know he (or she, as in Baby Elephant) is present. Side Glance vision is utilized especially when the small child is negotiating the campus alone, with a pocketful of Bazooka bubble gum or Mary Janes or B-B Bats, or worse still, with the sound of two coins (of any denomination) in his pocket hitting one another, that to a small child carries the auditory effect of giant cymbals clashing together in an empty auditorium the size of two football fields.

The last position of ocular gaze I call Corner of the Eye vision, which is a further refinement of Side Glance vision. It is absolutely essential in survival situations, when there is no means of escape, but nevertheless the frightened child must know which part of his head or face will receive the blow(s). Orphan kids who were subjected to transfer-truckloads of physical and mental abuse often could be observed practicing these protective ocular positions of gaze even in an open cow pasture, with nary a human within five hundred yards in any direction, with silent cud-chewing Holstein cows serving as stand-ins for abusive adults and dumbass Big Boys. Sometimes practice makes perfect. At other times it is just essential for survival.

And finally a word about God's greatest gift to small orphan children, the famed "Middle Distance." Every orphan kid quickly masters the fine art of determining the exact location of the famed Middle Distance, while being subjected to mental abuse, a vituperative term sugar-coated universally by such words as "a scolding" or "a talking-to." Every child incarcerated at Stalag Oxford learned, however, that any adult on campus possessed carte blanche permission to turn captious criticism into instant physical abuse. To make eye contact with your adult assailant could well be taken as a sign of defiance, insubordination, or nonconformity; thus in the interest of self-preservation it was best to quickly locate visually a point in space somewhere between the end of your nose and the planet Neptune, and await whatever abuse was certain to follow. And of course it helped tremendously if the boy quickly learned his "place." And I suppose it would help if I explained the phenomenon of "place," a concept firmly entrenched in Southern society, but which may not even exist in the remainder of Christendom.

Concerning "Place," "Or Else," "Boy" and "Young Man," and the Influence of These Concepts on Discipline at Oxford Orphanage

If we were to scoop up with a large flat coal shovel the menacing and demeaning terms most used by insulting and browbeating teachers, cottage counselors and work supervisors, and put them all in a few abusive and threatening sentences, they would likely come out like this.

> "*Young man*! You're getting too big for your britches. You'd better straighten up and fly right, *or else* I'm going to give you the whipping of your life. You'd better learn your *place*. You hear me, *boy*!"

Teachers, cottage counselors and work supervisors were wont to refer to a child as getting "too big for your britches," which is how we spelled the word "breeches" upon hearing the word properly pronounced.

I found that this oft-repeated catch phrase is apparently a Southern regionalism for a young boy or girl who had become insolent, disrespectful, smart-mouthed, ballsy, cocky, sassy, or rebellious, or who had begun to exhibit any one of a number of socially undesirable traits necessitating some form of "attitude adjustment" in an attempt to bring the errant child in line with "the accepted mores of society," i.e., those standards that grownups had arbitrarily set for small defenseless children but not for themselves.

Following no doubt what must have been years of sociological research and scientific investigation, the brilliant and forward-thinking Oxford Orphanage administration and staff had settled on a decisive, foolproof and time-tested solution to the problem. They simply extracted from the mothballs of pre-Freudian child psychology the old adage "Spare the rod and spoil the child," accepted it as the Word of God, and proceeded upon His authority to beat the living hell out of nine- and ten-year-old "troublemakers," and I, unfortunately, was one of those luckless wretches of whom the administration had selected to make an example, and, alas, to "put me in my place."

Thus each new child at the orphanage quickly learned his or her "place." If a child's conduct strayed afar from that expected of him or her in the rigid disciplinary social order under which we all lived, someone, perhaps an older boy or girl, perhaps one of the teachers or work supervisors, sooner than later put this straying youngster in his or her "place." This concept of "place" was quite narrowly defined in the social order that existed at Oxford Orphanage in the late '40's and early '50's.

Lasting character traits, including respect and discipline, were molded for a lifetime not out of books or lectures from grownups, or from Sunday school lessons-though we orphan kids certainly had our up-to-the-gills-and-then-some share of the latter two-but from the daily "interactions" that for us youngsters on the dairy meant doing what we were told by Mr. Davis and the older boys, and learning how, for lack of a more sophisticated term capable of a true characterization of our lives at that time, to "get along."

The hierarchy of authority (read as "power") at the dairy mirrored that of life in general at the orphanage. Should we superimpose the dairy "pecking order" on an American Indian totem pole, Mr. Davis would rest atop, about thirty feet in the air, and beneath Mr. Davis would stand the dairy boys, the oldest of these standing on the shoulders of the next youngest, and on down the line until, buried to a depth of never-to-see-the-light-of-day plus an additional thirty yards, would stand huddled together the quite apprehensive and equally vacuous "new" boys, a group that in the Summer of 1950 included Little Orphan Al.

Anyway, as concerns "place" and "or else," the older dairy boys had at one time been "new" dairy boys, and they had learned rather quickly, either by force or threat (probably both) that they had to do what the older dairy boys told them to do-or else.

The term "or else" as it was used at the orphanage, translated roughly to "if you don't do what I tell you to do, and don't do it quickly, and if in doing it you give me any 'back talk,' or if you 'sass' me in any way ("back talk" and "sass" are first cousins) then I'll beat you senseless with my fists." Oftentimes a lot of meaning can be packed into a few words. "Or else" worked wonders. One could almost look upon it as a sort of spoken "shorthand."

Thus order was maintained surprisingly well on the dairy (as on the main campus in general) by those two ingrained institutions, "place" and "or else." Into this hierarchical, industrial-sized blender add the orphanage staff's aforementioned "young man" and "boy," and you end up with complete order-of sorts. Beginning with the first day in the Baby Cottage, Walker Building and Annex (upon arrival, nearly all children were young enough to be assigned to one of these cottages) children were introduced to discipline by being required (read as "forced") to 1) do their assigned "duty," 2) eat *everything* on their plate, and 3) answer any adult with a respectful (and using the correct-read as "subservient") tone of voice, Yes ma'am, No ma'am, Yes sir, No sir.

And then we have the aforementioned equally demeaning insults, namely, "Boy" and "Young man," that have been used so often over the years to berate small children that they have become names.

Apparently Jews so overused the admonition "Young man!" that they made it a surname, e.g., "Herschel Youngman." And an Englishman stranded in Africa, by the quite unusual name of Tarzan O'Derapes, in order to cover his own dearth of airplane navigation and piloting skills, apparently so tired of chastising his dim-witted son he finally just named the poor lad "Boy." Anyway, so much for the historical aspects of these two terms.

One definition of the word "boy" found in Webster's New World College Dictionary, Fourth Edition, is "a patronizing term applied especially by Caucasians to nonwhites." Rest assured, however, that in my postwar orphanage youth, this derogatory word was applied in non-discriminatory fashion to us white orphan kids.

The demeaning word "boy" was used at Oxford Orphanage as what I call a "sentence-ender" or as the suffix to the equally demeaning "C'mere." Thus the spitting out by an older boy or work supervisor of the command "C'mereboy" was an order to the defenseless youngster (Walker Building, 1-B or 2-B) that the child was about as valuable as a used "balloon" or Musky dine hull, and that the boy had to report to the speaker immediately, . . . "or else."

Verbal abuse at Oxford Orphanage was often gender-based. When verbally assaulting an orphan boy or girl, female work supervisors, teachers and cottage counselors generally addressed the hapless child as "Young man!" or "Young lady!" However, male work supervisors, teachers and cottage counselors followed the verbal abuse of boys with the demeaning "Boy." Thus "Boy," and the equally caustic "Young man," were the most common terms of disapprobation used when biguns addressed us timid tykes at Oxford.

CHAPTER 53

Concerning Pseudo-Saints and Other Unwanted And Wearisome Theological Flotsam

Religious instruction at the Oxford Orphanage Seminary was indeed an enigma, a fascinating study in contrasts. As with other aspects of life in this morass of child suffering, the conflict centered around how to reconcile the admirable Christian virtues of love and charity with the reality of daily physical and mental abuse of children practiced openly by those same teachers, work supervisors and cottage counselors charged with demonstrating, and, better still, teaching, these tenets of Christian love and charity to homeless orphans. Truly a dilemma of grand proportions. To those children affected, it was downright frightening.

Religious instruction at Oxford centered around Sunday school, church and Sunday evening Vespers, though some might argue that the latter term is a redundancy.

Prior to 1951 Sunday school was held in the dimly-lit chapel of the ancient Main Building, and was conducted by members of the orphanage staff, including Mr. Currin, Mr. Talton and Gabe Austell, the high school football coach and science teacher. When construction of the modern and very beautiful York Rite Chapel was completed in 1951, Sunday school was held in that building.

Following completion of our Sunday school instruction, children from the Walker Building (boys) and the Annex (girls) to high school, assembled on the Main Road in front of the Main Building, where they formed a column of twos, separated by church denomination, for the march to church services in downtown Oxford.

If a child's parents were or had been say, Baptist, this religious preference was duly respected, and the child was taken each Sunday to the Baptist Church. The high school boys were still required to attend church; however, they were not required to march in line, and these boys were given much latitude in choice of churches to attend.

There were only four families at the orphanage whose parents had been Episcopalian. The Hacketts and the Provosts were two of these. Since there were rarely more than eight of us, on Sunday mornings we just tagged along behind the Baptists (lots and lots of 'em; they must breed like flies) and dropped off when we arrived at the Episcopal Church. Because our group was so small in number, no teacher or staff member stayed with us during the utterly boring sermon, so Coley Lee would twist my arm and force me to skip church with him.

Coley Lee and I would wander around town for an hour, hoping that Mr. Regan would not drive by and catch us. If he caught us, he made us run as fast as we could back to the Episcopal Church, where we spent the rest of the church service panting and puffing and catching our breath. The bastard had absolutely no sense of humor. But usually he did not catch us. I believe the final score in that little game of wits was Little Orphan Al and Coley Lee-178, E.T. Regan-5.

The penalty for skipping church too often and getting caught was that the boy had to march in line with the smaller kids. In the 1957 Log, page 65, there is a snapshot of the rear of the church line as it formed for the march downtown. The big high school boy standing alone at the rear of the line-looks a lot like me. When Coley Lee and I were in high school and were forced to march in line, in order to avoid the embarrassment associated with having to be supervised like nine-year-olds, we acted as though it was our job to help the staff member supervise the group of youngsters. Worked pretty well, too.

Until 1951 Sunday school and Sunday night Vespers were conducted in the Main Building Chapel, that easily accommodated the entire orphanage population. In 1951 the York Rite Chapel was constructed adjacent to 1-G. This beautiful edifice was spacious and well-lit, and in this regard was a vast improvement over the dungeon-like setting of the Victorian-era Main Building Chapel.

Prior to 1951, Vespers, like Sunday school, was held at 7:00 p.m. each Sunday in the expansive but dimly-lit first floor chapel of the Main Building. This was the most depressing time of the entire week for us orphans. Those kids whose parents had visited during Sunday afternoon, became gloomy and homesick during our standard peanut butter and molasses Sunday supper ritual; this depression carried over an hour later into an equally depressing and boring Vespers service.

During Vespers we children were quickly lulled into boredom bordering on stupefaction listening to the master hypocrite, the illustrious (at least in his own mind) Reverend A. DeLeon Gray, thrum on for an hour or so, about nothing of interest to any child assembled before him.

First of all, not one of the three hundred plus children sitting quietly (and in the Summertime soaked in sweat) before Mr. Gray, cared two hoots to hell about him or his sermons/lectures. We sat, yawning and dozing sleepily, not out of respect for Mr. Gray or of interest in his pseudo-religious gibberish, but out of fear of annoying him.

Second of all, he was talking way the hell over the heads of us kids; his sermons/lectures were geared to grownups, because he read from a canned script, just like his fellow hypocrite the Episcopal preacher. In the late 1940's and early 1950's there wasn't much of a market for sermons geared to an audience of several hundred snot-faced orphan kids.

More often than we might anticipate, Lady Progress carries in her sheath a very sharp double-edged sword. We kids eagerly awaited the completion of the York Rite Chapel in 1951. However, we preteen and teenage boys quickly became sorely disappointed.

In the century-old Main Building chapel, even a reasonably loud fart bouncing off the old oaken pews was dampened by the mass of orphan bodies packed together in the low-ceilinged chapel.

However, in the new, quite spacious and high-ceilinged York Rite Chapel, sound carried so well that the reverberation of a battery of unmuffled preteen farts glancing off the new oaken pews sounded as if the Boston Pops Orchestra was holding an annual Drum and Cymbals Competition. And we children could not cut up, fidget in the pews, or whisper dirty jokes. The only ones present who could get away with anything were the girls who, as I mentioned earlier in our story, had honed the art of pooting to the point that the damage done was audibly unnoticeable.

My too numerous appearances on Mr. Gray's List at ages nine and ten had quickly soured me on organized religion. This pseudo-saint bastard was a mild enigma at best, a fraud at worst. Thus by the time I arrived at 1-B in the Summer of 1950, after enduring the droning platitudes of Pig Talton and Mr. Currin (the latter never hit a child that I know of-a real gentleman) for an hour or so during Sunday school, we boys found no joy in the half-hour trek to the various churches located in downtown Oxford, only to sit quietly for another hour of the same monotonous banality at a different location, and by a different false-saint.

So each Sunday morning while sitting in the very last pew in back of the spacious Episcopal church, I put my time to good use. I daydreamed, planned, plotted and schemed about the various happenings in my life. I would project myself out of my commonplace, humdrum existence, and imagine other, quite distant, more pleasant surroundings.

I recalled the Saturday afternoon matinee B-westerns at the Paramount theatre in Kinston, and I daydreamed about being a cowboy. Not a cowboy "actor," mind you, but a real live cowpoke. A cowpoke is called such because he pokes the cows with a stick to prod them along while herding.

Except in my sanitized, idealized daydreams I always wore a white hat, carried two pearl-handled sixguns strapped to my hips, never got dirty, and my golden palomino (being only coincidentally named "Trigger") never needed to eat or drink. And even at a slow trot, my magnificent steed would leave both Seabiscuit and War Admiral sucking dust on a mile-and-a-half fast track at Belmont Park.

Even at an early age, my mind was trying to find some semblance, however slight, of order in this really screwed-up mess into which by circumstances not of my doing, I had fallen, or, better still, had been unceremoniously "dumped," for lack of a more appropriate descriptive term.

My own quite confusing views on religion evolved as a natural consequence of early childhood experiences with uncaring and at times abusive grownups responsible for my care.

At ages nine and ten, nightly Miss Hobson read to us Walker Building boys stories from her ubiquitous book of Bible stories, the supposed purpose of which was to teach us preteen boys, by example, the Christian tenets of love, charity, forgiveness and understanding.

Yet on a whim, each Saturday Miss Hobson sent about five of us frightened boys to the Business Office to be beaten by Mr. Gray. How is an unfledged, highly impressionable orphaned kid supposed to reconcile such blatantly contradictory and hypocritical conduct on the part of grownups?

When Miss Hobson confiscated a gift given to me by mama, refused to return the innocent, harmless gift to me, then sent me to Mr. Gray for "sassing" her when I demanded the return of my gift, how was I to find logic and learn Christian values from such confusing conduct and callous mistreatment by these two adults?

So how does a hurt and disillusioned child of nine reconcile the confiscation of a mother's gift by a cottage counselor who reads him supposedly "inspirational" Bible stories each night, with the consequent physical battering by a Methodist preacher, and believe for a moment the he should respect and trust the two blatantly hypocritical adults charged with showing him Christian love and guidance?

Given these circumstances, it is stretching logic and faith to unreasonable limits to expect this abused and thoroughly confused child to develop any emotions toward these two callous and uncaring grownups except mistrust, hate and contempt. A. DeLeon Gray routinely battered and berated nine-year-old boys on Saturday afternoon, and the following day preached from the pulpit his pious, pseudo-religious malarkey.

However, we Walker Building boys were not stupid. We understood hypocritical behavior in grownups, without being able to convey our understanding by using fancy words. There was not one among the nearly thirty boys living in the Walker Building in 1948 and 1949 who did not fear and despise old man Gray, who did not see through his unmitigated, ultra-thin veneer of phoniness, who did not know him for the child abuser he really was. And we carried in our young hearts this ingrained, conditioned disrespect and hatred until 1) our relatives took us from this loveless, harsh and uncaring environment, 2) we ran away from the miserable, unhappy, fear-filled place, or 3) against all odds, we finally graduated.

When we got to high school, we boys were not required to march to church each Sunday, unless we had been caught skipping church. So the first chance we got, Coley Lee and I decided to go church-hopping, and possibly spread our much-sought-after views on religion to the masses of Oxford heathen.

First we tried the Baptist church. This was by far the largest church in Oxford, but it could have used a decorator with a lot more imagination. I thought I was sitting in a large white box, and none of the town girls was pretty. And to top it off, all the preacher ever talked about was money, money, money.

Anyway, the Baptist church was farther from the orphanage than any other church, being located smack-dab in the center of the Oxford city business district. When attempting to skip church, we might as well carry printed placards on our backs that read "I'm a stupid orphan and I'm skipping church."

The Presbyterian church was directly across College Street from the Episcopal church. But the inside of that church was so dark it was downright scary. I kept thinking I should have brought my Louisville Slugger. Quasimodo must have been Presbyterian. Anyway, we lasted only one Sunday in that dungeon.

And that left the Methodists. Whatever screwy "Methods" these people used, they sure were strange. And there weren't very many of them, which wasn't exactly a strong incentive to keep going there. And Coley Lee said he felt at home in the Methodist church, which meant for damn sure I was not ever coming back there again.

So soon we were back at the Episcopal church. Anyway, at about that time the new pastor, whom I first thought was a pretty nice guy, somehow became sexually involved with one of the women in the Sunday school, and since I had a sixteen-year-old's crush on her beautiful body, I hated her and the pastor, felt betrayed, and stopped going to the Episcopal church's Sunday School entirely.

CHAPTER 54

Puberty

Until the age of eleven the only two uses to which I attributed my penis (known also among my preteen peers as a "whanger," a "tally," and a "dick") were 1) to use to do pee, which I did a lot, and 2) to swat flies at an extremely short distance, which I did, if at all, only seldom. My firm belief during that shockingly naïve stage in my young life was that babies were the end product of a man and woman kissing, and that the actual moment of conception was when, while standing fully clothed and close together, the woman raised one calf at the knee like a 40's "pinup" girl. At least, that's what they always showed in the picture shows, and if it was in a picture show or on a billboard, it had to be true.

And because during my entire three years in the orphanage no girl had ever offered her lips to me (let alone bend at the knee and still keep her balance) I felt reasonably certain that I would not have parenthood forced upon me at such a premature age. And for all my innocence, "sex" could have been a Southern cornpone mispronunciation of the word "six." "Give me sex of them there Mary Janes." In a similar vein, I would have supposed that "pornography" was merely a Southern synonym for the word "photography."

One night in the Fall of 1950, Witch Robinson had just released us from that interminably boring two hours called Study Hall, when I noticed several kids gathered at a table, giggling and pointing at what appeared to be miniature funny books. Drawing closer, I found that was exactly what they were and, since I enjoyed reading funny books, I started looking over the shoulder of Terry Johnson, only because he was doing more pointing and giggling than anyone except Coley Lee Hackett.

And it was a "funny" book, all right. No color, just black and white. The title on the cover was "Pretty Boy Floyd." Everybody knows Pretty Boy Floyd, I thought. Wasn't he the infamous American gangster? Except that, in this funny book, in addition to carrying a gun, Pretty Boy Floyd also "carried" a "whanger" that was about two feet long, and he waved it at a different big-titted girl on about every other page. I was mesmerized-like the other kids I had never seen anything like it before. My fascinating introduction to pornography at age eleven.

I then looked over the shoulder of Butch Mitchell, his eyes as big as saucers, and there, in vivid black and white, was Flesh Jordan, who looked a lot like one of my favorite funny book heroes. Except along with a powerful ray gun, Flesh also possessed a powerful penis "gun," that appeared to look a lot like Pretty Boy Floyd's gun, and he was doing the same thing with his as did the gangster. Wow! The Flesh Jordan I never knew!

And there were others. I remember thinking at the time that if my tiny little acorn was going to become a whanger that large, at what age was this phenomenal transformation predicted to take place, and what was I going to do with it when it happened. With all the worries I had at that time in my young life, up popped yet another one. I was already suffering the awful depression associated with penis envy from observing the two dairy herd bulls Ace and Vic perform, and now this!

Eventually, Pretty Boy Floyd and Flesh Jordan's lease ran out on my short term memory, and a year later, at age twelve, I left the gawking but for the most part inoffensive Witch Robinson in 1-B and moved up to Mrs. Ethel Dye's 2-B. I don't recall either of these cottage counselors whipping any child under her care. And since at that time ninety-nine percent of my luck could only be classified as "bad," had beatings been on the menu in 1-B or 2-B, I would have received my (un)fair share. Thus if I don't remember it, it didn't happen.

Anyway, in 2-B, just as in 1-B, the toilets and urinals were set off to one corner of the large bathroom by a single walled partition. I was twelve years old, and sometimes I would wake up in the morning with a (very short) stiff peepee, along with the associated full bladder. As soon as I did pee, my peepee went limp again. I never paid it any mind.

Then one day I was sitting on the toilet, with the increasingly present stiff peepee and just as evident full bladder, when suddenly I experienced this very strange, warm feeling in my groin and peepee, and when I looked down, there was some chalky white solid stuff coming out of the end of my little whanger. Scared the hell out of me! Then shortly after the "chalk" came out, the very strange warm feeling in my whanger disappeared, and I went limp again.

Because the strange episode concerned my private parts, I was too embarrassed to ask Mrs. Dye about it, and I wasn't about to report to sick call and ask the dreaded White Monster Tomblin nothing about anything.

So after supper that night I told my older buddy Javon Frye what had occurred. He had a good laugh, then informed me that what had happened was perfectly normal, and, by the way, it would happen again, so don't pay it any mind.

And it did happen again. And again. And again. I had finally reached "puberty," that stage of adolescence in which an individual becomes physiologically capable of taking part in the process of sexual reproduction. Sure was confusing.

I reached puberty at about the same time movements of the hips of teenage girls beneath their thin, tightly-fitting dresses elicited an instant increase in my heart rate, along with a simultaneous, quite weird twitch in my groin; my "peepee" overnight became a "dick," synchronously I developed a mustiness in my armpits, and I discovered, much to an almost uncanny mixture of ecstasy, pleasure, self-consciousness and outright shame, the phenomenon known to adults as "masturbation," but to young boys as "beating off" or "jacking off."

The loose-fitting trousers and stupid-assed "knickers" we wore during the late '40's and early '50's had deep pockets, and soon I noticed many of my preteen peers replacing our sacred "dabs" with twitching pants pockets, and I discovered soon thereafter the fine art referred to universally as "pocket pool."

The average "pocket pool" player could be spotted at forty paces, standing perfectly still, both hands just about up to his elbows in his front pants pockets, dreamily gazing off into the middle distance, wearing a Mona Lisa-like half smile, not taking part in the game of dabs or even in idle conversation. The only things moving were his pockets.

In order to be ready when I found the "right" girl, I set out at breakneck speed in an attempt to grow The World's Biggest Dick. A year later I had not made much headway, and became depressed, feelings of inadequacy and failure creeping into that filing cabinet of my mind. However, at about that time I did seem to notice that my right hand now appeared larger than my left, and suddenly I could whip just about any kid at arm wrestling.

By the age of thirteen I was stuck on girls. I had it bad. Really, really bad. I got to where I would follow the big girls around, unobtrusively (or so I thought) staring at all their protruding body parts, looking for nuances between the equipment of the blondes versus the brunettes versus the redheads. I liked them all.

Della Dean and Ann Howell made me hate myself for being born five years too late. Ruth Bostic made me wish I could get re-assigned to 4-G, so I could just watch her wake up every morning.

And Joan Johnson and Ann Hare drove me crazy with all sorts of weird imaginings. When I was nine years old, I would go to the Candy Corner to drool over candy I could not afford. At age thirteen I just went to drool over the memory of Betty Evans. She was soooo pretty.

When I was nine, I wanted to marry Emily Cole, with her dimples and hair parted down the middle, and buxom Retha Bostic, simultaneously or in separate ceremonies, but I didn't know exactly why. At age thirteen the reason came to me almost overnight, but by then they were gone, so the three of us, my sad heart, my groin and I, reluctantly began our search for love closer to home.

CHAPTER 55

Melda

And I didn't have to look very far. Thinking back, I first noticed Melda at the time the piece of chalky white stuff first found its way out of the end of my little dick, or whanger, or whatever little boys call it. I should explain what I mean by the word "noticed." Melda was my very "first." And Melda is not her real name. I knew her for a few wonderful years, and eventually she became, much to my dismay and regret, one of those beautiful orphans classified in the Annual Reports of the Oxford Orphanage as "number of pupils returned to relatives during the year." I have never seen her since she left, but neither will I ever forget her. I called her "Baby Doll."

What ruined me to begin with was seeing the pretty blond cottage girl (the one with the bouncing behind) naked in the shower when I was eight years old, squeezing that soapy blond "kitten" between her legs. Five years later, when I commenced in earnest my attempt to grow the aforementioned Olympic-sized whanger, I began to picture in my quite (over)active and equally imaginative mind what certain big girls looked like without clothes. Later I progressed(?) to fantasies involving naked big girls wearing only high heels or hats, and so on, until I figured one day that I was going to become the World's Biggest Pervert.

Thus what initially captured my attention about Melda was that she looked much like the blond cottage girl had looked five years earlier. I was hooked. No doubt about it. Yet even in that moment of untutored youth, I questioned whether the not unwelcome pressure I suddenly experienced just below my beltline was a newfound stir of virility, or if I had merely accumulated yet again the cyclically bulging bladder.

I used to follow Melda down the hallways in school, position myself for a long, drooling stare at her as we waited to go into the dining hall, and daydream about her constantly. I became the unofficial, self-appointed Campus Pocket Pool Champion, thanks to Melda.

Then one day a miracle occurred. One of my female classmates confided to me that Melda liked me. I was enraptured by this news. But I didn't want it to show.

"Oh, is that right?" I asked, trying to look as though I didn't even know any "Melda."

"So," my perceptive classmate replied, "You can stop sneaking peeks at her. Everybody knows you like her."

Melda was pretty. Her face exhibited a pure, innocent quality that made her seem so, well, pure and innocent. Her engaging smile made her appear almost fragile in a body that was anything but delicate. She was carried along by a smooth, willowy walk and reminded me always of a flower in early bloom. Her quiet manner and flowing motion accentuated the light bounce of her behind. Something about Melda just melted my heart and made me feel physically weak all over. She was one of those young girls who oozed sex out of every pore in her body. I was hooked. Permanently.

I had this almost uncontrollable urge to touch Melda's ass, so well-rounded and inviting.

This fixation, fascination and near obsession (all three) with Melda's behind occurred simultaneously, like I said, with that time in my life that I started to notice girls' "things," which itself arose simultaneously with my little dick being hard a good part of the time, day and night. And it did not matter that my bladder was full, empty or half-full or half-empty. It was even the more disconcerting because I could not mentally fathom the cause and effect of these physiological and emotional happenings in my young life. In other words, I was confused about sex. Very. I found myself at about this time following the big girls around campus, sneaking peeks at all their protruding body parts, while at the same time trying to appear unobtrusive. It wasn't easy to do, and anyway I wasn't very good at it.

In addition, at such a young and inexperienced age, I was afraid of the male preteens' universally dreaded nemesis, R-E-J-E-C-T-I-O-N. Melda could break my heart anytime she chose. I knew that as an immutable fact. I needed to research my chances of success a little more, because *rejection* would be final, no, even terminal. I would lose her forever.

As a twelve- and thirteen-year-old, I had great difficulty at times, a real wrestling match between the rationality and reality of my ego (Melda was too good for me; I could never hope to rise to the level of her expectations), and the rapidly emerging irrationality of instinctual and groin-controlled sexual impulses of my id.

I believe firmly that some actions we take in our lives are made without conscious knowledge, that our subconscious acts without asking the permission of our conscious. Perhaps this subconscious decision to cement the relationship between Melda and me was one of these strange events, but when the time came I allowed it to happen and was gratefully taken along for the ride. My relationship with Melda was one of the crossroads in my life, and I have always cherished those moments.

"It" happened on a cold clear night in October 1952, when we kids were milling about in the dark waiting for the six o'clock supper bell to ring. I noticed Melda sorta separate from the group of girls and move toward the shadows of the Main Building. As though taking some kind of telepathic, inexplicable cue, I instinctively sorta separated from the group of boys I was talking with, and suddenly there we were. I didn't know just what to say or do, so I just mumbled "Hi."

Melda said it for me. Without preamble, she leaned toward me so that, by design or chance, her very warm and full and undoubtedly beautiful left breast touched my chest, and whispered with a stream of hot breath into my left ear,

"Alton, I want to see you."

I had never before had a beautiful girl blow her hot breath into my ear. I wanted to ask her to repeat the statement about five hundred times.

"Well, here I am." Stupid. Stupid. Stupid.

"No, dummy, I want to *see* you," she whispered louder, her now fireplace-poker-red-hot left breast burning a hole in my shirt, and simultaneously, as though for emphasis, reached for my hand and held it tightly in both of hers.

Oh, I thought, could she possibly mean what I think she means? Stupid. Stupid. Stupid.

"Where can we go?" I asked nervously.

"Let's just wait here," she said. "And when everybody goes in to eat, we'll find somewhere to go."

So we waited in the shadows, and by that time Melda had pulled my hand and arm close to her hot belly, and in the cold October night, she felt sooo warm. I had difficulty grasping what was happening, but pretty soon the last supper bell rang and everyone flocked noisily into the dining rooms. Everyone except Melda and I. To prevent discovery we had to move away from the main campus, but we also could not go too far. So we headed hand-in-hand down toward the Industrial Building.

As we approached the dark, empty building, suddenly I remembered the first floor Mattress Room. At the same time Melda leaned toward my left ear, and with more of the same hot breath in my ear, whispered,

"Where can we go, Alton?"

Without answering her, I released my hand from hers, walked to the outside Mattress Room window, and tried to open it. It was locked.

Without pause, I closed my eyes tightly, turned my head to one side, then with the pad of my fist, bopped the window pane sharply, shattering it into shards. I quickly reached in, flipped the latch and pushed up the lower window sash. I hoisted Melda up and through the window opening, then quickly climbed in after her.

Her hips were sooo warm in the cold Winter night. And there before us, illuminated well by the moonlight, lay four mountains of mattresses, each stacked about ten high. Quickly climbing up the stack of mattresses closest to the window, I pulled Melda up beside me.

As soon as she reached the top mattress, she found my lips and kissed me hard and long. Was I supposed to swallow her tongue? Or was she just probing my mouth with her hot tongue to make sure I was not chewing Bazooka bubble gum on this momentous occasion? This was the first time a girl had ever kissed me, and it felt strange and downright wonderful. My dick got hard.

As soon as we parted, Melda knelt beside me and began taking off her clothes. I didn't move. Before I could get a firm grasp of what was going on, most of what Melda had on was off.

"Come on, they won't eat supper forever," she whispered, somewhat impatiently.

Come on? Was this my cue to do something? Come on and do what? So, following Melda's example, I turned my back to her and quickly took off my clothes. Was I supposed to take off my socks, too? Glancing out of the corner of my eye at Melda's feet, I followed suit and removed my socks. And as many young boys before my time, I timidly approached my initiation into the still confusing and forever unmastered world of sex with fingers all thumbs, at the moment of truth wondering, almost aloud, whether this was such a good idea after all. But Melda helped me.

Soon we were both lying naked way up atop the stack of mattresses. By that time my little swizzle stick was also up in the air, though to my dismay, not "way up." I could see Melda's beautiful body in the moonlight streaming through the large window, so golden and pure. She quickly grasped my hand and rubbed it slowly against her kitten, and suddenly my hand was warm, wet and slippery, and I wished at that moment I had had five hands.

After a brief moment, Melda put her arm under my back and deftly rolled me over on top of her, quickly reached down and pulled me inside her, and I discovered Heaven. Heaven was somewhere inside Melda. Suddenly Melda was squealing like a young stuck pig, and I found myself grunting like an old root hog, and visions of old Ace the bull with the young heifer, the old man and young girl in the back seat of the big black Ford sedan, and Pretty Boy Floyd and Flesh Jordan all flashed through my mind in a crazy blur. Then Melda, her body pressing hard against mine, yelled,

"No, don't stop! No, don't stop! No, don't stop!" And in about thirty seconds the whole wonderful experience was over.

Suddenly a terrible thought came to me. In her excitement, Melda had quite distinctly moaned "No, don't stop! No, don't stop!" There had definitely been no pause, as though if she had written out her cries, there would not have been a period between her words "don't" and "stop."

Like a light bulb suddenly turned on above my head, funny book style, I realized that the yelps of the teenage girl in the back seat of the big Ford sedan two years earlier had not been the cries of fear ("No. Don't. Stop."); rather, we had disrupted her cries of climactic ecstasy ("No, don't stop!). She had not been yelling obscenities at the old man whom Butch and I thought was "hurting" her, but at Butch and me. Stupid, clueless preteen orphan kids.

We lay naked, holding one another for awhile, until finally my heart returned to my chest and I could breathe without panting. As I lay close to Melda in the moonlight, the thought came to mind that for the rest of my life I would never forget this brief moment (that's about all thirty seconds is, a brief moment), and that I hoped Melda felt the same about me.

Finally we put on our clothes and just lay together for awhile.

"Can we do this again?" I asked expectantly.

"We can do it anytime you want," she answered, and kissed me tenderly on my lips. Then, almost as an afterthought (I thought) she added "But could we do it a little longer next time?"

"Okay," I replied, though not knowing exactly what she meant.

"That's fine," she said softly, "and we'll do it a lot."

Reluctantly, we climbed back down from our love nest of new mattresses, lowered ourselves out the window onto the ground, and I closed the window behind us. We parted before we approached the dining hall. As we stood in the shadows cast by the large pecan trees, Melda whispered to me,

"I'll see you tomorrow." We parted, not with a fiery Hollywood kiss, but with a long, loving hug, our bodies pressed together for a long time. I couldn't believe how hot was Melda's body.

As I walked slowly (suddenly I was very tired, but I didn't know why) in the shadows across the campus toward 4-B, I felt like the King of the Hill, the proud eagle perched on the topmost limb of the highest hundred year old oak on campus. I had reached that first milestone in a young boy's life; the experience, however fleeting, had been wonderful, and I knew even then that I had shared the moment with a young, innocent girl for whom I truly cared very much. And though I was tired, I wanted to do it all over again. Right then.

Suddenly, as I approached the cottage, a strange thought began to push its way into the corner of my mind. I got the very distinct feeling that, well, uh, I mean, uh, well, that Melda had done this before. But certainly Melda had been as pure as I. No, perish the thought. I must have been her "first." I had to admit, however, that she definitely knew how to do "things" I certainly didn't know how to do. And she did them fast. And she was good at it. Really good.

By the time I went to bed, my mind was one jumbled up mess. If I had not been Melda's "first," then who was he? I imagined Melda "doing it' with every Big Boy on campus. Then I imagined her "doing it" with Pretty Boy Floyd and Flesh Jordan, but not at the same time-my puerile mind could not comprehend such a thing at age thirteen-and suddenly I felt so inadequate.

My mind climbed onto that universal male rollercoaster whose cars are named Jealousy, Inadequacy, Uncertainty and Selfdoubt, and somebody turned the speed on "runaway."

Melda had seemed so open and honest and sincere to me, and her touch had been so gentle and warm. So, even at the young, immature age of thirteen, I knew I had to decide my approach to Melda. And subconsciously I decided this would become my approach to women for the remainder of my life. Trust and acceptance? Or suspicion and jealousy? My whole being struggled with, and was bitterly torn between, what would be my relationship with women.

Should I ask Melda if I had been her "first?" Should it really make any difference? If I had not been her "first," would it make her dishonest, or soiled, or tainted? Was I just being selfish?

For a thirteen-year-old boy who had just experienced love for the first time, these questions had a smothering effect on me. There was no answer, for I was simply too inexperienced to decipher the complexities of love and life.

By the time we were together again, Melda had sensed a cooling of my feelings toward her. I suppose I wasn't very adept at hiding my emotions. The night was rainy and cold, but Melda decided beforehand on that night. For the longest time I wondered why she always chose the night of our liaisons, and why she couldn't "do it" on any given night. Didn't make any difference to me-why should it to her? But again, I suppose at that time in my life, a "period" was merely a dot at the end of a sentence.

Slipping through the shadows cast by the giant oaks that seemed always to protect the campus, we made it to the Industrial Building, into the first-story window and up onto the pile of mattresses. That night, however, along with Melda, I hoisted up all the doubts I had carried with me during the two-week interval between our first meeting and that night. Melda kissed me long and tender at first, I guess still trying to dislodge that Bazooka bubble gum I seemed always to be chewing. I never thought a girl's tongue could stretch that far. However, because of my previously mentioned doubts, I could not respond. Unless you have the mindset of a bull, I learned, tenderness with a woman and emotional trauma are quite mutually exclusive entities.

"What's wrong, Alton?"

"I don't know exactly."

But I did.

"You know I love you, and I want you to love me."

This was going to be hard.

"But I have to know."

"Know what? Ask me."

Melda was rightfully puzzled. I felt like a fool.

"Am I the first boy you've, . . . uh, . . . uh . . ."

"First boy I've what?"

She was getting a bit impatient, or so I thought. I don't know, but women have a certain, well, impatience in their voices when they become impatient.

"You know . . ."

God, I felt like a complete fool. I just couldn't continue.

She held my hand tightly. Then she pulled my hand down between her legs and held it against her kitten. Melda didn't wear any panties, at least not when we met. Anyway, she didn't move for the longest time. Then I felt her warm body heave slightly, and she began sobbing quietly. After awhile she spoke, in a cracking, soft and quite sincere voice.

"Alton, you're not my first boyfriend. And you may not be my last. But what matters, the only thing that really matters is that we are here now."

She stopped speaking for a moment, and began crying and holding me tightly against her as if in an attempt to control the heaving of her body. I felt like a complete fool, as though I did not deserve this beautiful girl. Finally she continued.

"That's all I can say. I'm sorry you have doubts about me. If you don't want me, just let me know, and I'll never bother you again. But I really love you. Isn't that the only thing that really matters?"

That night, lying way up on that stack of mattresses with a wonderful and understanding fifteen-year-old girl, I made the decision that has blessed me all my life. That was the decision not to be a jealous person, to be happy with what I had in life, to accept the love of a woman at face value. I cannot really say that Melda taught me this, but she did set my mind to thinking about it.

My buddy William Bryant apparently suspected that some sorta hanky-panky was in progress. Don't know how he knew, but that's not important. Oxford Orphanage was a small 400-acre microcosm. Well, anyway, one day we were walking back to 4-B after supper, when William sidled up next to me to avoid being overheard by the other kids and said, in a rather conspiratorial half-whisper,

"Y'know, Alton, they have a way over at the hospital to tell if you've been doing it."

"Doing *what*?" I asked in innocent (which I was at the time) bewilderment.

"You know," he said, wearing that little stupid half-smile that kids bring out to sport around when they think they have "something" on you. And quickly he added "You and Melda." Damn. Damn. Damn, I thought. He knows. That stupid "innocent bewilderment" thingy blossomed rapidly into florid cheeks that I was certain my friend (friend?) could notice in the seven p.m. December darkness. I gave William one of my by then patented shut-your-mouth-or-I'll-kick-your-ass-to-the-moon glares, and he didn't say another word. But apparently he knew *the secret*, and it bothered me.

Now it was common knowledge that in our little "city" there were really very few secrets. What did cause me concern in this instance, however, was whether The Starched White Hound from Hell, Mrs. Tomblin, could really tell if Melda and I had "done it," and if so, what would be the consequences of being exposed.

That night in the shower I made a close inspection of my dick, but could not find any printed, engraved, handwritten, embroidered or stamped sign that announced to the world "I DID IT WITH MELDA," and the color of my (still not very large) pencil was its normal whitish-pink. Still, however, my relentless personal nemesis, John Q. Paranoia, ever on the alert to ambush me, took charge, and for all I knew, medical science had garnered all its financial resources into devising a foolproof, sure-fire test to determine whether little Alton Provost had "done it."

However, I was the doomed moth to Melda's irresistible flame, which is the most poetic way I can say that I wasn't going to stop "doing it" with Melda. Nosireebob. I had to think fast. And I did. Yes, that's it! The Balloon Boys. I had been a stupid Balloon Boy, and I still remembered that some of those "balloons" we had blown up with child-like pride in the Summer of '50, had still been in the original sealed packages.

So the following Saturday afternoon I set out on my own to the lovers' lane on the other side of the trestle, and scoured the ground in search of pristine, still-in-the-original-package balloons. My God, there were literally dozens of the well-worn thingies! It was like folks had held a Rubbers Convention on that little half acre of scrub pine. Maybe using a rubber at that location qualified you for some kind of drawing for a grand prize or something. I pictured in my mind dozens of large black 1948 Ford sedans rocking to and fro in unison, the sounds of old root hogs and squealing piglets filling the night. Used rubbers galore!

Finally I found one single solitary pristine absolutely unused, still-in-its-package rubber. One. But then again, one was all I needed. But I had accomplished only the first part (the easy part, I discovered) of my grand plan. Would I know how to use my new rubber? Would Melda know how to use it? Was there an inside and an outside to the rubber? Would I be able to wash it after I used it for the first time, and use it again? If so, how many times could I use the rubber before it wore out? From use? From washing? And what kind of soap do I use to wash the rubber? And how would I dry it after I washed it?

The questions were endless, all unanswerable. How could I find out the answers to this myriad of important questions? I was discovering in my Gauntlet of Growing Up, that for some odd reason I could not fathom, there seemed always to be an overabundance of questions and a dearth of answers to match them.

I suddenly recalled that a couple of years before, when all that chalky white stuff was extruded under the inexorable pressure of puberty, from the head of my little weenie, my friend Javon Frye had explained to me what it signified. So now I could ask Javon Frye Question No. 2, and by the time I graduated high school I could write a best-seller entitled *My First Thousand Really Stupid Sexually-Oriented Questions*. So I searched out my sex expert mentor after supper that night, and after laughing himself silly at my stupid (he thought) question, gave me the answers I so desperately sought.

"By the way, where did you get a rubber?"

"Found it."

"Where?"

"Over in the woods past the trestle. There's lots of 'em there."

"Okay, next time you go over there, get me a few of 'em."

"Okay, be glad to. New? Or used?"

"New, you dumbass. What would I do with a used rubber?"

I was about to answer, "Blow them up and become the laughing stock of the entire campus." But I didn't. Javon was my friend.

"Don't know. Okay, I'll get you some new ones. Thanks a lot for the advice."

Okay, now I had a rubber, a new rubber at that, thus enabling myself to thwart medical science and making myself safe from discovery by Mrs. Tomblin. The old bitch. So that night as soon as supper let out I found Melda and excitedly pulled her into the shadows of the Main Building.

"I got a rubber. A new one."

"So?"

"So old bat Tomblin won't find out."

"Won't find out *what?*"

I could tell that Melda was beginning to sound a teeny bit irritated, or so it seemed to me. I had learned by now that a sharp rise in the tone at the end of a question signified that the speaker, usually a cottage mother, work supervisor or teacher (and now Melda) was becoming frustrated with either my stupidity, or perceived lack of understanding, or that the speaker was having a bad day and wanted to vent his or her spleen on the Number One Whipping Boy at Oxford Orphanage, little Alton Provost.

"That we've been doing it."

"But how could she find out?"

More incredulity. Now a really, really high-pitched ending. I thought briefly that it might be better to let well enough alone. But I (stupidly) pressed on.

"I don't know for sure, but one of the guys was talking, and he said they could tell if a boy had been doing it."

"Well, if it makes you feel better, we'll try it."

"When? Now?"

I didn't want to seem too eager, but to me the (new) rubber carried the status of a new toy, somewhat akin to a Red Ryder BB Gun, or a little plastic toy that glowed in the dark, or an interesting game I would discover while shamelessly opening Christmas presents that really belonged to more than three hundred other kids. The rubber was new, and I couldn't wait to see how (and if) it would work. I had decided that if it did not work that well, or if Melda didn't like it, I could save the wrapper, wash it off and pass it off to Javon Frye (my friend) as a new rubber and thus save myself a trip to the Rubber Patch.

"We can't do it tonight, it's already too late. What about tomorrow night?"

"Okay, I'll see you before supper tomorrow night. And I'll bring the rubber. It's a new one." (Never let a girl you love think you are using a used rubber.)

"Yes, you said that. A new one."

I had trouble concentrating on anything that night and all the next day. Except the rubber, and how I would use it, and whether I could follow the set of rubber-handling guidelines Javon Frye had given me, and whether using the rubber would complicate my life with Melda, and on, and on, and on. This growing up business wasn't getting any easier. Seemed like every time I learned something new, there was something else new I had to learn.

Anyway, the next night before supper I eagerly joined Melda at our regular trysting place in the shadows of the kitchen. We held hands as we scampered from the shelter of one shadow to another while making our way to the shrubs in front of the Industrial Building. About every fifth stride I would pat my left front pocket to assure myself that the (new) rubber had not jumped out of my pocket, hit the ground and run away.

I pushed open the sash of the Mattress Room window and the three of us, Melda, the (new) rubber and I, scampered in. We quickly climbed up on top of the large stack of mattresses, and I hurriedly undressed.

And then and there I was introduced to the brutal and unforgiving Dilemma of the Male Species. I had been so worried about my (new) rubber and how to use it, and with all these doubts racing through my (limited capacity) mind, I just lay there beside Melda, holding my (new) rubber in one hand, puzzled as to why my limpid donger remained just that.

"What's the matter?" asked Melda.

"Oh, I see," she added, almost as an afterthought, touching my lifeless little thingy.

"What are we going to do?" I asked with shame and embarrassment.

"Well, first we're going to forget about the rubber."

She then quickly snatched my (new) rubber from my grasp, and flung it unceremoniously across the darkened room, where I heard my (new) rubber make contact with the wall. Now if she changed her mind, I'd never be able to find the darn (new) rubber in the darkness of the cavernous Mattress Room.

It all happened so fast. I couldn't seem to recall if my (new) rubber actually stuck on the far wall (heaven knows, Melda sure flung it hard enough); I remember hearing the "SPLAT" when the "balloon" connected with the smooth plaster wall, but do not recall any sound of it making contact with the hardwood floor. Does a (new) rubber make a different sound when it hits wood than when it strikes a plaster wall?

I do recall thinking at the moment that I would ask Javon Frye-he seemed to know everything, and his answers all seemed to be based on experience.

"But what if old bat Tomblin finds out that I've been doing it?"

"Forget about Mrs. Tomblin. Believe me, trust me. I love you and that is all that really matters."

That did it. Melda had again told me she loved me. Since my arrival at the orphanage in February 1947, Melda was the first person other than my mother who had ever said to me "I love you." Anyway, my limpid lizard suddenly came to life (almost) without Melda's coaxing, and for the next few minutes I felt as wanted and needed as I had ever felt in my life.

After we had finished our three-minute game of bumpy-bumpy, we just lay naked on the large mattress, and finally Melda said softly,

"What brought it to life?"

"When you told me you loved me."

"Can you tell me you love me. It would really help."

"Okay, Melda. I love you. I love you. I love you."

"And I'll let you know how much that means to me."

And we did it again.

That night I learned, at the young age of fourteen, how to say "I love you."

The smile in Melda's soft blue eyes seemed to convey an expectation of something better to come. Her quiet voice (except when I said something really, really stupid to irritate her) belied a strength of determination that I found admirable and for which I developed an abiding respect.

The novelty of sex was important to us two teenagers, but I believe the central theme in our relationship was based more on care and respect and togetherness.

When we were alone, we did our glorious thing, and then just lay holding each other. We never once talked about our lives or the orphanage. Our togetherness was ours alone, not to be soiled or tainted by anything or anybody else.

Melda became, by virtue of this "period" thingy, the social director in our little get-togethers, often planning our frolicsome trysts three days in advance. Melda was the perfect mortise to my eager tenon, and we practiced our limited-time engagements with great delight and abandon.

And speaking from experience, I know for a fact that just because one isn't (or ain't) good at performing a particular function, as in dabs, doesn't mean he should stop trying. And I wanted to try with Melda-a lot. I worked at it with a vengeance every chance I got, until I believe she canceled her order for that three-minute egg timer.

Our love nest remained the Mattress Room for some time, until one day we received help from one of my Angel Benefactors . . .

CHAPTER 56

My Angel Benefactors

M.D. (Mad Dog) Tomblin arrived at Oxford Orphanage in May 1924, and retired thirty years later, on December 12, 1953, when I was fourteen years old. This old biddy's scowling countenance matched to a "T" her dreaded thirty-year caveat to small children, "You don't live with your mother anymore. You live in the orphanage now."

Upon the old ogress' retirement, Mrs. Elizabeth Micou, like Mrs. Tomblin a Practical Nurse, quite ably assumed the duties of nurse and hospital supervisor. And things were definitely looking up in my life. By that time I had been hit below the belt in this damned place so many times that I had seriously considered wearing suspenders for the duration of my prison sentence, in hopes that my luck would change.

Elizabeth was a tall, very well built brunette with a warm heart, heavy shirt and a really well-shaped ass. I liked her-a lot. She was a kind, warm-hearted, pleasant woman whom I came to know quite well. Occasionally I would report to sick call complaining of a splitting migraine headache, and Elizabeth would admit me to the boys' ward for a day or two, just to allow me to recuperate from that dreaded disease, dislike of the predicament in which I had landed on February 15, 1947.

My ninth grade report card shows that I was absent from school a total of twelve days. I called these much-needed days of respite from the rigors of incarceration and forced labor, "mental health" days, courtesy of Florence Nightingale reincarnate, my Angel in a White Uniform, Elizabeth Micou.

In keeping with my sine wave existence in "this damned place," Elizabeth's departure after only a year should have ushered into the hospital top spot Lizzie Borden herself. However, for once my luck held, in the form of my second-in-a-row Angel in White.

Elizabeth Micou left the orphanage in late Fall 1955, and Mrs. Mary Pruitt Daniel assumed the position of hospital supervisor. Although quite saddened by Elizabeth's departure, I soon found that Mary Daniel was as kind, and above all, as empathetic to the orphans' plight, as her sympathetic and caring predecessor. So one bitterly cold December morning I found myself sitting with a mishmash of the usual preteen and teenage orphan hypochondriacs and goldbricks, on the painted white bench in the basement of the hospital, looking very sick indeed, clutching my patented "migraine headache" in both hands. I thought that I had with much practice perfected that "I'm about to die at any moment-please help me," look. I must admit that I was good. I mean really *good.* Even I at times marveled at my prowess as an actor.

However, when it came my turn to tell my sad tale of woe and hurt to this kind lady, I just couldn't bring myself to tell a lie.

So then and there I made the snap decision to be up front with Mrs. Daniel about Saint Elizabeth's allowing me hiatus from the daily drudgery of orphanage life. To my utter delight and surprise, Mrs. Daniel thanked me for being honest with her, and told me anytime I did not "feel well," to simply report to sick call.

"And you really don't have to sit on the bench looking all down in the mouth, Alton."

"I didn't fool you?"

"Not a chance. Now come on and I'll find you a bed in the boys' ward."

Damn. If people kept on seeing through me so easily, I might have to change my name to "Springwater" or worse yet, "Windowpane." And I thought I had perfected one of the best orphans' "down-in-the-mouth" acts around campus. I would definitely have to work on my facial expressions, especially those exhibiting hurt, feigned incredulity and disillusionment. But I would draw the line at "whining." Coley Lee and a few of the other yellow-bellied wimp peers of mine were masters at this game, but they had to use "whining" along with their lame excuses to avoid punishment. I was Little Orphan Al, and Little Orphan Al simply did not whine. Except, that is, as a very last resort. Very last resort.

Later on I confided to Melda about my conversation with Mrs. Daniel, and Melda immediately asked me if she could "get sick" too. Melda was not only beautiful, she was also quite perceptive, resourceful and inventive.

So about three weeks later, Melda and I showed up for after-breakfast sick call in the hospital basement, making sure nobody suspected anything, sitting about three persons between us, but unable to prevent sharing Cary Grant-Ingrid Bergman conspiratorial glances toward one another about every second and a half, I trying my best to look seriously ill, and Melda complaining to everyone around her that she had thrown up twice during the previous night.

Mrs. Daniel put both of us to bed (in separate wards, of course). That night I waited until about an hour after Mrs. Daniel had gone to bed, then crept stealthily across the hall to the girls' ward, whispered to Melda, and we walked softly hand-in-hand down the dark corridor to the playroom.

Now the playroom had one large padded couch and four equally padded chairs. We took off our nightgowns and screwed ourselves silly, trying out all five pieces of furniture in the room. By that time in our relationship I had greatly exceeded the thirty seconds I had lasted on our first night together way up on top of all those mattresses in the Mattress Room. I was up to about a minute and forty-seven seconds, and getting better all the time. Melda was proud of me. Flesh, Pretty Boy, Ace and the old root hog would have been proud of me.

After two nights of all that adolescent frivolity and monkey tricks, Melda and I figured we would be pressing our luck to try for a third, so we each told Mrs. Daniel we were feeling better.

So she discharged us the morning of the third day. As I was preparing to leave, Mrs. Daniel put her hand gently on my forearm, and looking into my eyes said in a soft voice,

"You really do like her a lot, don't you, Alton?"

Hesitating a moment, I knew that she knew, so I simply answered, "Yes, ma'am."

Mrs. Daniel smiled, never once taking her eyes from mine. Patting my shoulder, she said softly,

"You two be careful now."

"Yes, ma'am," I said, and walked out the front door of the hospital.

From time to time I visited Mrs. Daniel in the hospital, and we became good friends. If there happened to be any new kids there, I talked to them and tried to cheer them up, telling them that I believed their relatives would try to come see them "real soon." I explained to Mrs. Daniel how I had been treated by Mrs. Tomblin upon my arrival, and Mrs. Daniel assured me she would seek to console the new boys and girls in their hurt and homesickness. And she did. Mrs. Daniel was the exact opposite of Mrs. Tomblin and all the kids loved her.

In the 1957 issue of *The Log*, the yearbook of John Nichols School, beneath the picture of each graduating senior are listed such trifling and inessential trivialities as "Nickname," "Pet Peeve," "Favorite Sport" and other space-taking-up idiocies. I had selected as my "Favorite Vacation Spot," none other than "The Orphanage Hospital," and as my "Favorite Personality," none other than "Mrs. Mary Daniel."

This dear and lovely lady had allowed two teenage orphans in love a chance to spend some time together alone, without judging us in any manner, and the yearbook was my way of showing my appreciation for her kindness.

During the 1955-56 eleventh grade school year, I was absent from school a total of thirteen days. At night Mrs. Daniel and I would stay up late and talk and listen to the radio drama shows. In the morning I would sleep as long as I wished, and when I awakened the hospital girls would serve me breakfast in bed. Mary Daniel enjoyed the subterfuge as much as I.

If in the Hereafter I should be fortunate enough to be selected to go "up" instead of "down," I hope that if I ever show up for sick call one morning, my nurses will be Florence Nightingale, Elizabeth Micou and Mary Daniel.

Florence will ask me what's wrong. I'll complain that I have a splitting migraine headache, rest my head in my hands, and try my best to look down-in-the-mouth . . . without "whining." As Florence is showering loads of empathy on my poor soul, and assuring me she will take good care of me, Elizabeth Micou and Mary Daniel will look at one another, nod their heads in acknowledgement, smile knowingly, and wink. This would be Heaven.

CHAPTER 57

On Pecans, Salt, Tomatoes and Strawberries

We dairy boys loved tomatoes. And salt. A tomato is not a real tomato without salt. There were two sources of salt at the dairy. It went something like this:

We would swipe several salt shakers full of salt from the dining room tables, and keep them in the Little Dairy. We didn't hide them from Mr. Davis, because Mr. Davis liked salt on his tomatoes also. When the salt ran out, we just took the salt shaker back to the dining room and exchanged it for a full one. But we also were a lazy bunch of hooligans. One morning at breakfast Mr. Pruitt called for quiet and made a request that "somebody" return his salt shakers. We checked right after breakfast, and found that we had eight salt shakers in the Little Dairy. Feeling all guilty, that same day we took three of the empty salt shakers back, and traded them for three full ones. Screw Mr. Pruitt. If he wanted salt shakers, find his own. We "felt" for Mr. Pruitt; we just couldn't quite "reach" him.

One of the many advantages of working at the dairy was that under cover of darkness we could steal any fruit or vegetable we desired. Mr. Davis was well aware of this practice, and never once mentioned it. On our way to the dairy in the wee hours of the morning, we would make slight "detours" by the tomato vines and the huge strawberry patch, that ran the length of the concrete driveway leading from the farm proper to the dairy complex.

By "feel" and a little light, either flash or natural moon, we just plucked the ripest tomatoes we could find, wiped them clean on our shirt sleeves, took out our own personal salt shakers and Presto! a meal.

And we never ran out of salt, thanks to our supplemental source, the ubiquitous "licks" ("salt" licks to the uninitiated), large blocks of rock salt placed in the pasture for the cows to lick. "Licks" are really natural sodium chloride, occurring in solid form. But salt is salt, and the farm tomatoes tasted just as delicious with lick salt as with table salt. We just chipped off a chunk of rock salt from the nearest "lick," and carried it around in our pocket. To make a salty tomato, we just licked the chunk of sodium chloride, and then took a bite of the tomato.

Only a really stupid orphan (found perhaps among a group of dumbass Big Boys in 4-B) would attempt to steal tomatoes and sell them door-to-door off campus. In reality, the tomatoes would sell quicker'n some vegetables, but no half-smart orphan kid would tempt being caught hawking a shopping bag full of tomatoes to the townsfolk. Imagine that same dumb kid being forced by E.T. Regan or Tom Adams to eat that same bag of tomatoes! And without salt, even. Only thing possibly worse than that would be to be caught by Regan or Adams trying to sell a bagful of okra! This really was a dilemma of grand proportions, however, because due to its scarcity, okra would sell faster than any other fruit or vegetable out in town.

Nothing grew small on the orphanage farm; even the cow cakes were oversized. Not even strawberries. Still the largest and juiciest strawberries I've ever tasted. When used in the kitchen to make strawberry ice cream, the vanilla ice cream came out of the mixer not pink but deep red from the juice of these delicacies.

Utilizing the 4:00 a.m. pitch darkness as our trusted ally, at least once a week during strawberry season every dairy boy would get foundered on strawberries. And the townspeople living along the periphery of the campus scarfed them down as fast as we could deliver them. Before long I had developed my own personal customer list, and never again lacked for money to spend. Little Orphan Al, King of the Candy Corner!

In the 1957 high school yearbook, *The Log*, noted under my photograph in the space reserved for "Life's Ambition" is written "To finish college and become a successful businessman." Fortunately, I accomplished both these goals. And then some. However, I learned the economics of supply and demand, customer satisfaction and asset allotment on the streets of Oxford, with one eye constantly on business and the other (sometimes both) on the lookout for Tom Adams and Pappy Regan (the slick bastards).

We boys could sell our contraband, be it strawberries, peaches, Musky dines, pecans or whatever, on Saturday and Sunday afternoon, and the goods had to be as fresh as possible. Not a big problem with peaches and Musky dines; however, as you know, strawberries fade fast once picked, and quickly form rotting spots, that resemble to the buyer out in town, and have the same effect on business, as measles pustules on the face of a young white child. Talk about depressing sales! Try two-day-old strawberries!

Thus for Saturday afternoon sales, we had to "pick 'n steal" the strawberries on the way to the dairy in the wee hours of that morning. So, on the way to the dairy, one thief, er, rather, boy, armed with bag and flashlight, crept stealthily up and down the long rows of strawberries paralleling the concrete dairy-farm driveway, gathering the largest and ripest of the crop. His friend stood in the shadows of the corn crib near the top of the driveway, and "mudded" for the picker-thief. "Mud" was another nonce word in common use among the boys (and girls) at the orphanage. It simply meant to serve as a lookout for the express purpose of warning your partner-in-crime in the event the "enemy" (a word that included any adult) appeared on the scene while some nefarious, illegal and serious pilfering was in progress.

The "mudder" was more often than not the smartest of the strawberry thieves; his was by far the most critical job.

Anyway, the paper lunch bags full of strawberries were stored underneath the manure wagon (*nobody* would ever look for strawberries under there, and it was the coolest place around) to be retrieved when everyone assembled for dinner at noon Saturday.

The main campus that we had to cross to get to the periphery was just that during the week. But on the weekend, and carrying lunch sacks full of stolen strawberries beneath your shirt, that same main campus was transformed into a veritable minefield, the "mines" coming in the form of meaner 'n hell 4-B low-life raiders.

Once we had safely negotiated the minefield, we hid our strawberries in the bushes. Then we walked to the first house on the street, knocked on the door, and announced to the lady of the house that we were selling *fresh* delicious strawberries. Was she interested? If she was, we said we would be right back. We then walked a few doors down, ducked into the bushes, and retrieved our tasty fruit. Then, with no cars that looked like they contained the likenesses of the Evil Demon Twins, Adams and Regan, in sight, we hurried back to the customer's house to complete the sale.

The reward was well worth the effort. The allowance for boys in 1-B and 2-B was fifty cents a month, disbursed by the orphanage treasurer, Maurice Parham's secretary at the business office. To a hungry orphan staring longingly through the glass enclosure in the Candy Corner, having no money could be downright demoralizing.

The dollar earned for selling a bag of strawberries, or the fifty cents for selling a bag of pecans in the Fall, went a long way at the Candy Corner. Some of us always seemed to have candy money; others spent their half-dollar allowance in a day or so, and suffered through the rest of the long, long month.

As a youngster, the lesson I learned between the strawberry patch and the Candy Corner was that if I really wanted to have more than was given to me out of charity, I had to be smart enough to find a way to achieve my goals. By the young age of fourteen I felt confident enough to "think" my way out of just about any adverse situation, and to figure out a way to get what I wanted. Little Orphan Al was living proof that necessity really is the mother of invention. And of deception. And of subterfuge. And of artifice, swindle, evasion, lie, scheme and conspiracy. In fact, the word "brainstorm" was brought into this world on the farm and dairy at a place called Oxford Orphanage in the late '40's and early '50's, with orphan boys, some of whom I admit openly were a lot smarter and more devious and daring than I ever could hope to be, plotting and scheming their way through puberty.

Occasionally, during the Summer months and kids leaving for two-week vacations, Mr. Adams would shanghai some of us dairy boys to help pick the tremendous volume of crops produced on the orphanage farm each year. Alfalfa used as hay for the cows and mules normally yielded four cuttings per year. "Truck farming" is that term used when referring to the harvesting of vegetables for the market. Truck farming was performed on a grand scale at Oxford Orphanage.

Among the crops grown yearly were two kinds of corn, snapbeans, lima beans, tomatoes, cabbage, strawberries, squash, okra, beets, sweet potatoes, carrots, turnips, rutabagas, pecans, musky dines (muscadines), apples, peaches, cantaloupes and watermelons, plus I'm certain a few I cannot recall. I used to stand in utter amazement at the enormous quantity of any of these fruits and vegetables that spring from just a quarter acre of properly watered and fertilized soil.

How do you pick okra? Very carefully, and you'll do a much better (and less painful) job if you take off your socks and use them as gloves. And name one orphan dairy or farm boy who hasn't more than a few times pulled a turnip, or sweet potato, or carrot or beet out of the soft soil, wiped the dirt off on his pantsleg, and eaten the raw vegetable right then and there. No orphan kid ever went hungry. There was always an abundance of food around the farm.

And what we picked that morning we were likely to see on our plates that night for supper. Once harvested, the vegetables and fruits were transported directly to the large, one-story screened-in wooden building called the Vegetable House, located directly behind the kitchen. There a group of young preteen girls spent their days washing and cutting up the harvest, then carrying bushel baskets of these prepared fruits and vegetables to the kitchen for cooking.

Every boy from Walker Building through 3-B looked forward to the Fall pecan season, and even a rookie pecan-tree shaker in 1-B could tell at a glance the stage of ripeness of a pecan.

A ripe pecan will fall to the ground with the assistance of gravity only after the protective outer hull has died, turned from bright green to shriveled black, and the still-closed end of the outer hull cannot remain attached to the proximal end of the pecan. And a ten-year-old orphan kid could spot a lone pecan lying invitingly on the ground at forty paces, and swoop down on his prize quicker'n a hungry hawk on a field mouse.

There were several dozen pecan trees on campus. The Evil Empire's "Pecan Rules" allowed a boy or girl to claim any pecans found lying on the open ground. However, we kids were forbidden, under threat of an agonizing torture, to climb the pecan trees and shake the limbs, or to sling baseball bats or broomsticks into the trees in an attempt to assist Mother Gravity.

And to show just how seriously we always-hungry orphan boys heeded this threat, every single morning during Fall pecan season, you could look out behind 2-B and 3-B, and find six or seven brooms and Louisville Sluggers hanging in the branches of the pecan trees like Christmas tree ornaments, courtesy of inexperienced dead-of-night pecan thieves. Screw the Evil Kingdom and its stupid "Pecan Rules."

Knocking pecans out of pecan trees with brooms, sticks or baseball bats is indeed an art, and takes a lot of practice in order to master the craft.

So in order to be effective, you can't just throw the broomstick or baseball bat up high into the air and let it fall, where it will certainly hang up on some branches.

Instead, you have to sling the broomstick or baseball bat as hard as you can, at about a forty-five degree angle. Then the broom or bat will do its job and usually fall back to the ground.

In the late night darkness, why would we kids use brooms and baseball bats to knock pecans out of trees, when we could easily have climbed the trees to shake out a lot more of the forbidden nuts? It's a matter of self-preservation. That Devious Dickhead Duo, Tom Adams and E.T. Regan, were wont to make surprise spot checks, creeping stealthily out of the darkness between 2-B and 3-B. Try to explain to one of those two sadistic pricks why you're twenty feet up in a pecan tree at midnight, when you're supposed to be in bed asleep.

As the Rulers of the Evil Kingdom considered pecans much the same as potatoes and okra, Tom Adams was in charge of harvesting the annual pecan crop. Only now it was okay for that arrogant bastard to make preteen farm boys climb the pecan trees in order to shake out the nuts.

After gathering the day's crop of pecans, and placing the nuts in large tow sacks, the farm boys lugged the heavy sixty-to-eighty pound tow sacks of pecans up the steep flight of stairs above the main dining rooms, where the pecans were spread out on the basketball court to dry out.

After drying for a few weeks, a portion of the precious crop was used in the kitchen to make pecan pies for the children and staff, and the greater volume of the crop was loaded onto the farm pickup truck and sold to the few large grocery stores out in town. We never called them "supermarkets" in those days. What we today label "supermarkets," back then we just called "big" grocery stores.

During the Summer, (stolen) strawberries and picked blackberries brought us enterprising lads candy, picture show and hot buttered popcorn money; Musky dines and pecans kept my sweet tooth satisfied during the Fall.

The word "pecan" appears to have as many different pronunciations as letters, occasioned no doubt by the inability of Yankees to pronounce properly "PEE-can," instead preferring the sissified "Pe-KAHN." Californians don't seem to be able to make up their minds, and hill country folk from the West Virginia, Kentucky, and Southern Ohio coal mines wouldn't know a "PEE-can" from a "Pe-KAHN."

I was the most enterprising preteen purveyor of stolen Musky dines in 2-B, much too crafty to be caught by that loser E. T. Regan. Usually, that is.

CHAPTER 58

Musky Dines

Seemed as though as a youngster at the OODF (Oxford Orphanage Detention Facility), I never ran out of luck. Only trouble was, it was mostly bad luck. In my seemingly endless battle with certain cottage counselors and staff members, sometimes I won and other times I lost. Unfortunately, most of my victories were Pyrrhic in nature. A few of the "true" victories are worth mentioning.

While an inmate in the ill-famed Baby Cottage Maximum Security Unit, waddling around campus all day with toilet paper padding the crack of my skinny butt cheeks was worth the trouble to ensure no more brown smudges resulted in hairbrush burns from the Sadistic Darkhaired Teenage Bitch Cottage Girl.

And again, while incarcerated in Hobson's Hell Hole, otherwise known as the Walker Building, not having old man Gray tell the difference between the SPLAT! of his wooden board across Coley Lee Hackett's thin-layered trousers and the muffled THWACK! when the same large board hit my three pairs of boxer shorts plus three more pairs "borrowed" from my buddy Bill Herrington's cubby for the occasion, took all the fear out of making the weekly Mr. Gray's List.

These were two definite "W's" for Little Al. But still others were definite "L's," and still others were of the kiss-your-sister type of part-win, part-lose.

For example, consider my Musky Dine Pyrrhic Victory. Musky dines. We called this larger-than-your-average grape "Musky dines," and for years I believed this to be the correct spelling. I learned later the proper spelling to be "muscadine," but this enlightenment did little to lessen the unique taste of these musky grapes grown on woody vines indigenous to the Southeast United States. These luscious mouthfuls are also called "scuppernongs," named for the Scuppernong River that meanders through the northeastern part of God's Country. But for our story we'll settle on just plain old "Musky dines."

On the whole, we orphan boys led pinchpenny existences. Some boys settled for less or none-others sought outside sources of income. Little Orphan Al led the latter group. Ever the entrepreneur, I peddled my bags of (stolen) strawberries and (stolen) Musky dines to the townspeople who lived in the modest-to-well-to-do homes along the periphery of the orphanage campus. Almost directly behind the swimming pool, across the narrow one-lane rough paved road that led from the hospital and farm down to the Industrial Building, lay a large Musky dine patch.

Many years afore, sturdy wire had been tautly secured atop stout wooden posts about seven feet high, and the thick Musky dine vines were each season laden chock full of the plump, delicious yellow-green fruit.

The skin of the Musky dine is rather thick and rough, not as tasty as the skin of the regular purple or white grape, and just a few of the Musky dine skins would give a boy a good-sized stomach ache. So, to eat the Musky dine, you placed the large ball of fruit into your open mouth, pressed hard your thumb and index finger, and the meat of the Musky dine just popped out of the skin and into your mouth. Likewise, because the seeds were larger than regular grape seeds, you would just spit out the seeds. Even then, we boys had a tendency to founder ourselves on the tasty fruit, so an occasional bellyache was to be expected, and was a quite acceptable trade-off for enjoying the free feast.

Because of the location of the Musky dine patch, I sold my Musky dines to the folks living in the homes along that back side of the campus nearest the Industrial Building. I wasn't about to trek all the way across the main campus (day or night) loaded down with ten or so paper bags filled with my precious (stolen) contraband. Not enough oak tree shadows even on that expansive campus to hide from the vultures-lying-in-wait sonofabitchin Big Boys eager to confiscate whatever-it-is-you-have. That would be the suicide of navigating a minefield blindfolded with one hand tied behind you. I was a fast study in survival techniques. Once-caught was plenty enough for me.

During Musky dine season, on Friday or Saturday night (for sale on Saturday or Sunday afternoon) I would take a large bag down after supper, and fill the bag with the juiciest (by feel-not too hard, not too soft) Musky dines. With the disciplined stealth of a U.S. Army Ranger I would carry the heavy bag of "dines," along with a dozen or so brown paper lunch bags, over to the fence at the edge of the peach orchard, located directly behind the Industrial Building. There I hid my treasure in the tall grass, covering it with leaves and more grass. I had the uncanny ability to look at Musky dines and see dollar bills, one side of which was always green, that being to course the back ("greenback") side.

Of course, this was the easy part. The following day, Saturday or Sunday, once I was free in the afternoon, I returned to my cache of gold and filled two paper lunch bags full (always mounded over, so the townsfolk-that's what they were called in the Saturday afternoon B-western matinees at the Paramount in Kinston, and calling the people townsfolk brought back memories of happier times-would know they were not getting shorted) of the "dines."

Now, that sorry-assed E.T. Regan apparently had nothing better to do on Saturday or Sunday afternoon but harass (in the old French meaning of "to set a dog on") little ole defenseless Al Provost, so he and I (as well as he and several others just like me) played our little weekend cat-and-mouse games.

But I was far and away smarter than E.T. Regan, because I knew what the mean old bastard's car looked like, and from three blocks away I had quickly learned to spot it, because he always drove slower than a normal motorist would have, as though on the lookout for enterprising orphan kids trying to make a few bucks off stolen strawberries, peaches and Musky dines. Little Al was learning fast how to bamboozle the best, and old man Regan didn't stand a chance-as long as I could spot him coming down the street in that sneaky fifteen-mile-an-hour car.

I would fill two paper lunch bags with the dines, keep the rest of them in the large bag, and sell two bags at a time. If I observed Regan's car close by, I could always fling the dines across the grass and fold the bags and stick them in my pocket. I was good at this.

I was just a snot-faced young boy who was not the least bit satisfied with his lot in life up to that point. And I loved candy, as much as did any other kid in the orphanage. It was never my intention at that young age to stop by the Candy Corner every day before dinner, press my face against the glass pane encasing all those goodies and come away with nothing more than a drooling mouth and a pressed face.

No, I was determined to have the money to purchase what I wanted, and to share my purchases with my buddies. The first thing I thought of when we stupid-assed kids discovered all those used "balloons" in the woods was the stuff my pockets and take some back to my buddies. And I had. And they had blown them up, and later hated my guts for months. But at least I had had the best of intentions, that should count for something.

I could ascertain with my sharp-as-a-tack mind when was the best time of the day or night to steal Musky dines, strawberries, pecans or peaches, could navigate that human minefield of good-for-nothing scumbag Big Boys eager to confiscate with force or threat thereof, my earnings, and was astute enough at ages eleven and twelve to peg the high end of the going market rate for my stolen fruit and nuts, and push that rate to the limit. I considered myself an entrepreneur second to none, and I was proud of it. And I wasn't about to cut myself off at the knees by walking anywhere near 3-B or 4-B with money in my pockets. Day or night. Especially night.

By mid-afternoon on the particular Saturday in question, I had sold six paper bags full (mounded over, of course) of the Musky dines. The juice of the tasty, distinctive-smelling grape is quite sticky, so periodically I had to spit on my hands and rub them on my shirt to keep my hands clean. I had six well-earned, neatly-folded dollar bills (and as always, green side out for luck) in my sock, secreted there compliments of my best friend Paranoia (the Big Boys often roamed these streets on Saturday afternoons, searching for easy picture show and popcorn money), and a quick glance up and down the street revealed no E.T. Regan in sight. I was feeling pretty good, and guessed I had about three more lunch bags full of Musky dines left. Six dollars for all that work was more than worth it. So I scooped another bag out of my large sack, stored the sack in the hiding place under a hedge, and set out in search of my seventh dollar bill. Seven dollars to an eleven-year-old orphan kid was confidence, power and pride. I had earned it, and I was richer than most of the other kids by seven dollars.

Turning the corner onto a side street, I glanced down the sidewalk and stopped short, startled to see a much too familiar form approaching me. Damn! Too late. There was my own personal nemesis, E.T. Regan in the evil flesh, walking toward me wearing the only smile I ever observed on his stupid smug face in the ten years I knew him. The bastard had tricked me because he knew I would be looking for his car. Son-of-a-bitch!

And his rare smile was indeed a Victory smile. Touché! An expert in facial expressions would translate his gaze as "Got you now, you little bastard!"

I stopped dead in my tracks, and stood still, clutching the bag full of Musky dines under my arm, staring up into his gleeful face as he quickly closed the distance between us. E.T. Regan was very good at that "closing the distance" thingy.

"Whatcha selling today, boy?"

"Fuck you, you stupid sonofabitch."

However, I spoke these words to myself, wanting to say them aloud, but fearful Regan would slap me into next week right then and there on the public sidewalk. But I had the satisfaction of saying these words to myself, and by my silence he certainly understood. In our neverending battles with the teachers and staff, most of our victories were small ones indeed; we had to take what we could get. One of the best known small satisfactions was to see how many times we could repeat "Fuck you" to ourselves while staring intently into the eyes of a cruel cottage counselor or supervisor. It didn't really accomplish anything save a little comforting lift of our spirits. But any light, however dim, illuminates an orphanage.

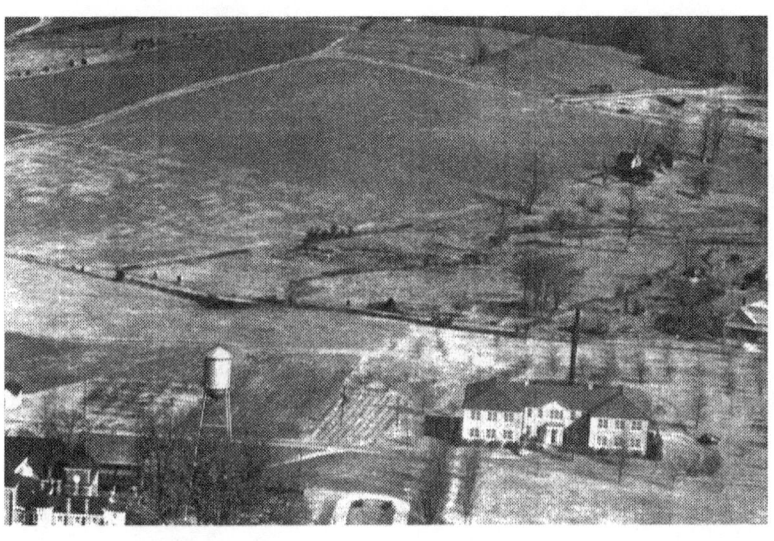

1951. Lower left (to left of water tower) is the large Musky Dine patch. Apple and Peach orchard is behind Industrial Building. Extreme upper right is hog pen. Just below hog pen is Beef Cattle Barn and pasture.

Failing to answer Regan's stupid question was in itself an insult to him, but he let it slide for the moment; he had better things in mind.

"Gimme that bag, boy," he ordered, reaching for my full (mounded over, of course) bag of Musky dines.

"Whadda ya get for this bag full, boy?"

"A quarter, sir." I lied by three-fourths.

"How many bags you sold?"

"None, sir." I lied by six dollars, but since I had already lied about the price of the bag full of Musky dines by three-fourths, I figured I was really lying by six times three, or eighteen.

Of course he didn't believe me, and my count of silent "Fuck yous" was by this time approaching ninety. I could count faster silently, less vocal cord energy and very little lip movement. And a lot of practice. *Sotto voce* is God's gift to young orphans.

"Empty out yer pockets, boy." This meant he did not believe me. I wonder why? I certainly would not have believed me, either. I was a sneaky, lying little shit, and he knew it and I knew it.

I emptied out my pockets. Nothing. (The money's in my sock, you stupid prick. And by the way, fuck you, ninety-three. Fuck you ninety-four.)

Finding my pockets empty, Regan accepted that I had not yet sold my first (and to him, my only) bag of Musky dines. Gullible dirtbag.

"You know you stole dem Musky dines, boy." Regan and his evil cohorts didn't ask questions-they made statements that we were supposed to take as questions, and defend ourselves accordingly. I use the word "defend" because every statement from Regan (or from Tom Adams, the sadistic dickhead) was an accusation.

I didn't answer. He was getting really upset that I wouldn't answer his statements (read that "accusations") though I was staring directly into his steel blue eyes. (Fuck you, one hundred twenty one . . .)

"Answer me, boy!" His voice boomed along the side street. I jumped when his voice rose those six octaves. Made him feel like he was frightening me. Sometimes it helped if you acknowledged the abusive adult scared hell out of you. But again, sometimes it didn't.

"Sir, if I stole 'em, then everybody else is a thief, too. All the boys pick 'em."

"But you're the only one selling 'em."

"What's the difference?" I asked, in innocent puzzlement.

He didn't answer, but instead handed the bag of Musky dines to me. I took them and held the bag under my arm. I couldn't believe my luck. I had apparently won our little battle of wits. The sonofabitch had backed down. But, he usually confiscated the booty. Was his return to me of my Musky dines a sign of total capitulation on his part? Perhaps my luck had changed finally. Perhaps old man Regan had finally realized that I was a power to be reckoned with. Or perhaps he suddenly discovered he was late for supper, or maybe he had to go to the bathroom, and just couldn't wait.

'Fraid not. Same luck. Only worse.

"Okay, boy, let's see here, now."

Apparently he was not late for supper after all, and did not have to go to the bathroom. He stood haughtily before me, arms akimbo, looking me straight in the eye. I didn't move a muscle. He looked downright unfriendly, bordering on adult-style "cruel," that was certain to turn "vicious" at any moment now.

With my side vision (every orphan kid quickly develops finely-tuned "side vision") I looked for any slight movement of his right shoulder; since he was right handed, if he was going to slap me silly, his right shoulder would have to move first, because his right hand and arm were attached to his right shoulder. Then, as though weighing my fate (which was exactly what he was doing), Regan sucked in a deep breath and spoke in an even, deliberate tone.

"Okay, boy, let's see here now." He was repeating himself. This was really serious stuff. The repeating-himself grownup always spelled trouble.

"Since you can't sell 'em, and you can't put 'em back on the vine, I s'pose the only thing you can do is, well, eat 'em."

I quickly looked down at the bag (mounded over, dammit!) of those large Musky dines, that appeared to double in size right then and there before my eyes, then back up at the gloating sonofabitch, standing triumphantly before me with this mouthy little half-smile on his stupid face. I didn't move. At all. Maybe if I acted as though I had not heard him, he would forget what he said. But he didn't.

"Well, let's get started, boy," he barked, letting me and everyone within a 200-yard radius know just who was in charge. Dammit! I got the distinct feeling that I was not in charge anymore. Had I ever been? Anyway, by now I had this *huge* bushel-basket full of Musky dines under my left arm, so I reached across with my right hand, took out one of the by now baseball-sized Musky dines, held it in my partially opened mouth, popped the meat of the fruit into my mouth, then threw the Musky dine skin on the ground before me. In my mouth I separated out the large seeds, and spat them also on the ground.

"Pick up that skin, boy."

"Sir?" I supposed he didn't want me littering the ground, which was perfectly understandable. So I picked up the skin.

"Eat it, boy!" he demanded sternly.

"Sir?" I implored, thinking I now realized what the bastard intended to do to me.

"Eat everything, boy!" he demanded.

"Seeds, skin, everything, boy."

"Yes, sir." Fuck you, two hundred forty seven . . .

I figured at that time that if I expected to live to see another dawn, I had better start doing just exactly as he instructed. So I started eating the Musky dines whole, meat, seeds and skin. And he just stood there watching me, enjoying every sickening mouthful I swallowed.

About ten minutes and half a bag of by now cantaloupe-sized Musky dines later, I was beginning to feel queasy, mainly in the area of my stomach. My chewing and swallowing had become quite labored and deliberate, slowing considerably, and I remember thinking I sure was glad I had been selling Musky dines and not squash or okra. It was time to admit defeat, and fall on his mercy, if the old bastard had any, or even knew the meaning of the word.

"I can't eat anymore, Mr. Regan," I pleaded. "I'm really sick." And fuck you, four hundred sixty seven . . .

Pausing before making comment, the gloating sonofabitch must have sensed I was being truthful, or else he noticed the skin of my face beginning to take on a greenish glow, so he said,

"Okay, boy, do you think you've learned your lesson?"

"Yes, sir." Fuck you, and fuck you again, four hundred seventy nine and eighty . . .

"Well, boy, give me the rest of the bag."

I gladly handed him the bag of Musky dines.

"Now, boy, you go on back to your cottage. And don't ever let me catch you out here again."

"Yes, sir." I turned, crossed the street, and started walking slowly toward the campus. By now I felt a wee bit unsteady on my feet.

But I sure as hell wasn't going to give the bastard the satisfaction of seeing me throw up. So I just held my breath. As I sneaked a peek out of the corner of my eye (every orphan kid quickly develops keen "corner of the eye" vision), the mean old bastard was getting into his car about half a block away. Good riddance, dirtbag!

"Son?"

"Son?"

"Son, over here."

I turned to see an elderly blue-haired woman standing on the front porch of the house where Mr. Regan had just humbled me.

"Yes, ma'am."

"How many more Musky dines do you have?"

"About three bags full, ma'am."

"How much for a bag?"

I thought for a moment. "Fifty cents a bag, ma'am."

"Bring all you have to me, son. I'll give you a dollar a bag. I don't like what he did to you. He's not a very nice man, is he?"

"No, ma'am."

I quickly retrieved my master bag of Musky dines from under the hedges, and raced toward the nice old lady's house. I gave her the rest of my Musky dines, and she gave me three crisp dollar bills. After quickly checking that they had one side green, I folded them and stuffed them into my sock, green side out for luck.

Then I looked up into the nice lady's eyes. She reminded me of mama, aged about thirty years. Kind. Soft voice. Sincere. Caring. I so much wanted to ask her if she would be my mother. But better not press my luck.

"What's your name, son?" She also called me "son," not "boy." What a difference a name makes.

"Al, ma'am. Al Provost." I really wanted this nice lady to remember me. And she did.

"Come back to see me when you have some strawberries."

"I will, ma'am. Thank you, very much. Bye now."

The widow, Mrs. Ethel Carter, became my best customer, and my friend. From that day forward, every bag of mounded-over fruit or nuts, I charged her fifty cents, not a dollar. Always give friends a good deal. It's the charitable thing to do, and it promotes business.

Begrudgingly, I must admit that my nemesis, E.T. Devious, whom I could usually outwit even on an off day, sure left me twisting in the wind on this particular Musky Dine Caper. But I still believe the score at that juncture in our "relationship" was Little Orphan Al-59, Dumbass E.T. Regan-3. At times even I marveled at my deviousness, cunning and rascality. My mind was at times not unlike a perpetual motion machine. It had to be in order to survive this repository of neglect and misunderstanding.

Now at this North Carolina prison farm foisted off on the public as an "orphanage," there were many enterprising preteen and teenagers who, like myself, earned a lot of extra money by selling pecans, blackberries and stolen strawberries and Musky dines. However, only the boldest of the bold, most daunting of the daring and the most stupid of the dumb, would ever attempt to sell . . . a pig. A pig? There was only one boy at the orphanage bold enough to try a stunt like that. And only one boy stupid enough to help him pull it off.

CHAPTER 59

The Tale of Butch's Pig in a Poke

In my youth, I always seemed to get mixed up with the wrong bunch of preteen and teenage felons. When we were in the Walker Building (ages nine and ten) and 1-B (ages eleven and twelve), I still don't know where Ersul Sowers and Blockhead Johnson picked up all those strange new words, that turned out to be cuss words, but every darn one of these newfound vulgarities exited my lips about six nanoseconds after reaching my inner ear. If you wanted the whole campus to know something, announce it within earshot of that stupid kid from Kinston!

Friendships were formed at Oxford based in large degree on having the same views as another child, or having suffered a beating with a group of your peers. Even while in the Walker Building, Bill Herrington and I read the front section of the Raleigh *News and Observer* and the Durham *Morning Herald*, because we both seemed to be interested in the world outside the hedges. In the Summer of 1950, after the Korean War started, every day Bill and I would follow the war in the newspapers, our mood, hopes and fears riding the tide of battle.

Van Edwards had befriended me that first traumatic day I arrived at the Baby Cottage, cautioning me that if I didn't do what Miss Minnie Warwick ("She's *mean!*") told me to do, I'd get a "whuppin." Sensing that Van's advice came from similar experiences, I heeded his counsel.

Sharing danger is probably the best cement used to bind a lasting friendship. Recall "The Return of the Balloon Boys?" That hairy-assed, mad-as-a-hornet pedophile pervert could have chased after Butch Mitchell as well as he chased me. And Butch tried his best to talk me out of stupidly climbing into that pen with Ace the Bull.

So I suppose if old Butch asked me to engage in some sort of illegal activity that might eventually blossom into a continuing criminal enterprise, could I in all honesty place restrictions on our friendship? Which brings me to the tale of "Butch's Pig in a Poke."

In my youth there were three significant events for which no accurate statistics were recorded, these being 1) the number of times I let the air out of Gray's, Regan's and Tom Adams' car tires, 2) the number of times I screamed "Fuck you!" (under my breath) while some sadistic lowlife teacher or work supervisor was physically brutalizing me, and 3) the number of piglets in a farrow (a litter of pigs) that was born and actually survived. And we were dead certain about that last statistic. Dead certain.

The one absolutely brilliant felonious scheme over which I cannot lay claim was Butch Mitchell's plan to sell unregistered, unnamed, uncounted and uncastrated three-month-old male piglets to the coloreds who lived in the run-down section of town about five blocks from the Industrial Building corner of the campus.

It was 1952, Butch and I were twelve years old, and were beginning our second year on the dairy. As explained to an open-mouthed Little Orphan Al, Butch's daring proposal for us to practically own the Candy Corner was bold beyond belief in its conception and almost foolproof in its execution. I begrudged my friend for thinking of it first. The scheme was hatched in Butch's brilliant mind in the following manner.

To avoid the heat of a hot June Saturday afternoon, a small group of us 2-B boys had trekked to a wide spot in the creek over beyond the railroad trestle, for an hour or so of swimming, and on our return were just moseying along trading nasty jokes and just as nasty farts, when we decided to detour by the pig farm to see the new baby pigs.

We picked up a few of the cute little baconettes, and they squealed and crapped. One of the guys clamped his hand over a piglet's snout, and the little devil squirmed and crapped, but its squeal was muffled somewhat.

Following this meaningless and innocent preteen diversion, we boys continued on our way toward the main campus. Pretty soon Butch tapped my shoulder and motioned me to lag behind the group.

"Y'know how many little pigs there are?" he whispered conspiratorially. Any preteen or teenage orphan boy's "conspiratorial whisper" could have only one meaning. If whatever the kid was asking was not illegal or against orphanage rules, there would be no need for the conspiratorial whisper. Dead giveaway. Every time. The "conspiratorial whisper."

"No, I don't," I replied, somewhat puzzled at Butch's question.

"Well, neither does Tom Adams."

Butch's matter-of-fact reply carried with it a degree of smugness that was clearly obvious when one orphan kid thought he knew something you didn't. Which, by the way, was exactly the case here.

"And if Butthead Adams don't know how many little pigs he's got, how's he ever gonna tell if some of 'em are missing?"

Butch's use of the plural instead of the singular might have slipped by most of our less intelligent and astute classmates, but not sharp-as-a-tack Little Orphan Al. Butch had not said "one of 'em," but "some of 'em," when referring to small domesticated animals that might or might not even exist, census-wise, that is. I was interested. Definitely interested. So I asked (in a conspiratorial whisper, mind you) the questions as they flooded to mind.

"Who we gonna sell 'em to? And how're we gonna get 'em off campus? Can't just pick us up a couple of the little buggers an' tote 'em away like we was carrying footballs or something."

"Don't worry, Al. We'll figure it out." I liked that about Butch Mitchell and Coley Lee Hackett. These two devious little bastards really didn't give a damn, and once they made up their minds, they'd figure out the details and fill them in to make the scheme work.

So over the next few days we two enterprising soon-to-be pig purloiners "figured it out," most of the mental work being done by ole Butch, who was not in the least skeptical about anything if there was money in it. And I thought I was a businessman. Musky dines, strawberries and blackberries were pennyante. This was the Big Time. This was serious. Getting caught doing something that in the World-

Beyond-the-Main-Gate might get us five-to-ten on a North Carolina prison work farm, might just get us a free ticket to the notorious Jackson Training School. So the two of us gave the possible consequences of our criminal enterprise some really serious thought-for about six-and-a-half seconds, that is. Fuck 'um! I still believe the term "Go for it!" was coined by Butch Mitchell. At times our two minds were as sharp as the Sword of Achilles.

Butch's Brilliant Blueprint for putting us, quite literally, "high on the hog" went something like this. First he would see if there was a market for small, live, uncastrated male pigs over in the colored section of town. We figured the colored folks would not squeal (no pun intended) on us to old man Regan or Tom Adams. There was certainly a market, Butch found out. I asked him how he knew there was a market. He said he just went over to colored town one Saturday afternoon, and the first ramshackle hovel he came to, he asked the old colored man sitting on the stoop, "Would y'all wanna buy a small pig that still had his balls?" The answer, Butch said, was a very quick "Yes." I asked one of the Big Boys one time why the colored folks wanted to eat pigs that still had their testicles. The Big Boy said the coloreds thought if they ate the pig's balls, that the coloreds called "mountain oysters," that was supposed to make the coloreds as smart as the white people. The Big Boy sounded serious, but I don't know if he was telling the truth, or was just "pulling my leg." I had my goddamn leg pulled so often by the Big Boys that I thought I would have to wear an elevator shoe on one foot to walk upright. Sometimes I wasn't all that bright.

The next decision was what price to put on each pig. Price. What's a stolen three-month-old piglet worth on the open market (or at least in the colored part of Oxford, North Carolina)? Butch asked twelve dollars. We got twelve dollars. That was easy. Should have asked for fifteen. But we were businessmen. Not dishonest and greedy businessmen. Just stupid. The goddamn pigs were probably worth fifty dollars each. Or more. Probably more.

But alas, just as any light, however dim, illuminates an orphanage, twelve dollars was a lot of money to us two preteen orphan pig-thieves, er, rather, porcine entrepreneurs.

So, how we gonna get them little pigs off campus? Gotta do it at night. What we gonna carry 'em in? Tow sacks, from the dairy. The sacks the feed comes in. How we gonna keep 'em from squealing? Tie their little snouts with twine. Sure weren't no giant rolls of "duct tape" floatin' round Oxford Orphanage in 1952. The little buggers'll shit all the way to colored town, but they sure won't make any noise doing it.

Anyway, back to colored town goes Butch, to take our first order. How many piglets they want? Three. That's thirty-six dollars, eighteen smackeroos apiece. Good for starters. There'd be more. You betcha.

How we gonna accept payments? C.O.D. We don't send no bills. We don't take no checks. Colored man asks Butch, what's "C.O.D.?" What's a "bill?" And for that matter, young white boy, what's a "check?" Our kinda customers. Colored folk with money to spend. What a market!

So, in the darkness of an after-supper Saturday night, off we went to the pigpen, pockets stuffed with enough stolen baling twine to hogtie the entire pigpen population, my sharp Barlow pocketknife, and three feed bags swiped from the dairy hay loft.

Y'ever try to steal three-month-old pigshit-covered piglets in the three-candlelight dimness of a half moon? Most sane persons haven't. So I chased down the first male piglet, grabbed it by its hind legs, flipped the little devil on its stomach and sat on it. While I clasped my hands tightly over its squirming snout, Butch tied the snout snugly, and we shoved the still-defecating, still-urinating little bugger into the tow sack.

Now, since the little devil wasn't yet a hog, we saw no need to hogtie it, so the gunny sack continued to move aimlessly around the pigpen while we chased down and literally "bagged" his two fellow "travelers."

Because I was a little bigger than Butch, and because he was the "brains" behind this enterprise, I agreed to tote two of the pig-filled tow sacks. So off we trudged in the half-moonlight, with the silent baby porkers trying to climb up our backs through the burlap bags. As we approached the perimeter of the campus, near the Industrial Building, the two sacks became too heavy to lug on my back, so I just dragged the constantly-moving swine-filled sacks on the ground behind me, and Butch followed suit. Our plan was proceeding well on schedule.

About a half-block past the campus fence we stopped to rest, and Butch, who had stupidly forgotten to tie the top of his tow sack, lay the sack on the grass beside him. And there went the captive little porker, scooting out of the bag in a flash, hoofing it down the dimly-lit Oxford street, darting back and forth like he was Charlie "Choo Choo" Justice side-stepping hapless Duke defensive backs in the open field, the only sound being the rapidly fading pitter-patter of its tiny sharp hooves on the asphalt. And in a flash he was gone. Immediately I started to mentally calculate what my share of the sale of now *two* baby pigs at twelve bucks each would be.

But Butch would have no part of the little devil's insolence. Right on its curlicue tail ran old Butch, yelling and cussing the escapee, chasing it into the bushes and across the street, zigging with every pig-zig, zagging with its every zag.

And suddenly the street fell silent. Quiet. Everything still. Then after about five minutes I saw Butch emerging from the darkness of the penumbra cast by the streetlight, walking down the middle of the street like he was Gary Cooper in *High Noon*, toting his little pigskin under his right arm like a football, laughing victoriously at having recaptured his errant piglet. Damn, I sure was proud of my friend! Restore them original three-pig sales and profit figures, you guys in Accounting.

Rebagging Butch's recaptured baby porker, we continued on to the "customer's" house. I waited in the bushes while Butch dragged the three constantly moving gunny sacks up the broken wooden steps in front of the small age-fading clapboard house. A smiling, wizened old white-headed colored man came out to the light of the front porch lamp, green money was exchanged sight-unseen for the moving burlap sacks, and my "business partner" rejoined me in the cover of the bushes.

We split the loot then and there, all of it in one-dollar bills. I was suddenly eighteen dollars richer, and with that thirty-six dollars Butch and I could just about clean out the Candy Corner at one whack.

On our way back to the campus, with the comforting bulge of eighteen neatly-folded greenbacks in my front pocket, the Chairman of the Board (Butch) and his Director of Sales (Little Orphan Al himself) began plotting their next "sale." We tried to determine how many piglets we could steal and sell before "Asswipe" Adams, as Butch referred to the farm manager, would notice an appreciable dent in the orphanage swine population and put an end to our little enterprise.

We agreed to top our sales off at a total of ten piglets, because ten was an even number. With our profit of sixty dollars each, I was going to see if I could locate and purchase a used Thompson submachine gun, for squirrel hunting. We were on a roll!

However, a few days later we were getting off work at the dairy about mid-morning, when word came that Mr. Adams had rounded up all thirtysome of the farm boys, and had put them to scouring the fields around the pigpen. Why? Seems as though that morning Adams had been down at the pigpen and discovered that three of his young piglets had apparently wriggled out through the fence, although nobody could find any holes in the fence.

Those thirtysome farm boys searched half a day for those three "escaped" piglets, and nobody ever found them. And old Butch was left shaking his head in awe and disbelief, that old Butthead Tom Adams had actually counted all those dozens of newborn piglets! Damn. So much for "dead certain."

CHAPTER 60

The Ditchbank Crew

To those older boys fortunate enough not to have incurred the wrath of staff members, teachers or the 3-B and 4-B cottage counselors during the week, the Farm Road was just that, a well-worn dirt road that started at the top of the concrete driveway leading to the dairy, and meandered an extra long country mile, across the railroad tracks and past the Thousand Dollar Spring, to where it terminated somewhere near the Farmer's Barn.

Preteen and teenage boys who during the week had either committed some sort of unpardonable or unforgivable sin (for example, Blockhead, Newton or Coley Lee) or whom the teachers, staff or cottage counselors had falsely accused of such breaches of strict discipline (for example, Van or Bill or Little Orphan Al) were either placed on Mr. Gray's Saturday Afternoon Flogging List or were slapped silly at the point of such infraction of the rules, or both.

It just so happened during that time at Oxford Orphanage there did indeed exist a group of older boys at whom, if Mr. Regan or Tom Adams had raised a board or his hand, might just get the board shoved down his throat-sideways. For this class of Big (Meaner'n hell) Boys was reserved the punishment of Oxford Orphanage's answer to a Georgia prison chain gang, the dreaded "Ditchbank Crew."

To this group of poor unfortunates and unjustly accused, the aforementioned farm road was not really a one-mile dirt road, but *two* miles of very deep and just as wide *ditchbank* that grew with weeds faster than it could be cleaned out.

The luckless older boys whose names appeared on the list of the Ditchbank Crew reported to the tool shed Saturday at one o'clock. The weather was not a factor, be it a blazing August sun or an ass-numbing cold snap in January. Shovels, hoes and sometimes pickaxes were distributed to the prisoners, and Mr. Regan or Tom Adams knew exactly to the foot how much of the ditchbank should be cleaned out by six teenage orphans in a certain period of time. No supervision was required. If the job was not completed from one o'clock to five o'clock to the satisfaction of Adams or Regan, the prisoners were automatically scheduled for a same-time-next-Saturday session.

The manual labor and harsh working conditions were not the only incentive to avoid the wrath of the staff. Saturday afternoon and Sunday afternoon were about the only times the older boys were "on their own," so to speak. I couldn't pick blackberries and sell them out in town to earn spending money if I was toiling away in the heat on a dusty red dirt road.

CHAPTER 61

My Seemingly Eternal Search for Identity

Fortuitous circumstances certainly not of my making had occasioned my being shunted off life's scheduled pathway and hurtled at the hyperspeed of Flash Gordon's (or Flesh Jordan) rocketship, seemingly without rhyme or reason, onto the spur track posted, in the Biblically-historical sense, "Job's House of Neverending Abuse, Longing and Regret."

It was as though I had been pre-ordained to languish for the greater part of my cherished youth in this Purgatory, this quagmire, this broiling sea of (damn) quicksand, and that this unfortunate interlude of my "second" life, that is, between 208 East Bright Street and young adulthood, should be spent in the evil clutches of petulant, damnable and disinterested grownups and in the company of more than three hundred similarly-situated unfortunates from broken homes.

Such were the depths of my disappointment, disillusionment and downright depression that at times it seemed as though I were merely offal on the giant technicolor panoramic screen of life, wastage discarded after the depredations of the hyenas and jackals that somehow had infiltrated the ranks of good and honest Christians. And at times random, fleeting, disjointed worries and fears bounced around in my confused young mind like agitated wasps inside that aforementioned closed tin can.

It was such that at times during my youth I experienced a detached, eerie sensation as though place and time were shifting sideways in real time, or that a strong wind was buffeting me from side to side, hindering my forward progress. Little Alton had fallen through the Looking Glass, tumbling headlong into a surrealistic, decade-long incubus. Oh, God, why me?

Upon being packed off to "this damned place" by mama at the angelic age of seven years, the precipitate shock to my mind (and body) was brutally abrupt and lasting, accompanied always it seemed by my equally resolute and mulish refusal to accept the notion that I could be an active participant in this postwar Southern ninety-nine percent tragic tragicomedy called "Oxford Orphanage." It was as though I were a B-western picture show director, viewing my life through the panoramic lens of a black-and-white motion picture camera. Seems as though this denial and disbelief have lasted a continuance without end.

And by the still-embryonic age of eleven, I was not yet with the worst behind me, was just opening Act II of this wretched Milleresque stage play marqueed as "Little Orphan Al Gets Shuffled to Hell and Back," and my pathetic life was "progressing" as one might expect, that is, if one expected me to get picked on, at, over and apart by a well-armed battalion of insufferable blackbooted, goose-stepping grownups and their evil deputies, the loathsome Big Boys, twenty-eight hours a day, seven hundred days a year.

My youthful search for "identity," for who I was and what I stood for, for what my place was in this highly-structured environment, in this diverse microcosm called "Oxford Orphanage," eventually was transformed into an adult pragmatism that has guided my life for more than half a century. And along the Pathway to Growing Up I missed by only a few clicks of Kentucky windage becoming a card-carrying, dyed-in-the-wool nihilist, occasioned by a frustrated and desperate response to maltreatment and neglect at the hands, quite literally, of oppressive and ill-meaning grownups.

I suppose I was ever searching for the mix that would validate the true meaning of my existence in this godforsaken place, would determine and give structure and reason to my "place" in my confused little world, would allow me to define with some minimal degree of logic and reason, who I really was and later would become. And all the while enveloped in that smoldering, smothering perplexity known universally among that fraternity of the world's orphans as "homesickness" and "longing." Orphans know exactly what I mean.

However, this obscured, quite ill-defined "identity" continued to elude me as though I were moving at a snail's pace toward a constantly out of reach receding horizon. Gradually, as I viewed the mistreatment of other orphanage children by staff and work supervisors, I began to internalize my thoughts and emotions, to adjust my attitude in response to my own persecution at the hands of these selfsame callous and uncaring grownups, searching for a response that would afford me hope, and add some small measure of order and rationality to my predicament. The search for . . . how should I say it . . . survival . . . comes to mind; I think I just wanted to survive this goddamn "orphanage" thing, and all the heartache and sorrow that accompanied it, and get on with my "real" life that surely must exist "outside the hedges." Odd thing about those ever-present hedges that delineated the periphery of the campus; seemed that as soon as I became tall enough to peer over the damn things, they grew a few inches higher. Egads! Even the blooming shrubbery was out to get me!

It was easy to spot me on campus. I was that stupid kid from Kinston, walking around on my tiptoes, craning my skinny neck skyward, searching for a glimpse of freedom. To me those harmless hedges represented double-stranded barbed wire, electrified with 20,000 volts. What a depressing predicament!

Prior to my being propelled at the speed of light plus an additional forty-five miles per hour toward Oxford Orphanage, our family had been close-knit, caring and loving. Following an extended period of deep-seated self-doubt, that lasted every bit of seven and a half seconds, I realized I had done nothing to "deserve" the physical abuse and mental torment showered upon my frail being by cold-hearted grownups and equally impenitent older children charged with my well-being. My crisis of confidence had passed in the swift blink of an owl's eye. This sense of moral insult developed as a tremulous orphan child became, without conscious design, the pawl to my ratchet wheel of life, ensuring that my direction of life in adulthood continued in a determined forward gear.

Contempt is a quite unwelcome emotion some youngsters acquire as a natural and logical response to physical abuse and mental degradation, and was the most difficult for me as a preteen and teenager to conceal. This strange sensation did not enter my psyche's menu spontaneously, nor was it washed ashore on the banks of the Provost gene pool. Rather, it was conceived at the hands (quite literally) of the callous, uncaring Edith Tomblin and her demon twin sister, the gargoyle Minnie Warwick, and hatched on the baseball field we Walker Building youngsters were forced by Bertha Hobson to cross on our way to A. DeLeon Lucifer's battering chamber on Saturday afternoons.

By age twelve my loathing for abusive cottage counselors and staff members had stuck to me like a just-thrown Junebug on a fresh cow cake, and after trying my best to conceal my feelings, and failing miserably in that regard, I made the conscious decision to flaunt my scorn and thus use it as part of my armamentarium in my neverending battle with belittling adults.

But alas, sometimes that which works too well for us often works against us. The scurrilous Tom Adams, fresh from years of honing his physical and mental abuse skills on the unfortunate inmates at a North Carolina training school, apparently could read contempt on my mind the moment he approached me while I was standing against the dairy barn wall with Frank and Butch on that fateful mid-morning in June 1951.

His scathing invective, after slapping me clean off my feet and bouncing me like a well-worn Wilson tennis ball against the whitewashed lower dairy barn wall, "I know you didn't say anything, but you were thinking 'dammit'" announced to me that he well understood my fractious attitude and would not tolerate such public display of unspoken insolence from me. At that seminal moment I realized I was beginning to exhibit outwardly my utter, pent up contempt for abusive grownups, and that my message was being heard. Damn, it felt good! My belittlement on that occasion was bitter indeed, the hatred boiling within me absolute and final, branded into my heart with the permanence of that selfsame brand into the rump of a West Texas steer. The stinging face I received from that bastard Tom Adams I wore like a badge of honor.

And inside a very brief span of time, artless, unworldly, naïve Walker Building and 1-B nine- and ten-year-old boys learned and practiced with a vengeance, the art of lying, cheating and stealing, oftentimes just for the sheer hell of juvenile nonconformity. We boys learned early on that the sweetest taste in the world was-no, actually not a peanut butter and molasses sandwich, after all-but REVENGE, most assuredly a major all-capper.

My life at Oxford was punctuated by a neverending procession of provisos and caveats and, try as I might, never could I convert the Chaos that was life in this foreign, inhospitable place, into even the semblance of a Cosmos. The pain seemed permanent. But as time passed and I grew older, and gained more confidence in my abilities, I realized I was spending somewhat less time inside my homesick skull, seemed to dredge up fewer unhappy thoughts and memories, and realized at last that my "situation," though still quite serious, was not glaringly hopeless.

And somewhere along the creeping timeline of my youth, perhaps at a point where preteen segued into stripling, fortunately I became as acutely aware of my potential as I had been of my limitations, and tried my damndest to expand and further the former while not dwelling for an inordinate degree of time on the latter. By age fourteen, I could almost taste survival.

CHAPTER 62

Chicken Farming

We kids ate fried chicken at least once a week, usually at Sunday dinner. Several crates of chickens arrived on Saturday to be served the following day. Eggs were also purchased from an outside supplier, and we kids ate a *lot* of eggs. The yearly expense of chickens and eggs was greatly alleviated in 1954 with the inauguration of a poultry program, eventually supervised by Mr. Godwin Noell, whose wife at the time served as 3-B cottage counselor.

In early Spring of 1954 Arnold and I were assigned to help Mr. Davis get the poultry program started. The old two-story Industrial Building, located beside the Snug House and outhouse near the dairy, had for years been used as a storage house for grains and potatoes. This building was converted into a "brooder" house, which is a heated enclosure for raising chickens.

Late one afternoon Arnold and I were instructed to meet Mr. Davis at the old Industrial Building, that we called the Potato Barn. Presently a large truck pulled up next to the building, filled with pasteboard crates full of holes, and we heard what seemed to be the excited chirping of a million cicadas, but, on closer inspection, turned out to be the incessant chatter of one thousand cross-bred baby pullets, that we called "biddies," since that is the name by which we referred to newborn chicks and annoying, elderly house (grand)mothers.

Arnold and I followed Mr. Davis upstairs and into a high-ceilinged, huge open room, covered in wood shavings. Several new heaters had been suspended from the ceiling around the room, close enough to the floor to warm a large area.

"The orphanage has decided to produce its own eggs," Mr. Davis announced rather proudly, and added "You two boys are going to help get us started."

So now I was a chicken farmer, and I got this strange feeling that we two boys knew about as much of what we were doing as did Mr. Davis. Anyway, he instructed us in the operation of the portable heaters, and soon we had the large open room at the temperature specified by our dairy manager.

We proceeded to lug the large cartons of biddies up the stairs, and once this task had been completed, Mr. Davis knelt down and began gingerly scooping up the furry little yellow balls of life and placing them gently onto the wood shavings-covered floor. Soon the floor of the cavernous room was filled with the thousand tiny biddies, scurrying hither and yon, inspecting their new surroundings and chirping as though begging for food. And almost immediately the little buggers began crapping-all over the place.

While Arnold and I looked around us in utter wonder, Mr. Davis announced what would be our part in this grand venture. The magical word "scutwork" immediately came into my mind's view. Until the thousand biddies were mature enough to survive in the normal temperatures, explained Mr. Davis, we two (lucky) boys would work alternate nights, from 6:00 p.m. until 8:00 a.m. the following day, at which time we would assume our daily routine until the following night at 6:00 o'clock. Our job was to maintain the space heaters and feed the biddies.

"All of them?" asked Arnold.

"Why wouldn't you feed all of them?" asked Mr. Davis, somewhat puzzled by the question.

"Don't know. Just wondered, that's all," replied Arnold.

Old Arnold was a wee bit strange at times. That's why I left his last name out of our little story. Wouldn't want his younger brother Robert to suffer any undue embarrassment. Anyway, on with our story. (But I still wonder why Arnold asked that question.)

Mr. Davis asked Arnold and me which of us wanted to take "biddie duty" the first night. I looked at Arnold, who immediately looked through the brick wall to a distance some three miles away, so Mr. Davis and I made eye contact (dammit) and I took by default "biddie duty" the first night.

The dry heat from the space heaters played havoc with my head and nasal passages, and by the time the sun came up in the morning I had the worst head cold I've ever had in my life. It must have taken a week or two for me to breathe normal again. My job was to regulate the heaters so as to maintain a constant temperature in the large room that took up the entire second floor of the Potato Barn.

The first time I lifted my foot to take a step through the swarm of yellow balls, one of the little devils zigged when it should have zagged; I heard a muffled crunch under the sole of my heavy leather brogue, and instantly the population of tiny (live) biddies was reduced to 999. It was going to be a very long night.

The salient question of the moment: What does a fourteen-year-old boy do with a dead biddy that he has sworn an oath to protect? He quietly kicks the DB (Dead Biddy) under a space heater table and doesn't ever mention it to anyone. Another fact of life, born of the necessity of the moment, somewhat akin to pouring hungry calves' milk down the drain in the Valley of the Shadow of the Mummy.

Determined not to completely decimate the plainly imperiled pullet population before sunrise the next morning, I began shuffling through the little furry yellow balls, and when you shuffle through 999 chirping, scurrying baby chicks, you shuffle through biddy-poo, lots of it, and come next morning my brogues were covered in the smelly goo.

Careful as I was, by daylight had Mr. Davis lined up the living and counted heads, the number would have come to 995, and had he searched with due diligence (try under the space heaters) he would have found five (reasonably) flattened yellow-feathered pancakes.

Arnold had the duty the following night, and the next morning at breakfast confided in me that he had crushed three biddies underfoot. Had I had a similar experience, he wondered?

"Who, me?" I asked, feigning incredulity.

"What did you do with the dead ones?" I added curiously.

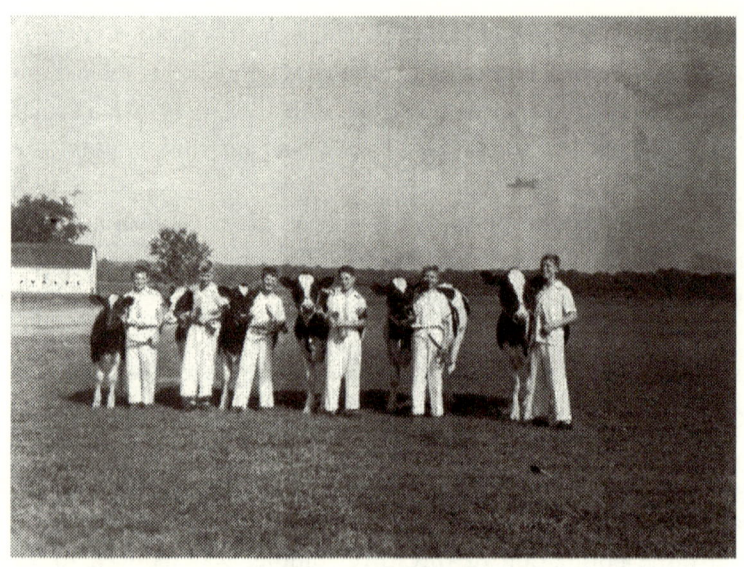

1952. Preparing calves for the State Fair. From left: Van Edwards, Butch Mitchell, Arnold Batchelor, Ray Moore, Coley Lee Hackett, and the author.

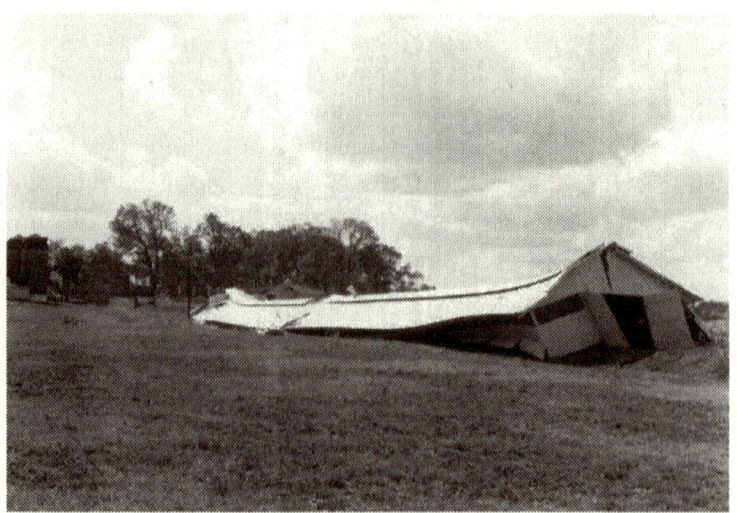

1954. The 1200-hen "laying house" constructed near the dairy in September 1954, and destroyed by hurricane Hazel a month later, on October 15, 1954.

"I saw a few dead ones under the space heaters," he said, "so I just kicked them under there." Great orphan minds think alike.

Put two club-footed fourteen-year-old kids in a large room full of a thousand biddies? What do you expect? Two things occurred on the farm and campus while Arnold and I were casually crushing chicks underfoot. The orphanage contracted to have a "laying house" constructed in a pasture near the dairy, with a capacity of twelve hundred cages. By the time this laying house was completed in early Fall 1954, Mr. Godwin Noell, who had been elected Chicken Manager (we boys immediately added the "S" word between "Chicken" and "Manager," making it either a two-word title or a three-word title), noted in the Annual Report of the Oxford Orphanage, that out of the original thousand baby pullets, "a hereditary failing took its toll, and we were able to cage 850 mature hens by early September." Hereditary failing? That club-footed little sucker, Arnold!

On October 15, 1954 Hurricane Hazel hit the area like a giant broom, and first among its casualties was the sprawling month-old laying house. Flattened it like a pancake in about thirty seconds. Mr. Adams had his farm boys crawl into the wreckage (OSHA? In North Carolina in 1954?) and the boys rescued nearly all of the hens. The laying house was completely destroyed, but within a short time another one was constructed, and before long the orphanage was producing a surplus of eggs.

The second notable farm event that took place in 1954 was the construction of an abattoir (slaughterhouse) behind the Vegetable House. It made the work of butchering hogs much easier and more sanitary, and when completed in early 1955 was fully equipped to handle slaughtered hogs, beef cows and chickens. The modern all-brick building contained large walk-in freezers and refrigerators for storage of meats. Construction of this modern abattoir allowed the orphanage to kill hogs and process the meat year-round and not just during the cold Winter months.

CHAPTER 63

Time and Unforeseen Occurrences

In 1872, halfway into that seminally humiliating and shameful chapter in Southern American history referred to by the victors as Reconstruction (1867-1877), the Oxford Orphan Asylum was established with the noble goal of providing Christian love, protection and education to literally thousands of homeless children orphaned by the ravages and excesses of the suffocating experience better known down South as the War of Northern Aggression.

Unfortunately, however, this commendable and aspiring goal became corrupted in the decade following the end of World War II by certain censurable, malevolent and perverted child abusers, to the extent that for hundreds of indigent, necessitous children who were warehoused at Oxford Orphanage during the decade 1947-1957, the orphanage, far from being a welcome haven from the disadvantages of a broken home, was de facto but another in that archipelago of prison work farms that dotted the North Carolina landscape during that era.

Time and unforeseen occurrences occasioned my accursed peer group to become trapped smack-dab in the evil clutches of the most fiendish manhandling, contemptible grownups east of the Inferno. The undisputed, glaringly disgraceful facts are noted herein.

Timing is of the utmost importance in the telling of my tale, the interval of which is the decade bookended by February 1947 and February 1957. The Reverend A. DeLeon Gray became superintendent of Oxford

Orphanage on November 25, 1946, inaugurating a period of permissive and systematic physical abuse and mental trauma against literally hundreds of defenseless, innocent children that continued unabated even after I left the orphanage in 1957.

The Bastard Abuser's appointment preceded by a mere two months my own ill-omened arrival at the foreboding Manderley known as Hicks Memorial Hospital on February 15, 1947. Fourteen months later, in early June 1948, due either to my age or my youthful incorrigibility, I was transferred in chains to Cell Block Thirteen (the infamous Walker Building), and the Warden, "Butcher" Gray, began his systematic flogging of us nine-year-old misfits that same Fall.

The sorry sonofabitch had at last found his (low)life's calling, so he quickly elevated his Satanic Abuse Hour to a weekly observance. Thus with great misgivings I became a reluctant charter member of that ill-fated beginning class of nine-year-old children to receive a thrashing by this abuser of half-pint supposed arch criminals.

And so that I might keep my Tale of Torment well-entrenched in its Count of Monte Cristo perspective, I stand on the authority commissioned to me by more than thirty similarly situated mates that Oxford Orphanage was indeed no "Boys' Town," and the counterfeit "preacher" A. DeLeon Beatumup certainly no "Father Flanagan," but was, in spades, the antithesis thereof. And more.

Our fervent hatred of this slick-skinned maize-eater was couched in the conviction of about thirty nine-year-old misfits that any "punishment" eagerly dispensed at one o'clock every Saturday afternoon was singularly disproportionate to any (real or imagined or reported) infringement of the rules either of the workplace or of social behavior.

These gross injustices foisted off on us wee ones served in great measure to heighten our acumen re more-of-the-same as we moved up from the Walker Building to 1-B and beyond.

The cycle of events through which each guileless, timid, apprehensive seven-year-old orphaned child passed during that pivotal stage in life known universally as "growing up" was illuminated at least for the interval between ages seven and fifteen by the constant daily realization that he or she was completely at the mercy of philistine, callous and uncaring grownup orphanage staff members. The one constant tangible intangible notion that pervaded our youth was that we had absolutely no control of our lives.

In reference to my decade spent cowering "inside the hedges," for some odd reason or other the portrait-like words idyllic, blissful and memorable have failed the inclusion test of my long-term memory. And as a purely practical matter, just how much mischief or laziness could a nine-year-old boy (or girl-the wee splittails fared no better than the little boys) possibly get into that would necessitate the infliction of physical brutality either as a deterrent or as a punishment?

According to the aforementioned timing, then, even boys just two years older than I, who were living in the Walker Building in 1945 and 1946, could not have suffered physical abuse by old man Gray, simply because Mr. Gray was not the superintendent of Oxford Orphanage at that time.

Anyway, at the time I began working at the dairy in June 1950, D.P. "Soapy" Peake had worked for Oxford Orphanage for thirty-eight years, most of those nearly four decades as farm manager.

During the five months between June 1950 and Mr. Peake's death on November 5, 1950, I spoke to Soapy on numerous occasions, and he was very nice to me and the other youngsters working at the dairy. Succinctly stated, none of us boys seemed to cower in fear in Soapy Peake's presence.

In January 1951 Tom Adams became farm manager, replacing the deceased Soapy Peake; just a few months later I was probably the first pitiable youngster slapped off his feet by that sick sonofabitch, and also the first mistreated boy to run from him after being struck by the sorry bastard, not necessarily in anger, but because physically and verbally assaulting small, defenseless children was part of his diabolic, heinous bent.

Again, any boys who were two years older than I, were not eleven years old when they worked for the despised Tom Adams; the main objects of his physical abuse were the hapless preteen boys. Plainly stated, Tom Adams was an evil-minded predator who should not have been allowed access to young boys. And Mr. Gray and Mr. Regan, the orphanage administrators, were fully aware of Tom Adams' quick temper and abusive nature, and these two paragons of kindness and understanding tolerated and encouraged such excesses.

Through our racing, timorous hearts almost daily ran the gamut of the emotions of misery wrought by pervasive physical abuse and/or threats of same, and the pangs of mental suffering, beginning at the moment of assault by the psychological denial that this unwarranted slap across the face, or leather belt across the butt, could be really happening.

Fast on the heels of denial and disbelief appeared the thought that certainly the abused child must have committed some serious breach of the acceptable social norm sufficiently gross that the child "deserved" the pummeling or battering. If the child at this point made the leap of logic and defiantly took umbrage at the abuse, he could "save" his sanity, and would eventually prevail over his tormentors. Thus the reason for the appearance of the names of five or six half-pint nine-year-old Walker Building recidivists on the weekly Saturday afternoon "Mr. Gray's List." Upon recognizing that our mistreatment was not deserved, our continued antisocial behavior, that manifested itself in general mouthiness and laxity in doing our "duties," was our youthful way of saying "Fuck you, buddy" to the pseudo-saint child batterer, the Reverend A. DeLeon Gray.

Every luckless, wretched preteen whose name appeared on the Summer or Fall Farm Work List posted in 1-B and 2-B trudged across the expansive baseball field to work each day in real and constant fear for his safety, and any boy who did not comply immediately to orders from the sadistic martinet Tom Adams received a lightning, vicious slap across the face.

As a direct consequence of this abuse, by far the greatest percentage of children who ran away from the orphanage and never returned, or who fortunately went home to relatives, was the group of ten-to-thirteen year old farm boys who labored in cringing fear of the despicable piece of human trash.

In order to understand the magnitude of Tom Adams' abuse and its direct and consequent effect on the number of boys who were either taken from the orphanage by relatives, or who ran away each year, approximately sixty preteen and teenage boys worked under the direct supervision and iron-fisted control of this pornographer and child batterer. Thus the pool of escapees was great indeed, and each year approximately ten more children were added to the bastard's menu. And he had help.

In June 1950 I began working at the orphanage dairy as one of the youngest dairy boys, at age eleven. A month later, on July 10, 1950, Bob Davis became dairy manager. A few weeks afterwards I became the first dairy boy to receive a whipping with the chunky dairy manager's leather belt, as "punishment" for failing to return a mother cow to her calf in the Green Barn following the previous afternoon's milking.

A simple verbal admonition was all that was called for in the situation, but Bob Davis, twenty-six years old and new on the job, chose instead to exercise his carte blanche authority given to him by Mr. Gray, to inflict at will, mean-spirited physical abuse on preteen orphan boys.

And so that we touch all the assault and battery bases, the orphanage administration, in order to supplement the teaching salary of the high school math teacher, Garland Talton, (un)affectionately referred to (behind his slick-skinned back) as "Pig" because of his uncanny facial resemblance to the funny book character Porky Pig, employed this abuser of young boys as a "straw boss" during the Summer months, working for Tom Adams supervising the younger farm boys.

Taking his cue from Tom Adams, and with the blanket authority from Adams, Gray and Regan, this piece of porcine trash use his ubiquitous five-foot-long tobacco stick instead of his open hand, to inflict abuse on any small, defenseless, frightened farm boy who wandered into his radius. Certainly a study of the attributes of human morals, behavior and character would not include Pig Talton, Bob Davis, Tom Adams, Regan and A. DeLeon Gray as examples. I was physically assaulted by each of these men, as were literally dozens of other children during my stay at Oxford.

So how does this crucial timing relate to our story, and to the direction my life took at age thirteen? And how does this timetable relate to the fact that more of the orphans in my age group managed to escape the abuse and degradation, either by running away or being taken by their parents or relatives, than graduated?

As of December 1948 Mr. Gray had been superintendent of Oxford Orphanage for exactly two years, and had been battering Walker Building boys for several months. This phony preacher's abusive conduct had just as much a deleterious effect on those boys who escaped his board as it did on those among us who routinely received such physical abuse.

Now the Oxford Orphanage administration, following numerous visits to the homes of these thirty Walker Building boys by the case worker, Miss Eunice Broadwell, had determined that the environment in which these boys lived was detrimental to their welfare, and consequently, the health and well-being of these unfortunate children would be best served by admitting them to the "care and protection" of Oxford Orphanage.

Of the thirty-two boys living in the Walker Building with me in 1948 and 1949, eighteen left the orphanage prior to graduation from high school. Only fourteen of the thirty-two graduated. Thus fifty-five percent of these needy youngsters left Oxford Orphanage before graduation from high school, to return to the same conditions from whence they were "rescued."

Some boys in the aforementioned group survived the ongoing, pervasive mistreatment and made it into high school before leaving the orphanage. The following children (boys and girls) entered ninth grade in August 1953, but did not graduate from John Nichols High School. All of the boys in this group lived in 4-B when Mr. Regan began his weekly beatings of these preteens and teenagers in 1952. The thirteen children who left the orphanage prior to graduation are Jimmy Frederick, Carl Holt, Alton Provost, Terry Johnson, Butch Mitchell, Ernest Perry, Ersul Sowers, John Williamson, Barbara Walton, Betty Jean Truitt, Joan Walsh, Iris Sheffield and Nancy Nethercutt.

Now, twenty-nine students started ninth grade in August 1953, and only sixteen graduated in May 1957. Thus in three years or so, again we lost forty-five percent of our class.

My earlier statement that the girls fared no better than the boys as relates to physical abuse and mental trauma is supported by the fact that of the thirteen high school students in my class who left the orphanage during the three-year period 1954-1957, five of these were girls. Based on the reasons for these children being admitted to Oxford Orphanage, twenty-nine of us should have graduated in May 1957. However, only sixteen went the distance and survived the abuses. And these statistics are typical for nearly every class of students during the decade I lived at Oxford.

The year 1955 was a representative period, and my sister was in that graduating class. I turned sixteen in April that year, and finished tenth grade a few weeks later. At the end of the year there were 320 children in the orphanage. Seventeen seniors graduated high school in 1955. However, somewhat more than half that number, or eleven children, ran away from the orphanage and did not return. Twenty-one children, four more than the number who graduated, were returned to relatives during the year.

These clearly undisputed and glaringly accusatory statistics represent an honorable and benevolent cause subverted and routinely corrupted by heinous criminals unleashed to prey on innocent, defenseless orphaned children. These abuses suffered by literally hundreds of disadvantaged children allowed by the State of North Carolina during the decade between 1947 and 1957 to be placed under the supposed "protection and care" of the evil administrators of Oxford Orphanage, were ongoing, pervasive and criminal by any legal standard.

In the United States and particularly the South, statutes defining and providing punishment for child abuse and cruelty to children have been met with continuing and disheartening stone walls. In North Carolina at mid-twentieth century likely these criminals sought to defend against outrageous acts of violence toward children by taking refuge in the nebulous concept of necessary corrective discipline.

Today all states have laws that punish one standing in loco parentis to a child, i.e., one supervising the welfare of, or having immediate charge or custody of a minor, who maliciously causes a minor (a child under eighteen years of age) cruel or excessive physical or mental pain. Cruelty to children statutes are designed to protect those who, because of their physical immaturity, are unable to protect themselves from the cruelty of older people, the hated and despised "biguns."

In all states, cruelty to children is a felony, often punishable by imprisonment for not less than one nor more than twenty years. Judged by these standards, the outrageous and malicious beatings by Mr. Regan, Mr. Gray, Tom Adams, Mr. Talton, Mr. Davis and a parade of cottage counselors, teachers and work supervisors at Oxford Orphanage during the decade 1947-1957, were guilty of countless acts of criminal assault, and thus would be classified under the law as criminals.

During my decade at Oxford Orphanage I personally witnessed and received numerous physical assaults by uncontrolled work supervisors, cottage counselors and teachers that included slapping across the face, punching with fists, kicking, beating across the butt, legs and back with wooden slats, leather belts and even a tobacco stick.

Preteen and teenage boys who attempted to escape this inhumane treatment were brutally beaten or slapped, often suffering the additional humiliation of having their heads shaved by the bastard child abuser E.T. Regan. One could spot immediately in a crowd of preteen or teenage boys who among them had recently run away, had been caught, and subsequently returned to the clutches of the turnkey.

It is important to review two seminal events previously discussed, and the effect of these occurrences on the statistics found in the Annual Reports of the Oxford Orphanage. Tom Adams arrived at Oxford in January 1951, and immediately began his indiscriminate physical abuse of sixty preteen boys, nearly every one of whom fell under the cruel bastard's absolute control. And late that same year Miss Mary Faison replaced Lynwood Halliburton as cottage mother of twenty-five preteen and teenage boys in 4-B.

And the following year, 1952, Mr. Regan began his systematic beatings of preteen and teenage boys in 4-B. Glaringly absent from the Oxford Orphanage Annual Reports for the years 1951, 1952, 1953, and 1954 is the number of students who ran away and did not return. This statistic was resumed in 1955, when eleven students slipped away after lights-out to return to relatives or make their own way in the world. Many of these boys who ran away simply never were heard from again.

The number of students who ran away each year represents those students who escaped the constant abuse and did not return. This figure does not include the approximately twenty boys and girls who ran away and were returned by relatives or picked up and returned by Mr. Gray or Mr. Regan after receiving sightings of escapees from police or well-intentioned citizens.

Of the statistics actually reported, the number of students who ran away and did not return was greater in 1950 (before the four-year omission) and 1955 (after the four-year omission). It can certainly be well-argued that the reason for the omission of this telling statistic for those four years was that to include such elevated figures would certainly have raised a red flag among at least a few of the Masons who actually read the Annual Reports of Oxford Orphanage.

These shocking figures represent the shameful truth that for the eleven-year period 1947-1957, only in the years 1948 and 1949 was the number of students graduating greater than the sum of the number of children who returned to relatives and who ran away and did not return. And during this eleven-year period, these two vainglorious administrators, Regan and Gray, relished in absolute and total control over more than three hundred children from broken homes.

Year	Returned to Relatives	Ran Away and Did Not Return	Total	No. Who Graduated
1947	19	5	24	22
*1948	16	4	20	22
*1949	7	3	10	26
1950	14	6	20	18
1951	13	x-9	(22)	21
1952	18	x-9	(27)	19
1953	20	x-9	(29)	20
1954	18	x-9	(27)	20
1955	21	11	32	17
1956	21	5	26	15
1957	33	3	36	16

For the years 1947, 1948 and 1949, both the number of students who were returned to relatives and who ran away and did not return declined each year, followed by a sharp increase in both these categories beginning with the aforementioned Reign of Terror of Bob Davis, Tom Adams and E.T. Regan in 1950, 1951 and 1952. Note also that the figures for both "returned to relatives" and "ran away and did not return" exactly doubled from 1949 to 1950.

In an effort to be generously fair, if we average the number of children who ran away and did not return for 1950 (6) and 1955 (11), give this average of nine per year, and add these nine each year for 1951-1954, to the number of students returned to relatives, we get the following.

Year	Returned to Relatives		Ran Away		Total Ran Away and Returned to Relatives	No. Students Graduating
1951	13	+	9	=	22	21
1952	18	+	9	=	27	19
1953	20	+	9	=	29	20
1954	18	+	9	=	27	20

In order to better understand these statistics, the column "Ran Away" means the number of students who ran away and did not return, and is a small figure compared to the number of students who vaulted the hedges in the middle of the night and either were returned by relatives, nabbed by police, or were observed by other persons who reported these on-the-lam orphans to Mr. Gray or Mr. Regan. Based on my own personal knowledge, an average of fifteen to twenty students ran away each year who were later returned, and nearly every one of these students who returned were greeted with a beating. Many students ran away several times and were caught and returned before finally making it to freedom.

The import of these figures is that two out of every five children whom the orphanage administration, only after careful and extensive investigation, had determined could not obtain adequate care in the environment from which they came, chose to return to this substandard setting, and relatives of these needy children chose to accept them back to live in these inadequate conditions, rather than remain under the so-called "care" of ignorant, uncaring and abusive teachers, staff workers and top administrators of Oxford Orphanage.

By what moral authority did the superintendent of Oxford Orphanage line up five or six nine-year-old children each Saturday afternoon, order these frightened boys to "bend over and grab your ankles," and proceed to beat them with a wooden board? Was there not some other way to discipline these young children than physically abusing them?

By what moral authority did the assistant superintendent of Oxford Orphanage order a thirteen-year-old boy to bend over the back of a chair, force the boy's head down by grabbing his neck, and then strike the boy sixty-one times on his back, butt and legs with a wooden board? This was not discipline. This was a criminal act of senseless brutality.

The foregoing statistics reverberate with a starkly cacophonous truth. Needy children do not seek to escape from love, affection and charity. Likewise, these same children will seek to flee abuse and fear occasioned by mean, contemptible and despicable adults.

Each year copies of the Oxford Orphanage Annual Report were distributed to each Masonic Lodge in North Carolina, to literally thousands of Masons. Yet not once during my ten years at Oxford Orphanage did any Mason ever look at the alarming number of students who ran away and never returned, and who were returned to relatives each year, and question students as to the reason for these children leaving. Each year the figures were there in front of them, the telltale signs of rampant abuse, of a system gone haywire; yet nobody picked up on it.

It was as though the orphanage administration, in order to maintain ironfisted discipline on North Carolina's warehoused unfortunates, had preached to the staff the admonition of Adolf Menjou's character in the picture show *Paths of Glory* that "the only way to maintain discipline is to shoot a man now and then."

Yet even during my oftentimes intellectually benighted youth I was determined to successfully negotiate this perilous minefield of grownup low lifes, muggers and maulers, and by sheer pluck, guts, intrepidity and youthful savvy, survive this hailstorm of perverse and pervasive adolescent human abuse and misery called Oxford Orphanage.

I learned early on, in the Baby Cottage and Walker Building, about making decisions. Left turns, right turns and detours in my young life were the result of my unconscious responses to those who (thought they) controlled my life. The salient, perhaps seminal difference in our lives then, is who makes the crucial judgments affecting our immediate (and at times not so immediate) future, ourselves or others?

Eventually my fear of mistreatment, and of arbitrary and capricious conduct on the part of those charged with my care, brought me to a critical juncture in my life. My general dismay and misgivings, accumulated in the few short years since my arrival at the orphanage, were tempered not only by the physical ill-treatment and bullying administered to me by those grownups to whom the Masonic Order of North Carolina had entrusted my care, but equally as much by the reprehensible and totally unwarranted mental abuse and physical mistreatment, dispensed quite indiscriminately and often, upon the vulnerable and fragile psyche of other boys and girls, orphans whom I came to accept as my brothers and sisters.

For seven wonderful years I had enjoyed the love and security of responsible parents. Abruptly taken from this protective environment, through no fault of my own, and shunted into the hands of oftentimes petty, captious and implacable grownups, was a traumatic and dehumanizing ordeal for me and for quite literally hundreds of defenseless children under the same or quite similar circumstances during my ten years at Oxford Orphanage.

Even as a young boy I observed three distinctly basic reactions of my peers to physical abuse, whether it be a slap across the face or a leather belt or wooden board across the back, butt or legs. Corporal punishment of adolescent and teenage children, though dispensed liberally, was never "justified." Children were physically punished (read as "slapped" or "beaten") for two reasons.

First, the small boy or girl had done something "wrong" in the eyes of the cottage counselor, teacher or work supervisor, that in the opinion of that grownup warranted physical mistreatment and brutality.

Second, inflicting a beating on a child, usually in the presence of other children, served as a certain deterrent, oftentimes announced as such, to the child's classmates, cottagemates or workmates, that they could expect a similar thrashing if they got "out of line," or if they committed the same or similar infraction of the rules as did the hapless victim of the instant assault.

Such callous and universally impenitent conduct by insensitive and unbridled counselors, teachers and supervisors was fostered and encouraged by the fact that we orphans had no recourse or appeal from this pattern of ongoing abuse. Though overlapping to some degree, the above-mentioned two basic reactions to beatings and abuses of children by orphanage staff members and teachers fell loosely into the following categories.

1. Resigned acceptance. Some young children, faced with the threat of physical harm from uncontrolled and vindictive grownups, simply withdrew, as a result of ongoing fear for their safety. These unfortunate girls and boys tended to become outwardly timid and diffident, quite often keeping to themselves, while developing few if any lasting friendships among their peers.

   Many of these children had suffered traumatic experiences prior to arriving at the orphanage, and, more often than not, had no siblings at the orphanage to whom they could turn for comfort and support.

   These emotionally-scarred, introverted and intimidated children remained this way throughout their years at the orphanage, were unusually quiet, and developed friendships usually with their own kind. Following eight to ten years of suffering, in all likelihood these children became timid, insecure adults. I empathized with these boys and girls as my peers, while growing up, and only pray that as adults they have somehow put their unhappy childhood behind them and found happiness. Many did not.

2. Defiant indignation. This second distinctly separate group of children, often at an early age, reacted to this undeserved and unprincipled physical and mental abuse with righteous anger and open resentment. Without truly understanding their emotions, these children were incensed and insulted by the flagrant injustice of being subjected to the crass humiliation of such physical and mental trauma. These were children who never cried out when being whipped or slapped, regardless of the severity of the punishment. Their shame at being traumatized in front of their friends only served to push to the forefront their rebellious indignation.

   This group of children appeared to possess a good self-image, and refused to be shamed into submission. Punishment of these defiant children served only to further enhance their resentment against unprincipled and unbridled authority. Children in this group tended to have enjoyed some semblance of a stable home life prior to the occurrence of circumstances that caused them to be sent to the orphanage.

These boys and girls recognized the gross unfairness of their mistreatment, and as they progressed into their teenage years developed an open resentment against those in authority at the orphanage. Children in this group tended to "talk back" to cottage counselors and teachers, take chances of getting caught, and if caught and punished, took the punishment in stride and continued their defiant ways. These children tended to carry this confidence with them when they left the orphanage, and to be successful in life.

3. Escape. This third category of responses to unwarranted manhandling and abuse by some members of the orphanage staff includes those children whose reaction to such untenable situations was to run away as fast and as often as it took to accomplish their goal of escaping the continuing mental and physical trauma of cruel and heartless grownups.

This group of children also includes those whose parent or other relative took them from the orphanage rather than have the child subjected to continual mistreatment. Many of these children fared well after leaving the orphanage, completed high school and college, and otherwise led productive lives.

On the other hand, some of these children were forced by cruelty of uncaring and abusive orphanage staff members to escape to the very dehumanizing family situation that caused them to be admitted to the orphanage in the first place. This latter group comprises the greatest travesty among the three general classes discussed herein.

I found Oxford Orphanage to be a curious contradiction, a singular incongruity, a unique and puzzling study in contrasts. The charming serenity of the beautiful, sprawling campus, the towering, majestic, almost humbling hundred-year-old oaks, the imposing Victorian Main Building with its surrounding elaborate white painted porches, and the placid, rolling hills of grain and farm produce, are part of a mosaic the likes of which are without parallel in my life.

However, the timeless beauty and welcoming tranquility of these four hundred acres, that was my home for ten long years, can never be reconciled, nor harmonized, nor justified nor explained by the traumatic psychological scarring experienced by nearly every timid, frightened and vulnerable child who entered with much foreboding the imposing Main Gate during those ten years. Just as thousands of children before and after me, I left a part of my young soul at Oxford Orphanage, never to be recovered during my lifetime.

The search for this part of a lost heart drives many who graduated, who ran away from the abuse, or who were returned to relatives, back in hopes they will yet find some part of their life, their youth, left behind. This sense of an unsalvageable adolescence is also what prevents many from ever returning.

By age fourteen I had developed an anarchic attitude re those charged with the responsibility of my welfare. I had fallen backwards through the proverbial Looking Glass, tumbling head over heels into an anfractuous, mysteriously animus-saturated childhood.

CHAPTER 64

The Crossroads of My Life

The opening of the heavy wooden front door of 4-B cottage begat a profound and ominous stillness that swept the night's study hall like a fast-rolling North Carolina coastal fog.

The palms of sixty teenage hands began to ooze sweat, sixty musty teenage armpits segued into clammy dampness, and the rates of thirty organs of circulation increased dramatically, in direct proportion to the mortifying fear occasioned by the dramatic intrusion into our lives by the universally despised and at the same time feared E.T. Regan.

The singular emotion engendered by the creak of that ageless wooden front door was fear, pure, unadulterated dread of grievous bodily harm and its certain accompanying pitiable humiliation. A time for long-practiced servile groveling for some of the 4-B unfortunates; a time for demonstrating rebellious scorn and truculent contempt from others of us.

Every teenager who lived in 4-B in 1953 knew this same fear, a fear as real as life itself. We will never forget the experience. Nor will we ever forgive the brutality.

Just as in the cases of Mr. Gray and Tom Adams, timing means everything. In 1950 Lynwood H. Halliburton became the cottage counselor of 4-B, replacing Eddie Harding. These men were capable of handling the discipline of thirty raucous teenage boys without assistance from Mr. Regan or Mr. Gray. However, sometime in 1952 Lynwood

Halliburton was fired, and Miss Mary Faison became the cottage "grand"mother of 4-B.

I moved up to 4-B in June 1952. I had just turned thirteen, and entered eighth grade that Fall. Mary Faison was one of those dodgy old spinsters who was completely out of her element in trying to supervise thirty, eighth and ninth grade boys, nearly all of whom since the arrival of the despised Tom Adams in January 1951, had suffered physical abuse and threats of same from the reviled and feared farm manager. Out of earshot, almost from the beginning of his time as farm supervisor, even the youngest boys referred to this former training school sadist as "that sorry bastard."

It has been said by one who professes to expertise in such matters, that the "present" lasts from six to twelve seconds, and that everything prior to that miniscule blink of time is the "past," and is stored somewhere in our memory. Perhaps.

Yet still it appears to me in a very broad sense that somewhere along the arduous path of life there exists a merging of my past with my present, where the former folds into and becomes part of the latter. Upon arriving at that critical point, my life, inclusive in which are my morals, ethics, character and the general perception of "self," became indelibly molded into what they forever would become.

This pivotal moment in my life, the experience in which the above-mentioned elements of psyche fused together to form the person I have remained for half a century, occurred in early Spring 1953.

At age thirteen I was in the eighth grade and well into my third year working at the dairy. I had experienced a growth spurt during these three years, so I had suddenly become taller than most of the dairy boys my age.

I had been moved up from 2-B to 4-B, where we bunked three or four to a room, depending on the size of the room. Because the dairy boys arose at 4:00 a.m., to trudge off to the dairy to milk the cows, in order not to disturb the other boys, we dairy boys bunked together in two of the rooms. Thus I ended up sharing a room with the older boys.

It was a change from being a big fish in a little pond (2-B) to becoming a little fish in a big pond (4-B), a momentary but universal experience that occurred every time a boy moved to a higher cottage, from the Baby Cottage up to and including 3-B. Same for the girls, from the Baby Cottage up to and including 4-G.

It was about that time in my complicated young life that I began to piece together the mysterious and wondrous relationship between the visual image of the curve and bounce of the high school girls' behinds and the simultaneous twinge in my groin. Cause and effect and Pavlov's dog all rolled into one confusing and inexplicable mess.

It was as though an entirely new phase in my life had opened before me. Sex. What a mystery! Jennie Mae was in my class, and all of a sudden we boys didn't have to follow the high school girls around. We had our own. The curve of Jennie Mae's ass was itself a fascinating work of art, and we seventh and eighth grade boys followed behind her in the hallways of John Nichols School, going from one class to the next, stepping all over one another in the process.

The natural consequence of this aforementioned hormonal awakening was that I arose each morning with a hard on, kept a hard on the entire day.

And had I not already discovered the wonders of jacking off, and after serious and concentrated effort, polished and refined the act to an art form, I would have fallen asleep each night with a hard on.

Of course, thirteen-year-old boys are so stupid that each thinks he is the only one possessed with the insight to have made this remarkable discovery. I was no different, and assumed naturally that the other boys my age would be at least thirty-five years old before they made the mysterious connection I had made. It was *my* secret, and I swore on a stack of funny books that I would not divulge it. Let my peers suffer in their ignorance.

Thus each night when the dormitory lights went out, I tried my damndest to grow a larger penis. At the rate I worked at it, I figured that by age fifteen I should hold some sort of world's record.

During this period, Miss Mary Faison was the 4-B cottage counselor. A good part of the time this eccentric old biddy was a few cards shy of a full deck. However, on those rare occasions in which she exhibited some lucid behavior, she was a vindictive, paranoid, despicable bitch who took delight in complaining to Mr. Regan that such-and-such boy had sassed or disobeyed her.

The boys' campus was well aware of Miss Faison's vengeful nature, and it was with this real fear of an unwarranted beating at the hands of Mr. Regan that I entered 4-B.

Mr. Regan's "visits," that literally struck terror in the hearts of us thirteen- and fourteen-year-old boys, went somewhat as follows:

About once each week, always during study hall, that lasted from seven until nine in the evening, the front door of the cottage would open, the Crotchety Old Bat would leave her seat she occupied while supervising study hall, and she and Mr. Regan would go into the small living room of her apartment. Mr. Regan did not come to visit. His sole reason for coming to 4-B at that time of night was to use his board to beat the hell out of any blameless orphan who had the misfortune of incurring the displeasure of Miss Faison. Thirty hearts would begin to race wildly, underarms and palms of hands would begin to sweat with fear, until some poor innocent child's name would be called out from the vindictive old bat's room.

Once a frightened child's name had been called, there was no recourse, there were no extenuating circumstances, there was no chance given for explanation or rebuttal of the cottage bitch's wild and false accusations. Nor were there alternative punishments considered. The helpless child knew that once his name had been called from inside the torture room, he was about to receive a beating.

No, this was the opportunity for a vicious, mean-spirited grownup possessed with unbridled authority, to vent those pressures and disappointments of his own personal life upon innocent and defenseless children. Brutal beatings administered to children, which in today's world would land him in prison for assault and cruelty to children, were in the orphanage in the 1940's and early 1950's accepted as a fact of life.

Charged by the State of North Carolina and the Masonic Order of North Carolina with the care and protection of orphaned children, this perverse, cowardly excuse for a human being chose instead to humiliate and brutalize these frightened and vulnerable young boys and girls.

Children called before Mr. Regan were accused, given no opportunity to defend themselves, then ordered to "bend over," and the beating would begin. Usually the frightened child would cry out in pain with the first blow; others, out of sheer defiance, held out as long as they could. The loud slap of the wooden board against the child's butt, legs or back could be (and was meant by the sorry bastard to be) heard by the other frightened boys assembled in the study hall, who softly counted aloud each blow, all the while fearing that their name would be the next called.

Following the beating, the crying child would be admonished that his (falsely accused) unacceptable conduct would not be tolerated, and the poor child, embarrassed, his eyes filled with tears, would take his seat in study hall.

Usually at least two unfortunate boys were brutalized and humiliated on each of Regan's "visits," and he was without doubt the most feared and despised common bastard on campus. The usual number of blows of the wooden board administered to a child was between ten and twenty, but more severe beatings were not uncommon. And Miss Faison relished clearly her role of accuser-without-justification. She gleefully stood no more than a few feet from Mr. Regan as he, also with great delight, commenced and continued his battering of the hapless child.

One night during study hall, Miss Faison brought a folded bedsheet into the room, got our attention, then unfolded the bedsheet and held it up in front of her. In the light we all could clearly see the sperm stains on the sheet, and there were a *lot* of sperm stains! Damn, I thought, maybe I wasn't the only kid to have discovered *the secret* after all!

Some of the guys started snickering and pointing to the sheet.

"Mrs. Minor (supervisor of the laundry room) told me to tell you boys to stop staining these sheets," Miss Faison's shrill, high-pitched voice admonished, gazing around the room as if she expected some dumbass kid like Blockhead or Coley Lee to raise his hand, stand up before God and everybody and say "I did it. It was me."

What the kids were pointing at and laughing was an especially large sperm stain in the center of the bedsheet. I mean, it was *really big*! It appeared as though one of the dairy bulls had jacked off on the sheet. And one of the boys sitting at my study hall table said as much, out loud, at which time the thirty kids present burst out laughing. And of course I laughed along with them.

Visibly upset, Miss Faison hurriedly rolled up her multiple-stained jack-off sheet and stalked out of the room, muttering under her breath.

During study hall the following night, the quiet was broken by that ominous sound of the front door opening, and as if on cue, everyone became real quiet. Miss Faison left her seat and walked into her living room across the hall. Presently the door to her room opened, and at the very young and innocent age of thirteen, my life changed forever.

"Alton Provost!" the old biddy's shrill voice boomed out, and twenty-nine pairs of frightened eyes turned toward me. I swallowed hard, my throat became dry and my vision blurred. I didn't move. I had done nothing wrong. Why was she calling my name?

There passed a seemingly eternal moment, frozen in time. Stark fear gripped me as though locking my body in a vise. I had difficulty breathing, and I could feel my heart thumping erratically in my chest.

"Alton Provost!"

This time the odious, aggravated tone of Mr. Regan carried throughout the house. Damn! In a dazed, surrealistic trance, I arose from my seat, crossed the room into the hallway, whereupon I looked across the hallway into Miss Faison's room.

There he stood, like Cerberus, the Hound of Hell, wooden board in hand, his face reddened with anger. And standing there beside him, shoulder-to-shoulder, was Miss Faison, the derisive look on her face announcing that this was vindictive payback time, and she was going to relish the moment.

"Miss Faison tells me you've been sassing her."

It wasn't a question, it was a bald accusation. But I answered nonetheless. Looking at the floor in front of me, I said,

"No, sir, I haven't been sassing her."

"Yes you have, young man," screeched the old witch, in her best practiced, polished accusatory tone.

"Boy, you've got a bad attitude," boomed this supposed protector of orphaned children.

"And I'm going to break you of that attitude right now. Bend over and face that door!"

I had lived at Oxford Orphanage for six years, and during this time I had been conditioned, as had literally hundreds of unfortunate children before my time, to accept physical assault and mental abuse as a fact of life. During this time I had never witnessed, nor had I ever heard of, any child who openly resisted this inhumane treatment at the hands of Mr. Regan, Mr. Gray or others.

Thus, fearing for my physical safety, but knowing I had no safe and viable alternative, I dutifully bent my body at the waist, closed my eyes tightly and awaited the bastard's brutality.

And the blows rained down, with a force whose purpose could only have been a practiced, orderly release of contempt, vindictiveness and malice. I refused to cry out, not wanting to give this cruel, sadistic bastard the satisfaction he so desired.

He started on my butt, but within a short time began striking the backs of my legs and my lower back. Suddenly I panicked, realizing he was never going to stop beating me, and I tried to raise my upper body. He quickly grabbed the back of my neck with his left hand, pushing me down, and yelled

"I'll tell you when to get up, boy!" and continued to hold me down with his left hand while battering me with his board.

At some point I must have feared not for my safety but for my very life, that what was happening to me was so undeniably wrong, that no adult had the right, whatever the circumstances, to batter and abuse young children in this manner. Without giving my actions any conscious thought, I suddenly threw my entire weight against the bastard, catching him off balance and knocking him against Miss Faison.

Mr. Regan ended up sitting in Miss Faison's chair, she lay sprawled against the wall from him pushing her, and the board lay harmlessly on the floor between us. He and I both looked first at the board, then at each other. Neither of us moved toward the board, though it was closer to me than to him.

The look on Mr. Regan's face could best be described as utter disbelief and shock. He started to get up, but instinctively I grabbed the board off the floor and raised it above my head. He just sat in the chair onto which he had landed, in shock, staring apoplectically at me holding tightly in my grip, hand raised, his instrument of hate that had suddenly become *my* instrument of vindication and revenge.

The venomous old bat cowered speechlessly behind the chair, her eyes open wide in sheer terror. For a brief moment, none of us moved. None of us said a word. It was as though we were in a play, and all the actors had suddenly forgotten their lines. I remember that even in the heat of the angered moment, I noticed how heavy was the board I held.

He did not move. Neither did she. Through blinding tears filled with vengeance and sheer hatred, I said, looking him squarely in the face,

"*You* are never going to touch me again. If *you* ever touch me again, I'll kill you!"

And at the moment I meant exactly what I said. And he knew it.

I turned to leave, but just as I reached the door, realized I still gripped tightly the handle of his board. I turned, flung the board underhanded against the wall just above his flinching head, walked slowly and deliberately out the door of Miss Faison's room, out the back door and down the concrete steps to the ground behind 4-B.

I quickly stepped under the back porch, grabbed one of the loose baseball bats, and walked about twenty yards from the rear of the cottage, trembling with fear and hatred, tears streaming down my face, clutching the baseball bat, repeating aloud in a low voice now filled with resolve and hate,

"Come on, you sorry bastard. Come on, you sorry bastard. Come on, you sorry bastard."

Presently I heard the front door of the cottage open and close, and Mr. Regan appeared, board in hand, walking from 4-B toward his house about seventy yards away. He stopped abruptly when he saw me in the light from the back porch of the cottage. I raised the baseball bat to my shoulder and said two words that to this day still warm my heart. My life had reached its turning point. I said clearly and firmly, making sure he heard me,

"Come on."

He paused for a brief moment. Then, wisely for him, he chose to continue walking toward his house. I stood alone behind the cottage until study hall was over, and out of interest and excitement, the other boys found me. They informed me they had counted sixty-one blows prior to hearing the rumble and my voice coming from Miss Faison's room.

My butt burned, the backs of my legs hurt, and my lower back felt bruised when I breathed. I felt as though my spine had been damaged. And I knew I couldn't stay any longer at the orphanage.

I walked across the campus to 4-G, knocked on the back door, and asked one of the girls to get Eoline for me. I briefly told my sister what had occurred, and told her I was leaving that night. I said goodbye to her, and walked back to 4-B, still holding onto my trusty Louisville Slugger.

I was getting a few belongings together, when Bobby Boyette and Javon Frye came into the basement. Eoline had contacted them in 3-B, and had asked them to find out what had occurred. But after I explained to Bobby and Javon that the son of a bitch had hit me sixty-one times with a board, and that I had pushed him across the room, they did not try to talk me out of leaving. They knew. They had been there before, and understood. I did not have any money, so Bobby gave me ten dollars, and I started walking north on the highway toward Virginia, a thirteen-year-old orphan kid running away from brutality.

At that time Bill, Kenny, Doc and J.B. all lived in the Washington, D.C. area. By that time all of my older brothers were married, and Bill, Kenny and J.B. had children. I hitchhiked through the night and the following day, arriving in Washington, D.C. at around midnight.

I contacted Kenny. He came down to the bus station and picked me up, and that night I stayed with Kenny and his family. The following day Doc picked me up. After I had explained everything to Doc, he had me take off my clothes and show him my backside. He immediately took me to a friend of his, a commercial photographer, who took a series of pictures of my backside. Doc had several eight-by-ten glossies made, and we sat down at his supper table and spread them out before us. The pictures appeared as though some sadistic bastard had hit a thirteen-year-old kid with a board about sixty-one times. The bruises went from nearly my knees to about halfway up my back. I looked downright awful.

We were alone in Doc's home. His lovely wife Alystine was still at work. I thought we would try to work out my situation. Doc became very quiet. Finally he spoke in a low voice, almost a whisper.

"Son, I'm sorry about daddy. I really am."

I looked across the small supper table into my older brother's eyes, suddenly brimming with tears.

"You don't have to explain anything to me, Doc. I know you loved my daddy. We all loved him. We don't have to talk about it."

"Okay, son, I just wanted you to know. If I hadn't done what I did, you wouldn't be going through this now."

"I understand, Doc. Just help me figure out where to go from here. I told the bastard I'd kill him if he ever touched me again."

"I know, son. I would have done the same thing."

"But I can't be a burden to my brothers, and I can't be a burden to mama. So what can we do?"

So, for several hours, long past the time Alystine had fixed us supper and gone to bed, my older brother and I sat at that supper table, planning and discussing and drinking black coffee and smoking Camels. The final plan went something like this.

Doc had ordered several sets of eight-by-ten photographs made of the results of Regan's backside artwork. Doc would keep two copies at his home, and put two copies in separate manila envelopes. Doc called them "gifts."

The following day I sat at the supper table while my brother telephoned Mr. Gray. All Doc told Mr. Gray was that he had me at his home in Washington, D.C., and that he would be bringing me back to the orphanage the following Saturday at 2:00 p.m.

The "conversation" was one-sided and to the point. Doc didn't "ask" Mr. Gray anything; rather, he told Mr. Gray what he was going to do. Then Doc cradled the telephone, looked across the table at me, smiled broadly and said, "Okay, son, that takes care of that. Now let's go fishing."

My brother and I spent the next three days fishing in the Atlantic off the coast of Morehead City, North Carolina, where Alystine's aging mother lived. We had a good time.

Early that Saturday morning we started out for Oxford. On the road, Doc explained it this way. If anybody ("I don't care who he is.") so much as touches me or takes any kind of reprisal against me in any way, "I'll see he goes to prison for what he did to you. You see, I have the proof, and every boy in your cottage is a witness." True.

I did not have to return to the orphanage. I could have stayed with Doc and Alystine and completed high school. But even at the young age of thirteen I refused to make my problems their problems. And I had resolved the direction my life would take. I had made this decision while walking north along the highway through Virginia, that I would never again run away from anybody or anything. Call it maturity. Or determination. Or resolve. Perhaps it was just plain old stoicism, in my case the indifference being to any attempt others may make to control my life.

At the appointed time on Saturday, Doc and I walked into the Business Office, and I pointed out Mr. Gray's office, the door of which was open. Motioning to a chair in the hallway, Doc said,

"Just wait here, son. This will only take a minute."

And that's about all the time it took. Doc walked into Mr. Gray's office carrying a manila envelope containing the photographs, and closed the door behind him.

"Keep your seat, sir, please," began Doc in a pleasant tone.

"I just want to show you a few photographs, and I'll be on my way."

I could hear Doc spreading the photographs out on Mr. Gray's large desk in front of Mr. Gray, who had yet to speak a word.

"What you see here, sir," began Doc in the same pleasant voice, "is the backside and legs of my younger brother. How would you feel if these were pictures of *your* younger brother?" It was a rhetorical question, of course. Doc did not expect an answer. Mr. Gray just sat there in silence, staring at the bastard Regan's handiwork.

After a long pause, undoubtedly for effect, Doc continued,

"Sir, you are the superintendent at this orphanage. I'm going to leave my younger brother here, under *your* personal care. I am notifying you here and now, that if any harm of any kind ever comes to my brother, I am going to hold *you* personally responsible." That disarming "pleasant" had segued into stern resolve. Still Mr. Gray did not respond.

After another pause, in which my brother was perfecting his "for effect" routine, Doc continued in a slow, even tone,

"Sir, you can have this copy of these pictures. I have several copies plus the negatives. I'm going to take my brother on down to his cottage. If I don't hear from my brother, you'll never hear from me again."

I heard Mr. Gray's heavy, high-back, brown leather chair push back, Mr. Gray stood and uttered his only sentence of the entire "conversation."

"You have my word, Mr. Provost, that this will never happen again."

Doc replied, his voice returning to "pleasant" mode once more,

"Thank you for your time, sir," and walked out of Mr. Gray's office, minus the manila envelope he had carried in with him.

"One last item, son, and I'll be on my way," Doc said as we got into his car. "Where does the son of a bitch live?"

I directed my brother to Regan's house, located at the front edge of the campus fronting College Street. The dirt and gravel campus road ran alongside the rear of Regan's house, and Doc stopped his car and turned off the engine. Reaching into the back seat, Doc retrieved a manila envelope identical to the one he had just given to Mr. Gray.

Without comment, Doc crossed Regan's back yard, climbed the steps and knocked sharply on the back door. Mrs. Regan appeared in the doorway, then disappeared, and presently Regan opened the door. Doc motioned him outside with a wave of his hand toward the grass, and the two men stood on the ground behind Regan's house. I observed that Doc was about a foot closer to Regan than one would normally stand when talking.

Doc took out the pictures and handed them to Regan, who looked at each picture. Doc then took the pictures from Regan's hand, carefully placed them back in the envelope, and gave the envelope to Regan. Doc then pointed to the car, where Regan could clearly see me sitting in the front passenger seat.

Doc said something to Regan, that I could not hear, because he got a little closer to Regan, as though telling Regan a secret, which I'm certain he was. Then my brother walked back toward the car and got inside. I wasn't about to ask Doc what had transpired. Nobody questioned Doc. If he wanted you to know something, he told you. And he chose not to tell me.

We drove back to the front of 4-B, and Doc walked me to the front door.

"Son, you know where a phone is located. If any son of a bitch ever so much as touches you, or takes any kind of action against you for what I just said to him, you only need to pick up the phone and call me. You'll be the last person on earth the bastard touches. And that's a promise."

Doc always kept his promises, so I knew well what he meant. Doc gave me a big hug, then got into his car and drove away. At the time, my brother was only twenty years old.

From that day forward, until I moved from 4-B to 3-B, Mr. Regan never again made a nighttime "visit" to 4-B, and Miss Faison never said two words to me.

At the time of my altercation with Mr. Regan in the Spring of 1953, I was just past the midpoint of my ten years in Oxford Orphanage. My first six years had been lived in extended periods of apprehension and angst, easily intimidated by certain bullying high school boys and equally hectoring grownups. This continuing pattern of inequity of treatment of younger orphans by these two intimidating groups gradually yet unalterably engendered in my young being a sheer hatred and disdain for imperious and heavy-handed treatment of younger orphans by those petty, mean-spirited lowlifes at whose beck and call we existed.

The bastard Regan's conduct was clearly outside the bounds of human decency, reprehensible even when judged by the stringent disciplinary mores of that era. My deep-seated hatred for Mr. Regan, that reached its peak on the night of his senseless act of brutality, continued until the day I left the orphanage, and beyond.

The decision I made in Miss Faison's living room that night in March 1953, that I never again would tolerate physical abuse in my life, be it at the hands of a sadistic animal such as E.T. Regan, or by older boys, carried with it the corollary that, you mistreat me at your own peril.

I was determined I would not carry throughout my life the psychological flotsam accumulated during my first traumatic years at Oxford Orphanage. Hereafter I would embark upon my own course through life, never looking back, from now on doing it my way, braking and accelerating, but at my own pace. This singular traumatic event was to be the hinge upon which my future eventually turned, the rock-solid newel on my spiraling staircase called "life."

My Cats

I'm a cat lover. Have been all my life. At age five I "owned" my first dog, you know, the one I locked in our garage that night, until mama switched me to effect the quick release of "my" dog. So that "ownership" lasted two hours at the most. Not being appreciated hurts.

When I started working at the dairy at age eleven, I began to understand cats, and because we tend to associate with our own kind, the defenseless mother cat and her litter of four kittens reminded me so much of orphans, that quickly I gravitated to favoring cats, and this desire to protect the small creatures has stayed with me all my life. I just wish I could get the little creatures to bark.

On the first morning back at the dairy following my return to the campus, I noticed immediately that the other dairy boys were unusually quiet, and that my friends acted collectively as though they harbored a secret they dared not divulge.

I had been gone about eight days by the time Doc brought me back from when I had run away, so dismissing my friends' apprehension as their puzzlement as to why I had not yet received the prescriptive thrashing and sometimes shaved head that awaited every youngster who ran away from the orphanage and had been captured or returned by relatives, I let it slide.

After breakfast I carried my usual portion of greasy bacon and small container of milk up to the loft of the Green Barn, looking forward to again feeding Mama Cat, as I called her, and her four kittens, as we dairy boys were wont to do for the past few years.

However, no family of expectant felines greeted me as I climbed the wooden rungs of the inside ladder of the barn to the loft. I called to them, but was answered by an eerie, disturbing silence. And none of my fellow dairymates had tagged along with me; that in itself was singularly perplexing. So I headed on down the sloping concrete driveway to the dairy.

Suddenly I saw Mr. Davis approaching me, and he held up his right hand, palm toward me, like he was acting like a traffic cop or something, so I took his actions to mean he desired to have a word with me.

However, my dairy manager was not smiling, that in itself puzzled me because during the past year we had become friends, and I had looked forward to seeing him again.

"I need to speak with you," he said, laying his hand on my shoulder and accompanying me slowly down toward the dairy barn.

Without preamble, and like a bolt from a thunderstorm, Mr. Davis said, "Tom Adams killed your cats."

I stopped dead in my tracks, my numbing mind unable to comprehend what Mr. Davis had almost matter of factly stated.

"Why?" I asked, in total disbelief. "Why would Tom Adams kill my cats?"

And then I calmly inquired, in a question to which one would attribute human, not small animal, motives and conduct, "What did my cats do to him?"

"He thought you would not be coming back."

"But what did my cats do to him?" I repeated, unconsciously ignoring a comment that offered no reason in logic or morals.

Small household pets, that is, cats and dogs, do not look upon us as humans. They believe humans are simply giant-sized dogs and cats, and their initial desire is to trust humans. If you put your face quite close to the face of a small kitten, the animal will look directly into your face, gazing back and forth from one of your eyes to the other, seeking comfort, communication and understanding. The kitten is seeking love, and this love transforms itself into trust that you will care for it, protect it and certainly not mistreat it.

Not long ago my wife's champion Persian gave birth to three absolutely lovely kittens. And today, half a century after Tom Adams' vicious, cold-blooded act of barbarity, every time I gaze into the trusting eyes of one of God's furry wonders, I imagine that selfsame creature gazing trustingly into the cruel eyes of that despicable bastard Tom Adams at the moment that vile, contemptible master of animal cruelty ended its trusting life with a .22-cal. bullet. Those four small kittens and the Mama Cat were of no harm to Tom Adams, and brought much joy to us dairy boys.

I began to cry, right there in front of Mr. Davis. The dairy manager continued, "He didn't think you would be coming back, and to Adams he just thought the cats were a nuisance. He shot them with his rifle. I just thought you should know."

Tom Adams was little more than a predator of small boys and a master of animal cruelty. That night I ripped to shreds the two rear whitewalls of his new Mercury, and for months afterwards, every time I saw him around the farm, I would spit into the air, in a show of contempt for the bastard. God, I hated this place.

CHAPTER 65

"Pig" Talton-My Second Test of Resolve

The first (unwanted) test of my conscious decision to refuse to accept further such degrading maltreatment was to present itself within a mere few months of my brother Doc's "visit" to Mr. Gray and Mr. Regan.

Certainly the most offensive and lamentable aspect of life at Oxford Orphanage during my ten year odyssey was the routine, accepted practice of widespread and indiscriminate physical abuse of the children, meted out at the whim of cruel and insensitive school teachers, cottage counselors, work supervisors and staff members including Mr. Gray, Superintendent of Oxford Orphanage, and Mr. Regan, Assistant Superintendent of Oxford Orphanage and Principal of John Nichols School.

Often brutal beatings of small children by grownups were elevated to the less socially repugnant terms of "paddling" (that carries the visual image of a child being swatted, as one would a fly, with a ping-pong paddle) "spankings" and "punishment" simply because the child, before and in preparation of receiving the sadistic, dehumanizing thrashing, was forced to "bend over" a table or chair for support, else the poor unfortunate would be required to pick himself or herself up off the floor following the force of each blow. I have related herein my personal experiences involving physical abuse at the hands of adults while at the orphanage, and my revolt of such treatment at the ages of thirteen and fourteen. Literally dozens of my peers could relate similar stories of their own experiences.

Garland Talton taught high school math, and was a (very) capable teacher. In addition, he served as a (fairly) capable baseball coach and a (who knows how?) capable assistant football coach.

I had been present several years before when one of the fourteen-year-old farm boys had told an off-color joke to the other boys in the presence of Pig Talton. Infuriated, Pig Talton ordered the boy into the large wooden tool shed, that had no windows, and followed the boy into the tool shed, with his ever-present five-foot-long tobacco stick in his hand.

Either Mr. Talton or the teenager had quickly closed the door; we never did find out who closed that door so fast. Instantly, it sounded like two bulls were fighting inside, and we could hear tools and bodies hitting the wood floor. After about a minute, things got eerily quiet. The door slowly opened, the boy walked out calmly, with nary a scratch on him, followed sometime later by Pig Talton, minus his eyeglasses, his shirt torn, clutching his arm.

Witnessing firsthand the teenage boy's deft handiwork, it quickly reinforced to us preteens why we stayed the hell away from 4-B. Some really mean bastards resided therein. "C'mere, boy!" was tantamount to receiving a death sentence.

Miss Gracie Critcher owned a very large tract of farmland outside Oxford, and for many years allowed the orphanage to grow watermelons and sweet potatoes on her land during the Summer. After these crops were harvested, the fields were leveled off using a tractor and harrow, and rye grass was sown as Winter ground cover.

One day in early June 1953 I was assisting Mr. Talton in supervising the younger boys, including my younger brother Pete, who was ten years old at the time. As usual Mr. Talton carried his trusty tobacco stick along with his foul temper onto the job that day. If one of the young boys did something to displease Mr. Talton, he used the tobacco stick as a prod to threaten or strike the child, depending on how foul was his mood at the moment.

In the middle of a field of dirt and small rocks, Miss Critcher had constructed a circular pond about one hundred feet in diameter, with a high bank around the pond. During a break Pete and the other ten-year-olds were standing on the bank throwing rocks into the pond. I was throwing rocks at a stand of trees about forty yards away, and not even in the direction of the pond.

Apparently Mr. Talton had told the youngsters to stop throwing rocks into the pond. I did not hear him, and anyway, my rocks were traveling about forty yards away, not into the pond. Suddenly I heard a loud voice behind me, almost a scream, barking, "I told you not to throw rocks in that pond!" followed immediately by the hard blow of a tobacco stick across the backs of my upper legs.

In one motion I wheeled around, drove my fist into his face, and we tumbled head over heels down the bank of the pond. I ended up straddling his chest, and quickly grabbed him by the throat with my left hand and raised my right fist into the air, prepared to hit him again if he moved.

Mr. Talton's glasses had been knocked off in the scuffle, and he looked up at me in utter shock, the disbelief on his pale face saying it all. The words I shouted in Pig Talton's face rang as clear a year later as the moment I uttered them, my face only a few inches from his, my voice shrill with hatred.

"You are never going to hit me again, not ever again, damn you! And you're never going to hit any of these kids with your goddamn tobacco stick, either."

He didn't move. Just stared up into my face, not saying a word.

"Now, I'm going to get up. I'm going back to the campus and tell Mr. Gray what you did."

Again he didn't move. Just stared at me, blinking.

Slowly I got up, almost hoping he would move or threaten me. He did neither. I picked up his tobacco stick and flung it as far as I could into the field, and slowly walked away, leaving the bastard on his back on the ground, and thirty preteen boys in silent wonderment.

I hitchhiked back to the orphanage, and walked directly across the campus to the Business Office. I knocked on Mr. Gray's door and he motioned me to enter.

I stood across the desk from Mr. Gray, and as calmly as I could, explained to him what had taken place out by Miss Gracie's pond. I was three months into my fourteenth year, and one thing I sure as hell wasn't. I wasn't afraid of Mr. Gray, or Mr. Regan, or Mr. Talton, or of any sorry son of a bitch in this world. If all three of these worthless bastards had been in that room with me at the time, I wouldn't have been afraid. I felt I had finally grown up, and fear of bodily harm left me forever on that day.

Almost overnight I had become the *enfant terrible* to the two top dogs at the orphanage, forever their nemesis, the proverbial hair up their asses, and they were powerless to do anything about it, to punish me in any manner whatever, simply because my brother Doc possessed "The Pictures."

This fact became as clear as Thousand Dollar Spring Water as I calmly related to Mr. Gray the details of my altercation with Mr. Talton. Mr. Gray did not raise his voice, did not appear in the least upset by what I told him, and was (almost embarrassingly) polite to me. He was so obviously out of character that the idea of The Pictures did not come to me until I had left his office.

Standing before Mr. Gray, I was surprised at his calm response to my account of what had occurred at the pond. He asked me if Mr. Talton had been hurt, and I replied that I did not think so. Then he asked if it would bother me if Mr. Talton continued to supervise the farm boys for the remainder of the Summer. I told Mr. Gray that as long as Mr. Talton had nothing to do with me, it was none of my concern. Mr. Gray assured me that Mr. Talton would not have any control over anything I did, then instructed me to report to Mr. Adams. I thanked him and left his office.

The immediacy of my response to Mr. Talton's unprovoked physical assault was a welcome confirmation of my determination, following my quite recent run-in with Mr. Regan, that I would never again accept physical abuse as a way of life at the orphanage. My resolve had been quickly tested, I had shown myself the courage of my convictions, and I was proud of the stand I took on that hot Summer day on Miss Gracie's farm.

As Mr. Gray had instructed, I walked into Mr. Adams' office, and there he sat behind his desk, facing me, grinning like a Cheshire cat, a just-opened Pepsi-Cola and a big Baby Ruth candy bar sitting on the edge of the desk in front of him.

"Mr. Gray just telephoned," he smiled broadly, "and told me I was to keep you two apart. Now let's hear the details. These are for you." He gestured toward the Pepsi and Baby Ruth.

Tom Adams didn't like Pig Talton very much. To Tom Adams, Pig Talton was a nuisance at best, an adult to keep occupied for three months during the Summer. Any fourteen-year-old kid who had worked on the farm picking beans, okra, tomatoes and other crops, hoeing the fields and chopping corn, knew one hell of a sight more about supervising preteens than Pig Talton ever would. And the teenager didn't have to have a tobacco stick with him to keep order, either. No, the older kid had "Or Else."

Anyway, I sat across the desk from Mr. Adams and recounted the incident. After I had finished, Tom Adams said,

"I knew one of these days he would hit the wrong boy with that damned tobacco stick. Don't repeat what I'm saying, but I'm glad you did it."

Mr. Adams continued, "It's difficult to keep you on the farm for the Summer and not have you run into him, and Mr. Gray wouldn't stand for any more trouble, he let me know. Got any ideas?"

After discussing the possibilities for a few minutes, I had an idea.

"I know the plowing is done by the colored men," I said, then added, "But if you gave me a mule and a plow, I'd be by myself, 'cause there's no reason for him to be in a field while it's being plowed."

Tom Adams nodded. During the next two months I confirmed what literally thousands of Southern country boys before my time had proved, that is, you can plant just as much corn in a crooked furrow as you can in a straight one.

Every morning at eight o'clock I showed up at the mule barn, harnessed a mule to a plow and went off to an assigned field, carrying a pail of water and ladle, the plow laid over on its side, the mule pulling the plow. Off I would trudge with one of the colored workers, and if Tom Adams had to find me, he just looked for the crooked furrows. Nobody complained, the colored farm workers told me I would get better with experience, and I spent the Summer learning more about colored folk than any other kid in the orphanage.

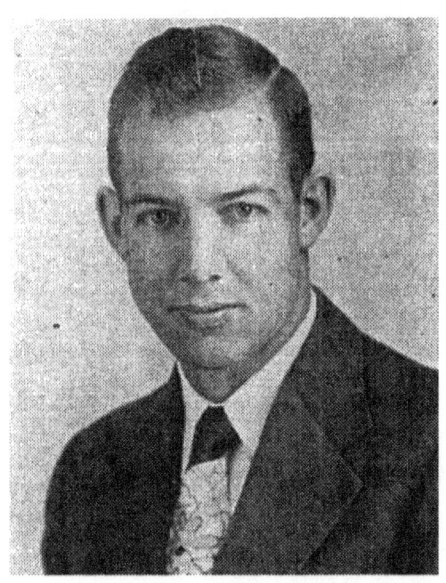

1951. Gabe Austell, Football Coach and Science teacher.

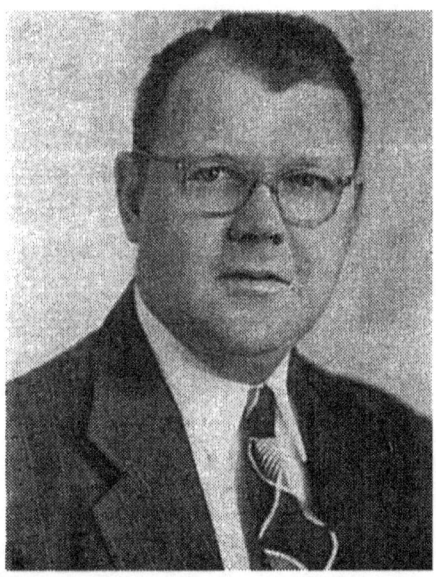

1951. Garland Talton, Baseball Coach and Math teacher.

During a span of six years, from age seven in 1947, til just turning fourteen in 1953, I had been beaten, slapped across my face or in some way struck in unwarranted and vindictive anger, by seven different grownups charged with my care and welfare. I had been slapped twice by Mrs. Tomblin, on my first night at the orphanage, at age seven, and again at age ten. At age nine, while in the Walker Building, I had made "Mr. Gray's List" on at least six different occasions, and had been beaten with a board each time.

In the fifth grade, at age ten, Mamie "Baby Elephant" Baldwin had slapped me and knocked me out of my seat after Leonard stole my spelling book. On the dairy at age eleven, Mr. Davis had whipped me with his leather belt for failing to return a cow to her calf one night.

At age twelve Tom Adams, the former Schutzstaffel from Jackson Training School, had slapped me senseless "for thinking dammit," while I was standing minding my own business in front of the dairy with some other dairy boys. He was not even my supervisor, and had no business at the dairy. The sadistic bastard had walked more than a hundred yards out of his way, simply because he was in a foul mood and wanted to slap a defenseless orphan kid.

The next to last assault was at the hands of that other sadist, E.T. Regan, who lashed me with sixty-one blows with a board across my back, butt and legs, at age thirteen. My life of physical abuse at the hands of grownups at the orphanage came to an end with Pig Talton's tobacco stick across my upper legs, when I was only three months into my fourteenth year.

I remained at the orphanage nearly five more years following the 1953 physical assaults by Mr. Regan and Mr. Talton. At Oxford Orphanage in the late 1940's and early 1950's, challenging the mistreatment at the hands of abusive adults was a rare trick, and usually landed the poor unfortunate kid in Jackson Training School. I had turned the trick twice in less than three months.

The group of boys most interested in the details of my defiance was not my cottagemates in 4-B, but rather the older high school boys in 3-B. Three years earlier, in 1950, one of the boys in 4-B had been removed from the orphanage and sent to Jackson Training School, and a couple of the older boys asked me if I thought Mr. Gray would try to do the same with me.

I had given the idea about as much mental thought as passed gas; Doc had the vivid black-and-white pictures of my battering by Mr. Regan, and Regan and Mr. Gray each had his own personal copy of the glossies. Doc's "any repercussions" meant exactly what Doc had said.

My refusal to suffer further mistreatment by the orphanage staff apparently earned me the respect of the boys' campus. During my remaining nearly five years at Oxford, not once was I picked on or ordered to do anything, or had my money taken, by any high school boy. I walked purposely across the main campus, down the hallways in school, and in my work area, with money jangling in my pockets. My refusal to knuckle under to mistreatment included older boys as well as grownups, and as long as I was on a roll, I felt I might as well go all the way.

There were a number of high school boys who could have kicked my ass from here to Sunday, but with a few exceptions I got along well with them.

And apparently the couple of bullies who even then were taking money from the younger boys and kicking them around here and there just to be mean, didn't want to be known as being the third leg of any hat trick. I had at last shed my hauberk of timidity, and determined consciously that from that time forward, any older boy who dared mistreat me during daylight would not make it across the campus after dark without a cracked skull.

And of course I became an instant hero to the younger boys who had been present that day on Miss Gracie's farm. For the remainder of the Summer, I never once saw Pig Talton's tobacco stick, and my ten-year-old brother Pete, who had been present that day, reported that Mr. Talton never mistreated another child that Summer. It's difficult to describe just how proud this made me. The only emotion that tops having a hero is being one.

Thus I spent the last two months of the Summer of 1953 working with the colored farm hands. Claud Satterfield was already an old man, his brown leathery face sun-baked from long years in the North Carolina sun, the creases of hard labor clearly portending that his youth was a long time gone. Claud referred to himself as an "ole coon," and all the kids were kind to him and the other colored farm workers.

Even I could tell the colored men didn't like Tom Adams, whose patently dictatorial tone of voice and total absence of empathy for, and condescension toward, those less fortunate than he, engendered in all who worked for him an instant dislike and mistrust. None of the colored workers would ever voice such an opinion; however, it showed clearly in the amount of praise they heaped upon the memory of the recently deceased Soapy Peake, who had been the farm manager for thirty-eight years at a time when Soapy and the colored farm workers were much younger men.

Henry Martin was the biggest and strongest of the five colored men. He smoked a pipe, and seemed to enjoy it immensely. Since no store owner in the town of Oxford would dare sell an orphan kid a pipe-I had already tried to buy one and the owner of the small store on the corner of Alexander Avenue a block from the main gate thought I was joking-I asked Henry if he would buy a pipe for me if I gave him the money.

I wanted to get the pipe, I explained in my most sincere manner to Henry, as a "present" for my brother, and nobody, absolutely nobody, would ever know he had purchased it for me. And by the way, my brother would also need a tin or two of Prince Albert tobacco. No, I explained, my brother could get his own matches. But thanks just the same.

Much to my surprise, Henry agreed to do me this big favor, and the following Saturday and Sunday I picked enough blackberries and at night stole enough strawberries, that by Sunday night I had earned the few dollars to give Henry for the pipe and tobacco the following day.

Wednesday morning when nobody was around, Henry took the "presents" for my "brother" from his lunch sack, and I was in business. I already had a pocketful of kitchen matches Eoline had swiped for me from the kitchen. I stopped for a break about two hours later, and couldn't wait to light my treasured Dr. Grabow.

Carefully I followed the Henry Martin pipe-lighting procedure I had observed so many times, and pretty soon I was sitting in the shade at the edge of the twenty-five acre field, leaning against a weathered wooden fencepost, smoking like I had been doing it all my life. And there I sat, with a beatific look on my happy face, drawing in the smoke, pushing my lips out, practicing blowing capital "O's."

Fuck Tom Adams. Fuck Pig Talton. Fuck the world. I believe "happiness" is simply a state of mind, and by this criterion I was indeed a happy lad. I had something I wanted, that nobody else had, and it felt good. The feeling of ownership of that Grabow pipe was the same sensation I had before my Red Ryder B-B gun rusted away in the waterlogged coal bin in the basement of 2-B.

When not using my pipe and tin of Prince Albert, I hid them in a corner of the Long Barn loft, and when I left the orphanage on February 15, 1957 I retrieved that pipe. I still have it in a drawer in my writing desk, alongside my daddy's personal ice pick that he kept atop our icebox at 208 East Bright Street, in the World's Foremost Tobacco Center.

Thus I had fashioned for myself a rather idyllic Summer, replete with plowing wobbly furrows, musings over my recent resolve concerning yet another vanquished overreaching grownup, and frequent smoke breaks with my pipe.

I long ago ceased smoking that pipe. Of course, I realized later that it never was the "smoking" that was important to me, not even the day Henry Martin brought me my pipe. The only thing of real importance was a fourteen-year-old orphan kid "owning" something of value that he could call his own.

At Oxford I was always reminding everybody that my hometown was known throughout the world as "The World's Foremost Tobacco Center." We know that because the billboards around town remind everybody of this, and to me, if it is important enough to be put on a larger-than-life billboard, it must be true. And I do have some support for my claims. The American Heritage Dictionary of the English Language, Third Edition, tells us this about Kinston.

"Kinston. A city of east-central North Carolina southeast of Raleigh. It is a tobacco market. Population 25,234."

By the time I started ninth grade in the Fall of 1953, the Talton and Regan incidents had roused in me an independence that served to efface the timid, fearful nature that had characterized my first five years at the orphanage. One of the manifestations of this transition was the unbridling of the five-year hope that mama would one day take me home to live with her.

My sudden self-direction occasioned by the traumatic events of the preceding Summer, while serving to boost my self-confidence, also had the effect of disengagement from the physical and emotional protection that returning home would surely give me. Plainly stated, from that point onward, subconsciously I did not *need* my mother anymore.

Why does any child need his or her parents? Mainly because our parents protect us from physical and emotional harm from those outside the home, and because they feed, clothe and shelter us.

Emotionally I had been toughened by my refusal to submit to the physical assaults from seven different grownups during my first five years in the orphanage. Physically, my brother Doc (Gray and Regan) and I (Talton) had let it be known what adults could expect if any one of these adults so much as ever touched me again. Food, clothing and shelter I could get at the orphanage as well as at home.

Thus in the sense of "need" as stated above, I did not "need" mama anymore. I still loved mama, and missed her greatly, and empathized with her ongoing suffering occasioned by the tragedy that had scattered our loving, close-knit family to the four winds of grief, but for the next five years not once did I ever plead with mama to take me home.

From that time forward, my recalcitrance seemed yoked to the degree with which I believed those entrusted with my welfare violated this trust. The more I sensed the inequity of the treatment of us young boys, the more intransigent I became, and the more vocal and belligerent were my objections to such treatment. I became the administration's worst nightmare.

Honor is an attribute that adults ascribe solely to adults. However, honor may well easily be a part of a child's psyche as he or she passes through early childhood and into teenage years. Unjustified and unwarranted corporal punishment of a child besmirches this honor, greatly restricts the child's emotional development, and leads the child to question his or her self-worth. This physical and emotional abuse, repeated often enough, cannot help but scar many children for life. Pity the plight of the orphaned child.

These altercations with Regan and Talton were eerily Frankensteinian in nature and effect. I had become the cornered possum of my youth; having been treed by these two callous and overreaching pricks, I had no place to turn, was given no honorable choice, no way out, no reasonable option. But fortunately for me, E.T. Regan and Pig Talton had slipped on their own petard, hooked forever on the horns of their self-created dilemma. And Little Orphan Al had eventually prevailed.

Ultimately, I came to terms with my (childish) dreams, (ridiculously unreasonable) hopes and (completely unfulfilled) expectations. The aforementioned events of the Spring and Summer of 1953 served to lend concreteness to my developing psyche, to enable me to define in some loosely tangible manner who I was, what I stood for, and to develop a set of unspoken rules that was to guide my conduct (or misconduct) for the remainder of my prison sentence, as well as help mold my character for the rest of my life. I gained from my experiences of abuse at the hands of grownups a finely-tuned empathy for those disadvantaged youths in situations similar to those that through no fault of my own, I was forced to endure.

CHAPTER 66

Why I Didn't Fumble the Football

Thoughts of my altercations with Mr. Regan and Pig Talton of the previous Spring and Summer, while not fading from memory, at least had been eased to rear compartments of my mind, replaced by my love for football.

After being knocked six ways to senseless by Blockhead Johnson and Red Albertson the first time I "carried" the football (that I really, really didn't want), I had developed a passion for the game, and during school hours, or when milking cows or even when playing "pocket pool," I would devise plays in my head, that always showed me carrying the football for an eighty-yard touchdown, stiff-arming each and every player on the opposing team, or throwing a sixty-yard pass (usually to myself) for a touchdown. For some odd reason, I was two feet taller than my (less athletic and not really needed) teammates, and even opposing players cheered for me as I scored touchdown after touchdown. At age thirteen, I was already a football legend in my own mind.

Coach Gabe Austell had heard of the disagreement between me and his assistant coach Pig Talton, and after the first day of football practice Coach Gabe had asked me to remain on the field for a few minutes. Well, not really. Ask me, I mean. Not in the meaning of "request." Can't picture Coach (Meanass) Gabe Austell "asking" anybody anything. We did as he said.

Gabe was a hardcase, but we could not have asked for a better coach. All he wanted to do was win. Several of us ninth graders practiced with the varsity, and we were considered to be varsity players. We played all the junior varsity games, and some of the varsity games as well. I was backup to my friend Jack Barger at quarterback.

Even as a ninth grader I was the fastest runner on the team. One day at practice Coach Gabe was working with his first string defense, so I was playing quarterback on offense. First play I called was a quarterback keeper around left end. Odis Hutchins snapped the ball, I faked it to the left halfback Bill Herrington going off left tackle, and took off like a scalded dog toward the sideline. Nobody on the first team came anywhere near me. And this was against the team that was to go on to win the North Carolina District II-AA Conference Championship that year. They must have just been having an "off" day. Leave Little (Fast) Orphan Al at quarterback and every day would have been an off day for those suckers.

However, Gabe Austell was, in a word-upset; in two words-crimson livid! Following a few choice expletives and threats yelled at the top of his lungs, Coach Gabe let the offense rest while he ran his hotshot "championship" defense ragged with hundred-yard wind sprints.

During a five-minute break before practice resumed, Jack Barger came running over to me, panting like a bloodhound that had just lost a race to a jackrabbit (which he had) and let me know,

"Al, you're a nice kid, but if you do that one more time, we're going to kick your ass from here to Sunday."

Discretion being the better part of valor (especially at Oxford), I ratcheted down my sprint speed from eighty miles per hour to two-and-a-half miles per hour, and most of the slow-footed "first string" bumpkins still couldn't catch me. In a footrace with these turkeys, likely I could drop back two furlongs and still be six lengths ahead at the finish line. Admittedly, however, some of these hotshots were so slow, it'd take them two days just to run out of sight.

Anyway, I reported to Gabe as ordered that first day after practice, and the coach asked me point blank if he was going to "have any problems with you and coach Talton?"

I looked the mean sumbitch in the eye and replied "Not if he don't ever hit me with no tobacco stick again."

Coach Gabe's reply was short and to the point.

"That's not going to happen. Now, get on to the locker room."

What I liked about Gabe Austell was that he was a man of his word. I knew everything would be alright. And it was.

The two best ways to get on either of Gabe Austell's "bad" sides (the mean bastard didn't seem to have a "good" side when it came to coaching football) was 1) to fumble the football, regardless of which team recovered the fumble, and 2) to allow a pass receiver to get behind you when running out for a pass, regardless of whether he caught the pass or even had the ball thrown to him. The poor pass receiver could have gotten past you, then fell over and died right there on the thirty-five yard line. Didn't make no difference, you still had to answer to Gabe. And I used to get nervous just being on the same football field with Gabe Austell. And I sure wasn't by myself in that regard. Nosireebob. Thus my "Four Plays of Fame" were really Coach Gabe's fault.

Anyway, at midseason of that Fall 1953 year we made the trip to Raleigh for the annual Orphanage Bowl game between Oxford Orphanage and Methodist Orphanage, played at North Carolina State's stadium. Several thousand spectators attended this game each year, mostly college kids taking a break from their studies. There was a lot of pride on the line, so the game was as serious as death to both teams.

During the year Coach Gabe would allow me and the other five Freshmen who practiced with the varsity, to play a few plays each game. Though we six boys were listed on the varsity roster, we played all the junior varsity games on Thursday. So usually we six boys dressed out for two games each week. We were proud of ourselves.

For me the Orphanage Bowl began as the other games had from the beginning of football season. By the end of the first quarter, I had thrown seven touchdown passes, one of these a trick play, a spectacular 85-yarder to my favorite receiver, namely myself; the score was a lopsided 48-0 (we had missed an extra point because our kicker had been busy applauding my great play) and we were trouncing the inept and thoroughly outclassed Methodists.

However, by the middle of the second quarter I had awakened from my first-quarter flight of fancy; we were barely ahead 13-7, and it looked as though I'd spend the night warming the bench. We may have won the conference title that year, but those Methodist orphans were tough as nails, and they hit hard.

All of a sudden I heard Coach Gabe's booming voice barking "Provost!" and I jumped from my warm spot on the bench and reported to him. When Coach Gabe talked to you, you looked him in the eye. He had this fixation on you that told you he meant every single word he said. Plainly put, Gabe Austell was a mean sonofabitch, and nobody disputed him.

Coach Gabe also had this odd habit of grabbing you by the nape of the neck and squeezing hard while he was lecturing you, as if to remind you that if you screwed up, he could snap your skinny neck like it was a toothpick. And he would've done it. Mean bastard.

His gaze boring through me, Gabe said evenly,

"Provost, you go in for Barger. And look at me now. You'd better not fumble the goddamn football. Now go!"

Talk about the heat of the battle! I didn't practice with these seniors. The backs were accustomed to taking handoffs from the famous Jack Barger. If I fumbled the ball, the unforgiving Gabe Austell would kill me, right there on the fifty-yard line in front of thousands of screaming fans. There was only one way not to fumble the football, and that was not to ever hand it off. My mind was made up before I reached the huddle.

Gabe didn't call the plays. He left that responsibility to Jack Barger. And he was also leaving the play-calling to me, because I was the quarterback. Talk about a vote of confidence!

In play-calling the "Split-T" formation, the quarterback is the No. 1 back, left halfback No. 2, fullback is No. 3 and right halfback is No. 4. The "hole" between center and left guard is the No. 1 hole; between the center and right guard the No. 2 hole, etc. So a play called "21" would mean the quarterback hands off to the left halfback going between center and left guard.

In keeping with my "not fumble" promise I had just made to myself, the first play I called was "Eleven, on two." I got up under the center, squeaked "Hut one, hut two," and when the center snapped the ball, I lowered my head, held onto the football (why did the game ball always seem larger and slipperier than the practice ball?) with both arms, and burrowed my way between center and left guard, gaining about six yards.

I always thought there were supposed to be only eleven players on a football team, but that night Methodist Orphanage must have cheated; there were 37 players on their team, and 36 of them hit me head-on. Rattled my head inside that cheap football helmet, too. Anyway, I hadn't fumbled the ball. Back to the huddle.

With the other players looking expectantly at me, I said,

"Twelve, on one."

Back under the center.

"Hut one."

The center snapped the ball. Off I ducked between center and right guard. This time a five-yard gain. A first down in two plays. Move them chains, you chain-gang you. Back to the huddle.

"Thirteen, on two."

"Hut one, hut two."

Another six-yard gain off left tackle.

Back to the huddle, bruised but determined.

"Hey, kid, you gonna run the goddamn ball every time?"

Looking up, I replied firmly,

"You're goddamn right I am. Now, fourteen, on one."

Another five yards. Another first down. Move dem chains again, please. I was on a roll. I was getting my guts kicked out, but I was having a great time doing it. I had not fumbled the football, and in four plays had gained two first downs. I was elated after that fourth gain. And this was no daydream. This was the real thing, the big time. I imagined I would run the quarterback keeper 27 straight times, and we would win the Orphanage Bowl by the lop-sided score of 48-7. I would be the hero, and my old dairy buddy, Jack Barger, would warm the bench for the rest of the year. I was even beginning to wonder if it would affect our friendship.

I looked up from the huddle expecting to really trick those dumbfounded Methodist orphans by calling "Eleven, on two," when I heard Jack Barger's excited, irritated voice,

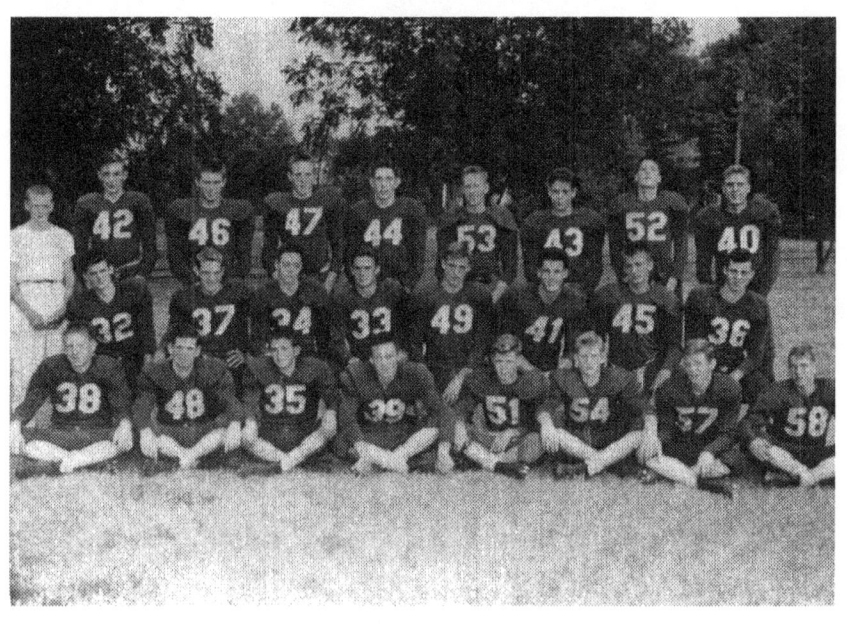

1953. Oxford Orphanage "Red Devils," North Carolina District 3-AA Conference Champions. The author (no. 58) is on bottom row, last player on right.

"Provost, get the hell out of here. Coach Gabe wants you, you goddamn glory hog."

Alas, here was my answer. The irritation in Jack Barger's voice, and the name-calling. My fears were realized; my heroics had indeed affected our friendship. Well, fuck you, Jack Barger.

Rushing to the sideline, I reported to a, believe it or not, smiling Gabe Austell. I didn't even know the bastard could smile.

"What the hell you doing running the ball every play, Provost?"

"You told me not to fumble the football, coach. And I didn't fumble the football."

And then he caught on.

"Good boy, Provost. You did good. Now go sit down."

I was one happy kid! And I hadn't fumbled the ball. What a great feeling. Given a choice of having my head kicked in by 37 meaner'n hell Methodist orphans, or being murdered on the way back to the locker room by Coach ("Don't fumble the goddamn ball, Provost!") Gabe Austell, which would you choose? Little Orphan Al weren't no one-trick pony. Survival was good!

Back on the bench, I made a mental note that Oliver Gibbs had missed yet another crucial extra point, and to remind him that I had told him a hundred times about not hooking the ball like a darned soccer player. And I do recall that when I got after Oliver about it, he had asked me what in the world is "soccer."

Throughout my lifetime, the closest I ever came to belonging to a brotherhood, of enjoying a sense of camaraderie, was when Coach Gabe allowed several of us Freshmen to play on the varsity football team. Coach Gabe treated us Freshmen as though we were Seniors, and made us a part of that unforgettable 1953 Conference Championship Team.

A half century later, on October 12, 2002, we all met at the orphanage on homecoming weekend to honor Coach Gabe. I had not seen most of the players during that fifty-year period, and was pleasantly surprised that the older boys remembered me and called me by name the moment I met them again. Only at that memorable reunion did I fully realize what that association had meant to me. In my motel room that night, at the end of the festivities, I admit to shedding a few tears of nostalgia. These thirty or so men were truly my brothers, and I will never forget them.

Six months after the reunion, on April 29, 2003, while working in his garden, Gabe Austell died of a heart attack.

Sadly there is a postscript to this story. At our October 12, 2002 reunion, on a table in the basement of the York Rite Chapel lay a nametag for each boy invited, that included a photograph of the boy. Bill, Van, Newton and I looked over the nametags, and I picked up one of a member of our class, and remarked,

"No way in hell is he gonna show up here."

And he didn't.

In the Fall of 1953 Gabe Austell taught our Freshman Science class in the basement laboratory of John Nichols School. We were fourteen years old.

One afternoon we were gathered around a table as Coach Gabe explained a chemistry experiment to the class. One of our best friends moved behind two of the girls in order to get a better view of the experiment, and as he did, one of the girls moved forward to allow him to pass by. I saw everything that occurred. Our friend never touched either of the girls.

Apparently believing the boy had touched the girl who had moved forward, without warning Coach Gabe attacked the unsuspecting boy, slapping him four times in the face as the boy fell back reeling, the coach all the while screaming and cursing the startled teenager.

Our abused friend never even attempted to explain his innocence to Gabe Austell, because to do so would certainly see the abuse repeated. So the battered lad just accepted the physical and verbal assault, as he had been conditioned to do so for many years.

Gabe Austell was but another heartless grownup given unfettered rein to abuse at will defenseless orphan children. The boy graduated high school in 1957, and to my knowledge has never returned to the orphanage. The 1953 physical and verbal abuse left a scar that has not healed in half a century.

CHAPTER 67

The Secret of the "Red Bread"

James Milton Pruitt joined the orphanage staff in 1946, the year before I arrived at Oxford. Mr. Pruitt had been a "town" boy, so his return to Oxford Orphanage following a tour in the Pacific during World War II was a homecoming for him. We kids addressed the quiet, soft-spoken gentleman as Mr. Pruitt; the staff called him simply "Milton." For thirty-four years Mr. Pruitt was the supervisor over all food preparation facilities and operations, and at that time a total of approximately three hundred forty students and forty staff members ate three meals each day, seven days a week, in the large family-style dining rooms. He knew us young ruffians for the thieves we were, never held it against us because he realized stealing food from the kitchen at midnight was for us boys a diversion and nothing more. We liked him for that. Mr. Pruitt died on April 24, 1997, and an awful lot of people really missed him. The job Mr. Pruitt held for all those years fell eventually to a classmate of ours, Hazel Strum (Davidson), sister of my most dependable football teammate, Lawrence Strum. I don't think we ever heard Lawrence speak a word on the football field. He was all business, and anchored our line as well as anyone on the team, giving his hundred and ten percent on every play. His sister Hazel was (and is) just as dependable.

During my ten-year stay at Oxford, the institution was pretty much self-sufficient, notable exceptions being during the early years, dough for making bread, eggs, and butter, that was obtained in large, one-pound blocks from the U.S. Government. We grew most of our own vegetables, and slaughtered hogs for meat, on the approximately three hundred fifty acre farm and dairy. A few crops, among them watermelons and sweet potatoes, were grown off campus, on land leased from Miss Gracie Critcher.

The Food Department of the orphanage, the second largest building on campus, was located just behind the Main Building. We referred to the entire building as the "Dining Room," and it housed the kitchen, four dining rooms plus a faculty dining room, refrigeration rooms, freezer facilities, a smokehouse and other storage areas. Built in 1894, the massive two-story all—brick structure with a full basement had additionally housed the Masonic Temple. The dining rooms and kitchen had been used for these purposes since 1894.

In 1933 the building was condemned as unsafe for use for any purpose. However, the grand edifice was spared the demolition ball by placing steel beams between the old Masonic Lodge on the second floor and the large dining rooms on the main level, in order to give the monstrous building more structure and support. Once the second floor ceased being used as a Masonic Lodge Meeting Hall, it was converted into a basketball court.

The building itself was older than the North Carolina Board of Health. However, since the state Board of Health had been organized, the building never passed a single safety inspection. In 1955 the Board of Directors of Oxford Orphanage decided to dismantle the building and replace it with a modern fireproof dining room and kitchen, as soon as funds became available. These structural hazards, however, did not affect the cleanliness and functioning of the Dining Hall, and it remained the center of life on campus throughout my decade at Oxford.

All our bread was baked from scratch in the bakery, located in the basement of the massive kitchen and dining room facility. In the making of bread, the bakery boys poured the flour and other ingredients into a large metal hemisphere, open at the top, and this mixture was then kneaded into a uniform mass by a curved, revolving metal arm.

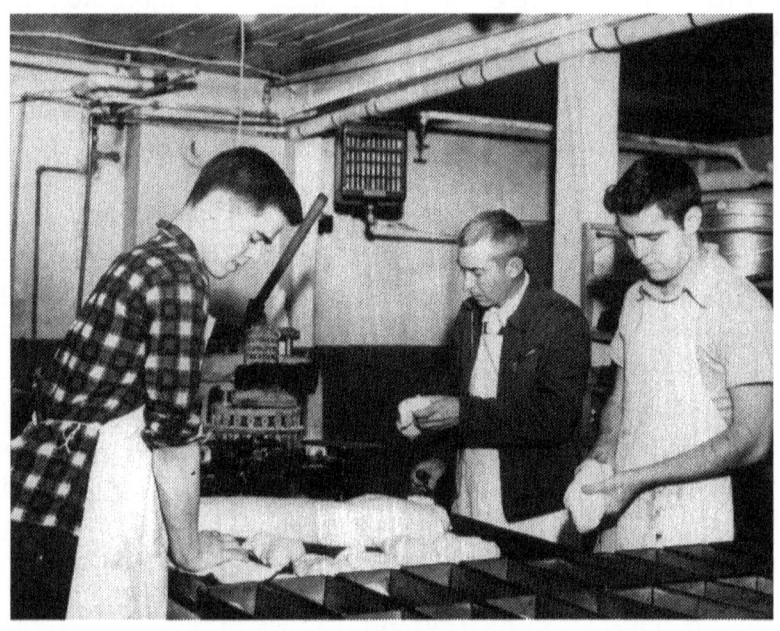

1954. From left: Jeff Pargoe, Milton Pruitt and Frank McMillan.
Preparing dough for making bread in the bakery in the basement
of the kitchen-dining room complex.

Once this kneading process was completed, the mass of dough was placed on a table, rolled to the prescribed depth, cut into the desired length, and placed in the bottom of individual metal compartments. The trays of dough were then placed in the oven, and under intense heat the dough would rise to fill the form of the oblong containers, shaped miraculously just like a loaf of bread.

These baked loaves were then fed into slicers and the sliced bread was placed neatly on stacked breadracks. Three hundred and forty hungry orphans and forty staff members consumed a lot of bread.

Toast for breakfast was prepared by the kitchen girls, and every girl at the orphanage eventually was assigned for a year or more to work at the myriad of tasks involving food preparation. To make toast, first large blocks of pure USDA Grade A surplus butter were melted in a metal pot. The required number of slices of bread, usually more than a thousand, were placed side by side on large metal trays.

Next the young kitchen girl, using a small basting brush especially designed for such food preparation, dipped the brush into the melted butter and basted each slice of bread. The trays of "painted" bread were then heated in ovens, and once done, these absolutely mouth-watering slices of pre-buttered toast appeared as bright yellow moons painted on square amber canvases.

One hot Summer morning in 1954, because we were not yet living in enlightened times, thus I could not have been "hanging out," I was killing time with my two bakery buddies, Frank and Charlie, in the basement of the dining room complex. Frank and Charlie were busy kneading the dough in the large metal hemisphere, that we orphans just called a "tub." At times the bakery boys would assist the metal kneading arm by leaning over the side of the metal tub and pounding the dough with their fists.

Sounded like fun to me, and I could imagine the tub of dough was Tom Adams' stupid face. I was about up to a good rhythm, as though I were hitting a punching bag, when suddenly my right elbow preceded my fist, and my forearm made full-force contact with the sharp edge of the metal tub. Immediately blood gushed from the large cut in my forearm, and sprayed all over the dough in the tub.

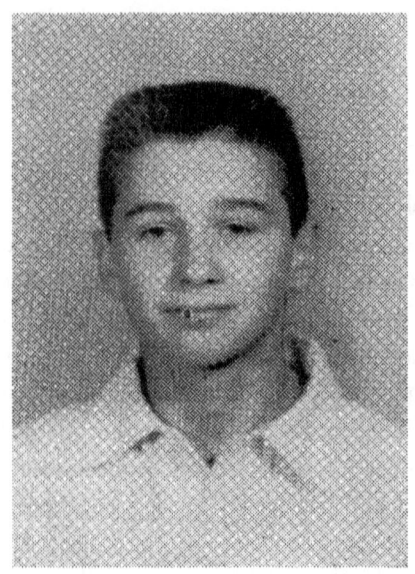

Butch Mitchell. Friend and Partner-in-Crime.

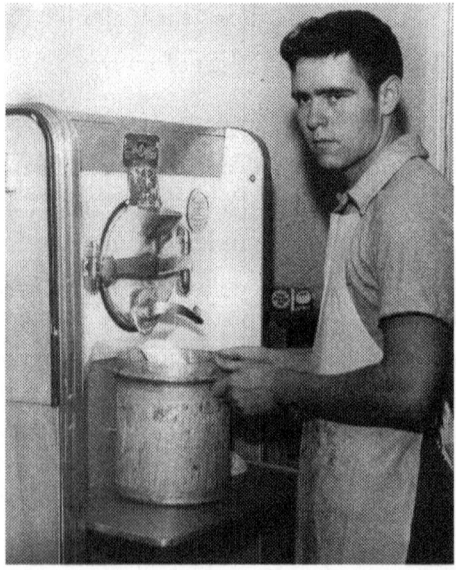

1954. Frank McMillan making ice cream in bakery of kitchen-dining room building.

I screamed in pain, and Charlie and Frank came running. Seeing the blood covering the tub full of fresh dough, Frank started helping me stop the bleeding, while Charlie began doing his best to sop up the blood, that was rapidly seeping into the mass of dough.

We three boys were faced with one grand dilemma. If we threw out the huge tub of kneaded dough, how were the boys going to mix another large batch of ingredients without Mr. Pruitt discovering what had occurred? And because the blood had soaked into the porous dough, how would Charlie and Frank explain the new "red bread" to Mr. Pruitt and three hundred orphans?

The final vote, that carried by the overwhelming majority of 3-0, was to just bake the bloody bread and hope for the best. True orphans' reasoning. Decisions that made our country great. Meanwhile, Charlie tied a pressure bandage on my bloody arm, and I hurried over to the hospital and told the nurse I had fallen down and cut my arm. She closed the cut with four stitches, and nearly fifty years later the scar is still visible.

As for the new "red bread," Charlie, Frank and I held our collective breath. But apparently nobody noticed the discolored bread, and we three breathed a big sigh of relief. So three hundred orphan kids and about a dozen or so staff members got to taste Little Orphan Al's blood, and I could swear that for a few days after consuming that batch of bread, all the kids appeared somewhat more intelligent, industrious and respectful. Except Charlie and Frank. And to the best of my recollection, the three of us kept our bloody secret.

But here we are into perspective again. The only boys who worked for Mr. Pruitt in the massive kitchen-dining hall complex were the three or four teenage bakery boys. Thus the kitchen manager supervised mainly thirty or so preteen and teenage girls. Just as with other staff members, Mr. Pruitt's control over these young girls was absolute; the quiet supervisor's quick open hand was well known on the girls' side of the campus. However, because Mr. Pruitt's fits of ill temper did not affect us boys on a daily basis, many of the boys were unaware of his proclivity for abusing young girls.

CHAPTER 68

Hot Buttered Popcorn and Its Influence on Segregation in the South

"Five orphan tickets, please sir."

It was a gray December Saturday afternoon in 1955, the speaker was my buddy Bill Herrington, and he was addressing a distinguished-looking mustached gentleman nattily dressed in a businesslike gray tweed jacket, sporting black horn-rimmed spectacles and a circa 1940 red bowtie.

Deftly tearing off five blue tickets from a ticket roll, the Orpheum picture show "official" presented each of us a ticket with the solemnity of a college president presenting diplomas on graduation day at Duke University thirty miles down the road. Bill Herrington, Newton Wilder, Red Albertson, Van Edwards and I graciously accepted our tickets, and I asked the "gentleman" if he could just bill the price of the tickets to our "good friend," Pappy Regan, as usual. This comment elicited a burst of laughter, the loudest guffaw coming from the smiling "gentleman."

This was a one-act play scripted on innumerable occasions in my last two years at Oxford, during which time the five of us boys never paid for a ticket to the Orpheum. We lucky lads had, as the saying goes, "a friend in the business."

The (tongue-in-cheek) "gentleman" was no gentleman at all, but better than that, he was our good friend William Arthur ("W.A.") Wilson, a "town" boy who attended school with us. W.A. was a veritable genius at math, to the extent that when our math teacher, Pig Talton, was required to be absent from school, W.A. quite ably took his place as our schoolmaster, though he was only one grade ahead of us in school. My favorite author of all time, Chuck Dickens, would have called W.A. a "bright lad," and would have claimed that our friend would have "great expectations" for the future.

On many a Sunday after church had let out, W.A. would stop by 3-B and pick us up in his car, and the six of us would go joy-riding around town and the Granville County countryside, invariably stopping for Moon Pies and RC Colas at Red's Three Way Stop at the northern edge of town.

However, we had become best friends long before W.A. started his part-time afternoon and weekend job, that involved being the ticketmaster at the rear door of the Orpheum, that had opened its doors for business in 1943, and was still the only picture show in the small town of Oxford.

The Orpheum's continuing popularity stemmed from the fact that if you didn't like what was playing at the Orpheum, you could take an hour-long drive to Raleigh or Durham to find the next-closest picture show. So, the Orpheum "packed 'em in" so to speak.

Any Southerner (and probably Northerner as well) born before 1950 probably understands why our good friend W.A. was selling picture show tickets at the rear door of the Orpheum. As of the time I left Oxford in February 1957, picture shows at least down South were still segregated, and the rules of deportment were strictly observed, to the extent that the term "zero tolerance" may well have originated in small-town Southern picture shows in the postwar years.

Southern segregated picture shows of that era were generally laid out as follows. The Paramount on Queen Street in Kinston, as well as the Orpheum on Hillsboro Street in Oxford, had a balcony at the rear of the picture show that consisted of an upper floor of seats that jutted out over the rear of the main floor, and was enclosed by a railing.

Colored folks were allowed to pay to see the picture show, as long as they remained unseen and unheard by the white patrons. In fact, many white patrons never even knew that coloreds attended the picture shows.

About half an hour before the picture show started, our good friend W.A. Wilson would seat himself at a small portable table at the back door of the Orpheum. He collected the price of the ticket, gave a torn-off stub to the colored patron, and the customer ascended a steep flight of stairs located just inside the rear door, that led to the colored balcony.

The colored customers did not bring their babies and small children to the picture show, because they could not control crying babies and boisterous preteens. Plainly stated, if the coloreds talked or laughed aloud, or threw or dropped by mistake any item over the railing of the balcony and onto the white patrons seated below, the Orpheum management (meaning W.A.) cleared the balcony immediately. No warnings. No explanations accepted or even listened to. No second chances. No disturbance of any kind was tolerated. Period. The coloreds were expected to police their own.

At times we boys would just stop by to visit W.A. while he was on the job, and often we chatted briefly with the colored customers. Occasionally one of the five colored farm workers would show up, and once we boys showed recognition, W.A. would allow the colored farm worker into the picture show at no charge. W.A. was a nice guy, one of "our own."

The Orpheum picture show was built in 1943 by Mr. E.G. Crews, and was located directly across Hillsboro Street from the historic Granville County courthouse. W.A. was the assistant to Mr. G.P. Duffy, a dapper, quiet man in his mid-forties who, year-round, Summer or Winter, was dressed in a tweed coat, dark trousers, white shirt, colored tie and a black Fedora sporting a wide brim. Mr. Duffy took up tickets from the white patrons from his position just inside the swinging double doors of the picture show.

World War I was not called as such before World War II came along. The first war was simply called "The Great War." Hard contact lenses were never called "hard" contact lenses before the advent of the "soft" contact lenses; the original lenses were simply called "contact lenses."

Likewise, the word "segregation" had no meaning to our lives down South at the time I was at Oxford. We had no cause to question the status quo, and any sign of what we look upon today as "discrimination" was not consciously thought of as such at the time. Not by white people anyway.

But make no mistake about this fact-the colored folks had no desire to sit in a picture show with white people. No, the only thing the coloreds coveted that the white folks had was the hot buttered popcorn. White people are sometimes dumber'n dirt clods. They associate the stereotypical Southern colored man with greasy fried chicken, and it's always with the chicken *leg*. Ever seen an advertisement showing a colored person eating the white breast of chicken? Neither have I. Neither has anyone else. It's always the chicken *leg*. The South is probably full of "closet colored chicken breast lovers."

However, Southern colored people loved one thing more than they ever loved chicken *legs*, and that was hot buttered popcorn.

Stupid white Southern politicians could have delayed racial integration for at least another half century if they had just allowed the coloreds to buy hot buttered popcorn and cold soft drinks in picture shows. Shortsighted asses!

Heat rises, and on any given day the coloreds probably started hating white people as soon as the sharp aroma of that good ole hot buttered popcorn wafted in through the swinging lobby doors, quickly filled the main picture show and rose inexorably upward to permeate the *balcony*. Must have been an absolutely mind-numbing, unbearable, torturing experience for those poor colored folks.

If you enumerate all the bitterness and deep-seated envy engendered by the denial of hot buttered popcorn and ice-cold Pepsi-Cola to a balcony full of colored men, and multiply all this pent-up hostility by the tremendous number of picture show houses in the South, it's a wonder of wonders how the South remained racially segregated past 1950. Integrated picture shows surely must have brought a tremendous increase in hot buttered popcorn sales. The greatest thing that Americans who didn't grow up in the South between 1940 and 1960 missed was just that, not growing up in the South between 1940 and 1960. I wouldn't trade it for all the gold in Fort Knox. And if mama hadn't packed me off to the orphanage in 1947 when I was just seven years old, it would have been even more interesting. Southerners possess a rich and diverse heritage that can never be understood or appreciated by non-Southerners. Any culture capable of producing, in the same era, chitlins, grits, lard and the "Moon Pie," could only be the forward reconnaissance team of an advanced civilization.

In retrospect, we kids lived in a different world, being spared the oftentimes bloody (and deadly) racial strife that characterized life in the South during the decade 1955-1965. Words such as "freedom march," "civil rights movement," "sit-ins," "bus boycott" and "separate-but-equal" were quite foreign to us.

CHAPTER 69

"Come Here, Football!"

John Nichols School was a part of the Oxford City School System. The high school boys and girls referred to the school building itself as John Nichols High School; however, the school building housed all twelve grades. And because John Nichols School was a North Carolina public school, families from out in Oxford were allowed to enroll their children in the school.

There were several good reasons for town parents to enroll their children in John Nichols School. One of these reasons was that for their children from fifth through twelfth grades, they had to attend school four hours each day, compared to the six-hour school day for Oxford city schools.

North Carolina state law required all children to attend supervised class instruction six hours per day. Because the orphanage children from fifth grade through twelfth grade had to work half a day, the school day was only four hours long. The additional two-hour requirement was fulfilled by a supervised two-hour "study hall" that lasted from seven til nine o'clock each evening during the school week.

The two-hour study hall accomplished another purpose-it forced the children to do their homework. The study hall was supervised by the cottage counselors, who insisted on complete silence during the entire period.

The town kids likewise were supposed to observe at home the two-hour requirement, but they were not bound by the rule unless their parents enforced it. To most of the high school town students, the mandatory two-hour study hall was an open joke, and they were free to take half a day off to work or do as they pleased. During the time I was at Oxford, fully one-fourth of the students who made up the student body of John Nichols School were "town" kids.

Most of the town children were good students, however, and we treated them as though they were our own brothers and sisters. Some of them attend homecoming and are active in alumni affairs. It was a delight to know them.

Children of the orphanage staff also attended John Nichols School. Troy Regan, son of my own personal nemesis, was a good friend. However, he was not allowed to do things with us outside school and sports activities, and Troy spent many a Saturday and Sunday afternoon at home when he could have been stealing and selling strawberries and Musky Dines, blowing up "balloons" on lovers' lane, playing touch football or roaming the woods with his friends. Troy knew well the hate-hate relationship between his father and me, yet to his credit he refused to allow the situation to interfere with our friendship.

Troy was on our high school football team, the Red Devils. Our locker room was located in the basement of the Industrial Building, beneath the Laundry Room, all the way across the campus from the football field, and we had to go by the kitchen on our way to the Industrial Building after football practice each night.

The steep outside stairs leading to the rear of the kitchen-dining room building were really two sets of stairs, with a landing halfway up. If you walked up the first set of stairs and faced straight ahead, you were looking into a large window that opened onto the staff dining hall.

The time was the Fall of 1955, and I was a Junior in high school. We older boys would get one of the dining room girls to unlatch the window at the stairway landing, and after football practice and showering in the locker room, we would run up the stairs in the seven p.m. darkness, fling open the large window, climb in and raid the kitchen of fresh bread, ice cream, milk and anything else good and tasty and absolutely free.

It was all just in fun, no harm was done, and it was as much a diversion from our daily humdrum orphans' existence as it was the food. Anyway, one dark night on our way from football practice, we were just walking along planning and plotting and scheming about our heist for the night, when Troy asked us if he could raid the kitchen with us. Sounded like a good idea to us; his daddy had not caught us in about six or eight months, and it was all right with us if he wanted to join the fun.

Anyway, to do this right, we could not all just bunch up at the window on the landing like we were the Keystone Kops or something. We had to go one at a time. There were four of us, including Troy.

I told Troy to stick close on my heels, but to give me a few seconds to fling open the dining room window so nobody would spot us. As we approached the open paved clearing between the dining room-kitchen and the shadows, I suddenly sprinted across the lighted area, bounded up the first flight of stairs three at a time, pushed open the unlocked window sash, and scampered inside the large pitch-black rectangular staff dining hall.

Parting the drapes that covered the large window, I peered out into the lighted area to see Troy sprinting toward the stairs. However, as he jumped from the landing and grabbed the window ledge to hoist himself up, I reached out to grab his arm to assist him, when I observed a large form emerge swiftly from the shadows, bound up the stairs, yell "Come here, football!" and somebody pulled Troy's extended arm from my grasp. It was as though the other person and I were having a tug-of-war with Troy's body, and I had lost. Jerked old Troy right off the window ledge. God, that must have hurt! Now Troy was taller than I was, but skinny as a rail. Even today I can hear every bone in Troy's upper body scraping against that window sill and the only sound out of the terrified kid was a surprised grunt, then his upper body disappeared into the void of night. It all happened in a blinding flash.

I heard a sharp "SPLAT!" as old man Regan slapped the snot out of his own son, then heard him exclaim "Troy! What are *you* doing here?"

Later I asked Troy what he had answered his father, and Troy said he didn't get the chance, because his father had slapped him senseless with a couple more backhands. Apparently his father's question had been somewhat rhetorical in nature.

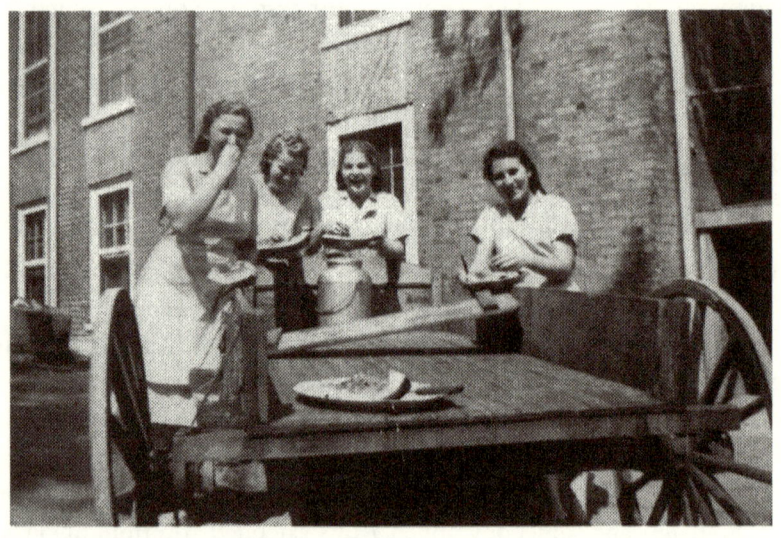

"Big Girls" foundering on watermelon at the dairy milk wagon outside the kitchen-dining rooms. Note milk can and wagon tailgate. At far right is stairway landing from where E.T. Regan snatched his son Troy on the night of our aborted raid on the kitchen.

I said "Later I asked Troy . . ." Obviously I did not wait around to "face the music." I couldn't help my friend Troy, so I bounded across the dining room darkness, miraculously not colliding with any tables or chairs, and escaped out the front dining room door.

I hoofed it on down to 3-B, and waited on the front concrete steps for the certain arrival of E.T. and his battered, frightened son. This would be the first time I would get to test first-hand my brother Doc's warning of a few years before. So I took out my trusty Barlow pocketknife, given to me years before as a present from my brother Bill, that I kept sharp as a razor blade, and placed it beside me as I sat on the concrete step. Just in case.

Presently I observed Regan's car pull up to the curb in front of 3-B, and I walked down the steps and confronted him on the sidewalk, holding my Barlow's handle down by my right side and slightly behind me. I felt safe holding the knife in my right hand, because I doubted the angry bastard would extend his hand toward me and say "Hey, it's good to see you, Al. How have you been?" In other words, I wasn't likely to be shaking hands with this prick.

Glancing to Regan's right, I noticed my wide-eyed, scared-out-of-his-wits friend cowering in the back seat of the car, and I could tell he was worried he had caused me trouble for wanting to come along with us on our "raid."

As for me, afraid of Troy's father? No chance in hell of that happening. I was several years past being afraid of his father, or anybody else for that matter. My brother Doc was not one to make idle threats.

I had no real intention of using my Barlow. It was a "just in case" type situation, if things suddenly got out of hand here. I believe what I am trying to convey here is that at this juncture in my life, I really didn't give two hoots to hell about any grownup assaulting me. It just never would happen again.

Pulling up short about four feet from me, a quite visibly shaken Regan demanded, without telegraphing any anticipated blow,

"Why did you let Troy go with you?"

"Because he wanted to, sir. We didn't twist his arm," I replied, in as calm a manner as I could muster. Then I added, in an attempt to mollify the obviously shaken bastard who had just slapped his own son silly.

"Mr. Regan, we weren't harming anybody. All we were after was some fresh bread and milk. We weren't stealing anything." In point of fact, occasionally Mr. Pruitt would catch some of us around the kitchen at night. He knew what we were up to, and he only shooed us away. Raiding the kitchen at Oxford Orphanage was a pastime engaged in by every orphan kid who ever lived there during my time. It was on par with climbing the high water tower or swimming in the pool at night, both of which were strictly forbidden, but I never heard of any kid getting punished for engaging in these two teenagers' diversions.

"But I don't want Troy hanging around with you boys. You all are a bad influence on him."

"Troy is a good friend of ours. But you never let him go to the picture shows with us, or even play touch football with us." Or steal and sell Musky Dines, I thought. I would ask Troy later about Musky dines.

"And he's not going to. I don't want to see you around my son anymore. Do you understand?"

"Yes, sir. I'm sorry you feel that way." And fuck you, No. 78 and 79.

Without further comment, Regan turned and walked toward his car. As he got into the driver's seat, Troy turned his face to the window, smiled, and I saw his hand and wrist come up from the bottom of the window, and he gave me a knowing wave of his hand.

Stay away from Troy? No way in hell. Troy was our friend. We just didn't bound up any more stairs and through any open windows together. In the days to come we kidded him about being slapped silly by his father, and told him now he knew how it feels to be an orphan. And we remained close friends until I left the orphanage in February 1957. As a favor to Troy, we taught him all the cuss words we knew, that he never would have picked up in his own household.

I left the orphanage on February 15, 1957, and graduated high school in Kinston in May of that year. On the morning of my classmates' graduation, I stopped by Raleigh and picked up Butch Mitchell, who also had not graduated from John Nichols High School, and we drove to the orphanage to see our former classmates graduate.

Anyway, after I left the orphanage in February, I enrolled in the high school in Kinston to finish out the year. It was the beginning of baseball season, and the team needed another pitcher, because one if its pitchers had been declared ineligible because he had exceeded the age requirement. So I became the team's second pitcher. We played sixteen games that Spring, I pitched in seven of them, and won five. I was awarded a letter in baseball, and the school gave me a nice school jacket. They were nice people, and although I was only at the school for about three and a half months, the students and faculty treated me as though I had gone to school there for four years.

Anyway, when Butch and I arrived for the graduation of our class, I was wearing my school jacket with the large yellow letter and baseball on it. I got close enough to my friend, E.T. Regan, for him to get a real good look at my jacket and letter. We did not speak, but I saw him get a good look at my jacket.

As I was chatting with some of my former classmates after the graduation ceremony, Troy came over and gave me a big hug. Then he slipped into my hand a small card, saying, "Put this in your pocket. Good luck to you," and left. When Butch and I got in my car to leave, I took the card out of my pocket. The card was a miniature diploma from John Nichols High School, one that the school gave as a memento to the graduating seniors. So the school had already made up the diploma when I left Oxford on February 15, 1957. Troy apparently could not swipe the real diploma, but he had taken the card-sized one. It was a nice gesture on a friend's part, and I still have the card today. Anyway, what are friends for, except to swipe miniature high school diplomas and (attempt to) raid kitchens together? E.T. Regan died years ago, but no doubt his last thought on this earth was of him slapping the pee out of his son outside the kitchen.

CHAPTER 70

But We Really Weren't Running Away

Butch Mitchell and his sister Jo Ann were from Raleigh, and during the time we were at Oxford, their mother still lived in the capitol. Butch and I were fourteen years old, and had just started ninth grade in the Fall of 1953.

One Friday night Butch got a hankering to visit his mother in Raleigh. Of course, we were strictly forbidden to leave the city of Oxford, and it was understood that if a child did leave the city limits, he or she would be "running away." Therefore, if the child were "caught running away," he or she would "suffer the consequences," one of which was always a severe beating by Mr. Regan or the other sadist Mr. Gray.

But, we really weren't running away. And Butch assured me nobody would miss us for the weekend. Sounded reasonable to me. But then again, Butch had this almost uncanny ability to make any chancy, illegal and foolhardy scheme appear perfectly logical and innocent. After all, only a few months before, Butch's "Baby Oinker Caper" could have landed us in the infamous Jackson Training School on a charge of "grand theft-pig." And about a year later I reached the same conclusion about Butch as I had about Coley Lee, this being that these two junior hardened criminals just didn't "give a happy damn" about anything that smacked of authority.

And as I desperately needed respite from all the "orphanage" trauma that was crowding my life in ninth grade, I readily agreed to accompany Butch for the weekend trip to the capitol. After all, we really weren't running away.

We had to work Saturday morning, so it was already late afternoon when we walked out the front gate like we were going to the picture show, except where College Street dead-ended at Hillsboro Street, we took a right (to Raleigh and Durham) instead of a left (to the Orpheum picture show), and pretty soon we were jerking our extended right thumbs in a southerly direction.

We weren't there very long until a kindly old white-haired man and his wife pulled their car to a stop on the shoulder of the highway just in front of where we were standing. Leaning across his wife, the old man asked Butch, who had poked his head in through the passenger side window,

"You boys from the orphanage?"

How could he possibly have thought that, I wondered. Stupid old man, of course we were from the orphanage. Where else would we be from? Old people sure get stupid fast. Damn!

"Yes, sir," replied Butch.

"Where you boys headed?"

"Raleigh, to visit my mother."

"Sure you boys aren't running away?"

"No, sir. We really aren't running away. We're just going to visit my mother in Raleigh," pleaded Butch.

After a long pause, the old man said, "Okay, you boys hop in, as long as you're not running away."

You ever get the feeling when you start out doing something that wasn't your idea in the first place, that somehow or other it just wasn't going to work out right? Anyway, at about this time I was getting just that feeling, like sixth sense or something, that I should have turned left at Hillsboro Street and gone on to the Orpheum anyway. Alone.

Butch and I were being chauffeured for the two-hour jaunt to the state capitol, we found out early on, by "Horace" and his wife of at least half a century, "Gertrude." Horace's nearly shoulder-length snow-white mane matched Gertrude's, and they looked an awful lot alike, so in addition to the couple's professed positive marital status, Butch and I suspected they might also be brother and sister which, in North Carolina during the early part of the twentieth century, well may have been the case. One never can tell. But they seemed happy, and that had to count for something. Shouldn't it? Not if they're committing incest, you say? Okay, whatever.

Seemed as though Senility, the Fifth Horseman of the Apocalypse, had grabbed Horace by the nape of the neck and was not gonna let go. The poor guy ran off at the mouth nonstop the entire trip, and at first we wondered why he seemed to be yelling at us, until Butch noticed these two large contraptions protruding from the octogenarian's middle ears that looked very much like a pair of Delco spark plugs.

In response to his finding, old Butch slowly put his hand on the door handle on his side of the back seat, preparing to make a swift exit from the moving vehicle should Horace prove not to be of this world. After all, we were just a few years into that 1947 Roswell, New Mexico little strange men from space thingy, and were living in uncertain times.

But I assured Butch (and myself) that I had noticed those really weird "plugs" in a Collier's magazine advertisement, and I thought these thingamajigs were called "hearing aids." Butch wasn't impressed; thought I was making up the part about hearing aids, said they still looked like "Delcos" to him, and kept his hand on the door handle "just in case".

At least old Butch wouldn't have been hurt seriously if he had to escape from the moving vehicle. About ten miles south of Oxford, approaching Creedmoor, I became quite concerned about our (lack of) land speed, and peering surreptitiously over Horace's right shoulder, noted that the speedometer on the dash of our 1949 metallic green Studebaker was registering a steady twenty-three miles per hour.

In our oft-benighted youth we kids could hardly tell the difference between an octogenarian and a nonagenarian; we also had great difficulty determining whether these old Southern Methuselahs were eighty, or ninety, years old. Horace's senility and Gertrude's anility had long since crawled beneath the thin, wrinkled and liver-spotted skin of these two old kindhearts, and Christian passivity and a post (Civil?) war upbringing appeared to be the angle iron that held together their existence.

And communicating with Horace was getting on my nerves. As was his humming of *The Battle Hymn of the Republic*, over and over again. And the old codger had about as much white hair growing out of his ears as I had on my head. Ohmigod! Here I was taking a daytrip with two, no, three really weird people, while my hero Lash LaRue was outdrawing some scrungy desperado at the Orpheum.

"Why are we going so slow," I yelled into Horace's right spark plug.

"Huh?" came the reply from the driver's seat.

"Why we going so darn slow?" I repeated, yelling even louder.

"No, it's not going to snow," Horace assured me.

Well, that was a conversation-ender for sure. Weren't gonna get anyplace talking to this geezer. Could I be the only sane occupant in the car? The only part of this Roadway Tragicomedy in One Act played by Gertrude, Horace's wife/sister, was to repeat "Yes, Horace," every time her husband/brother yelled anything. This seemed to assure Gertrude that Horace was still alive behind the wheel of their automobile, that resembled a giant Junebug and was traveling at about the same rate of speed. Of course, back then none of us had ever even been on a "four-lane" rural road, and didn't have the slightest inkling of what a "divided highway" was, so all the other southbound vehicles were passing us on the left (and right), and blowing their stupid horns at Horace. The poor sod doubtless never heard a one of those blaring, irritating horns. One man shook his fist as he came alongside Horace to pass us, and old unassuming Horace just returned the irritated motorist's "wave," smiling like they were old friends or something. This wasn't working out so well.

If it's true as they say that "ignorance is bliss," then old Horace had a Schlage deadbolt lock on "bliss." And in a lucid moment, if our driver had such an experience, he no doubt wondered why the stupid orphan kids sitting behind him thought it was going to snow.

It was long past nightfall when the two old fogies let us out on a street corner about twelve city blocks from Butch's house. We walked to a nearby café, where Butch telephoned his mother. No answer. She must be out shopping. Let's have some dinner. Looks like a nice café, and we're kinda hungry, what with listening to Horace's yelling for a couple of hours.

We ate. By that time it was getting on toward ten o'clock. Butch phoned home again. Still no answer. So we started walking the twelve long blocks to Butch's house.

It was nigh onto midnight when we arrived at our destination. Let's ring the doorbell. No answer. Let's knock. Same negative result. Let's go around the house and try the back door. Nope. We weren't getting anywhere. Let's try a side window. So we both cupped our palms and peered in through the window into the darkened living room. I was attempting to push up the lower window sash, when the stillness of night was broken suddenly by,

"What're you boys doing there?"

The squeaky voice from toward the front of the house sounded like it came from a teenager, and what he was doing really hacked me off, so I snapped back,

"Quit shining that goddamn flashlight in my eyes, you dumb idiot!"

"I'm a cop, dammit. Ya'll stop right where you are!"

In a *Man Against Crime* television show, my hero Ralph Bellamy would have added "Or I'll shoot!" However, this was a stupid twenty-year-old-at-the-outside Raleigh, North Carolina rookie cop working the night shift. Probably never had even shot his weapon, ever. He was still speaking soprano.

"I live here," stammered Butch, his shocked, quivering voice almost making his words appear a question rather than a statement.

"If you live here, why're you boys breaking in through the window."

I really didn't care for this punk's condescending tone of voice and air of superiority. But I let it slide for the moment. If the smartass young cop didn't have a gun, he never would have caught me in a footrace through the mean streets of Raleigh. I was fast.

But he did have a gun. So I decided to stay put . . . for the moment. I still had options. I was Little Orphan Al. I always had more options than Carter had Little Liver Pills. Butch finally recovered from his initial yellow-bellied shock to make up a lie.

"We weren't breaking in, we were just looking in."

I still couldn't tell whether Butch was making statements or asking questions. Neither the young cop nor I could tell whether Butch was really certain of what he was saying or doing. Which didn't help our case none. But Butch was correct. We were just looking in. Then we were going to break in. But for now we were just "looking in," or something like that.

"You boys come on out to the sidewalk," Boy Soprano ordered, waving his stupid flashlight toward the front of the house. Once the fool had stopped trying to blind me, I saw that his free hand was resting on the butt of this huge holstered revolver. If they ever made a picture show entitled *Wyatt Earp as a Stupid Child*, this kid cop could have had the lead role.

When we got to the sidewalk, we spotted a Raleigh police car on the street. Child Cop ordered us to "wait right here" and went over and called the police station dispatcher on his radio, informing the dispatcher that he had, as I recall, a "143," that in police jargon in Raleigh, North Carolina in 1953 probably meant "two probable runaways from Oxford Orphanage trying to break into a house that the frightened one claims belongs to his mother."

Butch seemed scared out of his wits. I also recall thinking just how comical was this whole farce. Not many months prior to this escapade, I had survived the brutality that was E.T. Regan and Pig Talton, and one thing I certainly wasn't, at age fourteen, was afraid.

I was not afraid of this snot-faced young cop, or the Raleigh police force, or anybody else. I just hoped, however, that the house we were just about to break into was indeed Butch's house. If not, we were in a bushel of trouble. If only we had gone to the Orpheum . . .

Anyway, Child Cop asked Butch his mother's name and telephone number. He then gave this information to the dispatcher, who confirmed that the information was correct. The three of us seemed relieved.

"Where do you boys live?"

"In Oxford," Butch offered, rather meekly.

"Oh, you boys are from the orphanage?"

"Yes, sir," replied Butch, just as meekly.

"Then you boys must be running away." It was a statement, a forensic conclusion arrived at by a trained criminal investigator. Child Cop's deductive reasoning and perceptive insight into the criminal mind was indeed mind-boggling. I was singularly impressed. The young jerkoff could put two and two together after all. But before I could tell the cop how stupid and childish I thought he was, ole Butch said, rather meekly, since by now my frightened buddy had cornered the market on "meekly,"

"But we really weren't running away."

That did it. All that wimpcrap from Butch was getting on my nerves. Child Cop weren't much taller than I, and I probably outweighed him. So I said, rather unmeekly,

"Listen, officer, we weren't running away from anything. We just came to visit Butch's mother for the weekend. We are in high school, and are allowed to go home on the weekends. We didn't know she wouldn't be home. Just leave us here and we'll wait for her on the porch." This lie was one of my many "options" referred to above. It would either work or it wouldn't.

Didn't work. Never hurts to try, though.

After thinking over my lie for a moment, Child Cop responded, almost with apology,

"You boys better come on down to the station, since we don't know when your mother will be home."

So we climbed into the back of the patrol car, and soon we were sitting in the police station waiting room. Child Cop went into a room off to the side of the booking desk, and Butch and I waited, as several young colored men, who appeared as though they were drunk and had been in a fight, were booked in at the front desk, then taken off stage left. Then we heard the loud "CLANG" that sounded an awful lot like a jail cell door closing in a B-western Sheriff's office, and I figured the colored drunk rowdies had been locked up safely for the night.

After awhile an older cop came out of the side room, and introduced himself as "Sergeant Baker." I took his word for it, since he had three sergeant's stripes on his sleeves. I had not seen any stripes on Child Cop's sleeves.

"Officer Abel tells me you boys ran away from the orphanage." It was a statement, but he obviously expected an answer. Abel? Baker? Is this some sort of joke, I thought? I half-expected "Charlie" to show up any minute now, with "Delta" and "Echo" in tow. And this "running away" business was beginning to frazzle my patience. I'd better set 'em straight, once and for all, right then and there. Understanding is good. Finality is good. Vacillation is bad. Misunderstanding is bad. And this comedy was fast becoming a tragedy, fraught with vacillation and misunderstanding.

For a newly-minted teenager my patience was seemingly infinite, but it was being sorely put to the test by the juvenile actions of my obtuse young comrade and this Southern cast of the Keystone Kops.

"Sergeant Baker, we're not running away from anything. We're in high school, and we are allowed to go home for the weekend. We just came to visit Butch's mother, and she was going to take us back tomorrow."

If it's true that we will go to hell for lying, then I know where I'll spend eternity. Yeah, me and a couple thousand Oxford orphans. And each of us will swear to the devil that we never told a lie. And the devil will not believe us any more than Sergeant Baker was believing me now.

"Anyway, she's not here now, so you boys'll have to stay here tonight, and we'll call the orphanage in the morning."

I didn't answer. Sergeant Baker seemed to be a nice guy, and I wasn't going to talk him out of anything, since he seemed to outrank everyone else there, and his weapon was just as big as Child Cop's. At least the sergeant had the courtesy not to rest his hand on the butt end of his gun. Child Cop was still resting his hand on his gun. It must have been glued there, or else he was one really insecure cop.

Receiving neither comment nor question, Sergeant Baker continued,

"I don't know where to put you boys, so it looks like you'll get to spend the night in jail. That okay with you boys?"

"Do we have a choice?"

"No."

"Okay, then I guess it's okay with us."

"Good."

Sergeant Baker, whose last conversational exchange contained absolutely no logic whatever, gave Butch and me each a sheet, blanket and pillow, and showed us to a jail cell on the side of the jail opposite from where they had locked up the three drunk colored men.

After we heard the "CLANG" of our cell door, Sergeant Baker said,

"I'm not going to lock you boys in. There's a bathroom down the hall. If you need anything, the midnight shift will be on in awhile."

Sergeant Baker paused, then added "And you boys stop running away." I was about to tell this Sergeant Baker what he could do to a rolling doughnut, but he had slipped away down the hall. Like I said a half dozen times already, we really weren't running away, but it seemed as though nobody was going to believe us anyway. Talk about stereotypes!

Suddenly, Butch got up from his bunk, went to the cell door, grasped a steel bar in each hand, shook the bars violently, and said in a gruff-voiced half-scream,

"Let me outta here, ya dirty screws. I ain't no stoolie!"

"What the hell you talking about, Butch?" I asked, quite puzzled at his sudden strange behavior. He couldn't have already gone "stir crazy," hell, we'd only been in the (very small, confined, bars-enclosed) prison cell about thirty seconds at the most.

"Nothing," said Butch. "I heard James Cagney scream that line in a picture show one time, so I wanted to see how it felt."

Then, following a (very) brief interval of sanity, Butch asked,

"You heard them colored guys yet?"

"I ain't heard nothing. We supposed to hear the colored guys?"

"Yeah."

"You want to tell me why, or are we going to play guessing games?"

"Everybody knows the cops beat the colored guys with rubber hoses when they get 'em in jail."

Butch stated this staunchly immutable fact while looking in the direction the cops had taken the colored drunks, like he likely would hear at any moment solid black rubber truncheons, standard issue for mid-twentieth century redneck Raleigh cops, making solid contact with the heads of three drunk colored guys, followed rapidly by the certain yelps of pain from these same inebriated prisoners.

But it was an interesting concept, I thought. Back on East Bright Street during pre-orphanage times, when the colored guys talked about rubber hoses, I naively assumed they were going to water their lawns. But come to think about it, none of the colored men had grass in front of their shacks, it was mostly dirt and trash and tobacco juice. I'm certain the colored men in Kinston would think a "lawn" was when you "borra" money.

"You see that in a picture show, too?"

"Yeah."

If this "strange behavior" crap continued, I was going to ask the sergeant for a cell of my own. We had only been locked up for a few minutes, and already ole Butch was losing touch with reality. And I would definitely ask the sergeant to lock Butch's cell door for the night.

But then again, I thought, in Butch's favor was the fact that he hadn't told everyone in the orphanage who would listen, that Raleigh was The World's Foremost Tobacco Center, like that stupid kid from Kinston.

By this time, from sheer mental and physical exhaustion, Butch and I fell asleep on our metal bunks. Presently I was awakened by the "CLANG" of our cell door opening and, looking up, I saw a different cop with the same number of stripes on his shirtsleeves as had the perceptive and insightful Sergeant Baker, enter the cell and exclaim loudly,

"What the hell are you boys doing in here?"

At the same time, he turned to the stripe-less young officer standing behind him, and asked the officer, "Who put these kids in this goddamn jail cell? Jesus Christ, what's wrong with you people?"

Then to us, in a softer tone, the (apparent) night shift sergeant said, with a wave of his hand,

"You boys come on out here. Let's go down to the courtroom, and you boys can spend the night there. Bring your bedsheets and pillows."

Once we got to the small courtroom down the hall, the sergeant said,

"Sergeant Baker tells me you boys ran away from the orphanage. That right?"

"No sir," I replied, "we really weren't running away."

"What happened, then?"

So I briefly explained everything to him, the whole truth, including the blatant lie about us being in high school and having permission to go home on the weekends.

After hearing my tale of woe and misunderstanding, the sergeant nodded his understanding and empathy.

"Well, you boys just sleep here on the courtroom benches tonight, and in the morning we'll have some breakfast and I'll call the orphanage."

The sergeant awakened us early the next morning, the cook brought us jail breakfast on metal trays, that consisted of scrambled eggs, toast, bacon and milk, and afterwards we sat in the courtroom until about noon when Mr. Regan arrived to take us back to the orphanage, from which we most assuredly had *not* run away.

While sitting on the courtroom bench waiting for Mr. Regan, Butch expressed his concern that Regan would give us a whipping. I assured Butch that no harm would come to us.

"How can you tell?"

"I just know. Trust me, he'll never touch us."

Regan escorted us to his car, and opened the back door like he was a stupid valet or something. As we started to get into the car, he said,

"What are you boys running away for?"

"But we really weren't running away."

And I told Regan the whole story. And he didn't believe me. But he never touched us, because my brother Doc still possessed "The Pictures."

Mr. Regan stopped his car on the circular driveway in front of 4-B, and as we exited the back seat, he said,

"Now, you boys go on back to your cottage, and don't ever let me catch you running away again."

And as I walked away from the car, I turned, looked the mean old bastard in the eye, and said,

"But Mr. Regan, we really weren't running away."

He didn't answer me, but as he drove away, I knew he didn't believe me. But the only thing that matters now is that you believe me, when I tell you in all honesty that "we really weren't running away."

A parting word about my little wimp-buddy Butch. If he ever again mentioned that we should go to visit his mother in Raleigh for the weekend, it would take a team of proctologists and surgeons to extract my brogue from his rear. And he'd better start being a little more assertive when dealing with stupid kid cops and other overreaching grownups. Butch had better straighten up and fly right. Or else.

CHAPTER 71

Life Becomes a Little Easier

My last few years at Oxford passed with relative freedom from harassment by grownups. I played varsity football for four years. In 1955 the Masons constructed a modern basketball gymnasium on the site of the football practice field adjacent to the school, complete with "glass" backboards and retractable bleachers. I became a co-captain of the orphanage's first modern-era conference basketball team.

I played right field on the varsity baseball team my Freshman and Sophomore years. Archie Capps and a few of the lesser (in terms of athletic ability) players couldn't hit southpaws worth a flip, so Coach Talton asked me if I would become the sorta unofficial team batting coach, especially since the majority of my teammates' batting averages started with a big fat "point zero," followed by two numbers each of which was no greater than five. I did what I could to help out the team. Unappreciated, as usual.

Anyway, we traveled to "away" games on a converted school bus. Now, in 1955 North Carolina the speed limit for school buses was 35 miles per hour. On any street or road. Period. One sunny Spring afternoon we were returning from a game with Roxboro, where I went four-for-four with two towering 450-foot homers, Archie Capps and Bill Herrington went their usual embarrassing zip-for-four, and the rest of the team fell somewhere between "zip-for" and "two-for." I told

Archie and Bill it might be better for the morale of the team if they sat at the back of the bus. Our catcher, Charlie Gibbs, was explaining to Odis Hutchins and Red Albertson, since we had lost the game to Roxboro by a score of 9-4, that, unfortunately Steve Faucette had not hurled a shutout. Pretty soon we were going to run out of room at the back of the bus.

After cresting a long hill, the road dropped sharply on the downhill trod, and when the bus leveled out at the bottom of the hill, we heard the familiar wail of a siren that in that era could only be attached to the top of a patrol car driven by a Royal North Carolina Redneck Mountie. To this day the biggest, meanest overweight cops I've ever seen were those goddamn 1950's-era North Carolina highway patrolmen. I've watched as civilians crossed the street just so they wouldn't have to meet these mean bastards on the sidewalk. And that's the truth. Scary, it was.

Figuring the siren didn't concern us, old unassuming Coach Talton just kept on driving the converted school bus, until the patrol car pulled alongside the front of the bus, the cop screamed a string of obscenities at old Pig Talton, and the coach pulled the bus onto the side of the highway.

The patrol car pulled off the two-lane macadam behind us, and a grossly overfed Mountie (reminded me of Wun Hung Lo) with some effort extricated himself from the vehicle, approached the driver's side window, and the following verbal exchange ensued.

An Indignant Coach Talton: "What's the problem, officer?"

A Confident Redneck Mountie: "Do you know how fast you were going?"

A Slightly Confused Coach Talton: "Uh, I'm not sure, officer."

Overfed Highway Patrolman: "You were going 38 miles per hour. You were speeding, sir."

A Now Really Confused Coach Talton: "But the speed limit is 45 miles per hour."

Increasingly Irritated Mountie: "Not for a school bus, it ain't."

A Suddenly Confident Coach Talton: "But this is not a school bus. It's a baseball team bus."

Red-Faced, Visibly Upset Mountie: "What color is the vehicle, sir?"

The grossly overweight cop spat out the words color, vehicle and sir like he didn't like Pig Talton's attitude one bit.

A Once Again Puzzled Pig Talton: "Why, it's yellow, of course."

Confident, Arrogant Mountie: "Yer damn tootin' it is. If it's painted yellow and looks a lot a school bus, buddy, the speed limit in this state for school buses is 35 miles per hour. So you, sir, were speeding."

And our coach remained very, very quiet while the grossly overweight, smug-faced Mountie wrote ole Pig Talton a speeding ticket for going 38 miles per hour in a school bus that really wasn't a school bus. The stupid cop better be glad Pig Talton didn't have his trusty five-foot-long tobacco stick with him, that's all I can say. And as we continued on our (under 35 miles per hour) journey home, Bill Herrington tried to ask me what had occurred, but I couldn't hear him from his seat at the rear of the bus.

For reasons known only to himself, I am certain, Coach Talton insisted on giving a pep talk to each player before the boy went to the plate to bat. Didn't matter if you were the first player to bat in the first inning, you still got the lecture. Never could quite figure that one out. Oxford Orphanage seemed to have an unfair share of grownup yahoos that I couldn't figure out.

We boys showed our defiance against abusive grownups on campus by counting the number of times we could mutter "Fuck you" under our breath while being "put in our place."

But our beloved Coach Talton deserved better treatment than this denigrating slur. Instead, because we thought it appropriate, we kids substituted "oink-oink" for the usual "Fuck you," and astute young grammarian that I was, I quickly discovered that, because the words fuck, you and oink, in addition to being monosyllables, are all one-syllable words, the time elapsed for the two slurs was exactly the same.

Without a great deal of fanfare, my group of high school friends tried to put an end to the abuses of the 4-B boys, and this cut down on some of the ingrained pattern of 4-B boys picking on the younger kids.

And I am proud that we 3-B boys did not become hated "Big Boys." Those poor preteen boys caught enough abuse from Gray, Regan, Tom Adams, Bob Davis and a host of other cottage counselors, teachers and work supervisors. I felt sorry for the younger boys.

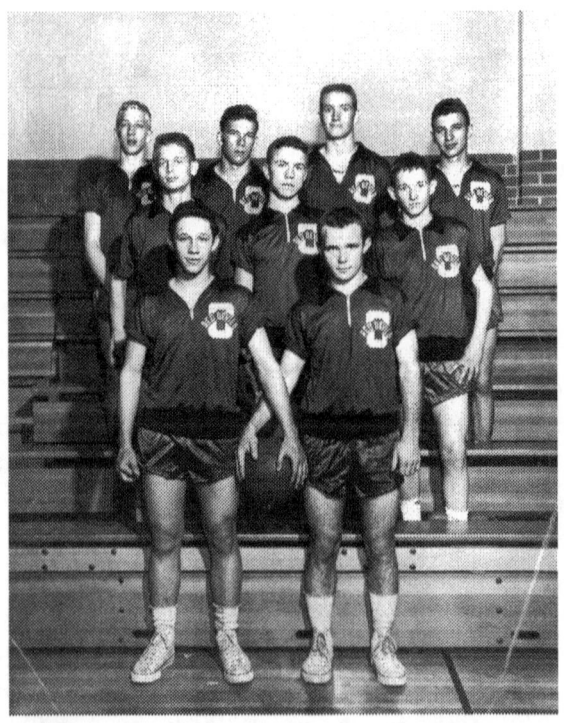

1955. Oxford Orphanage's first modern era basketball team. First row: Paul Tausch, Van Edwards. Second row: Charlie Burton, Laylon Jordan, Larry Mumford. Third row: Troy Regan (Mr. Regan's son), the author, Red Albertson, Dalma Evans.

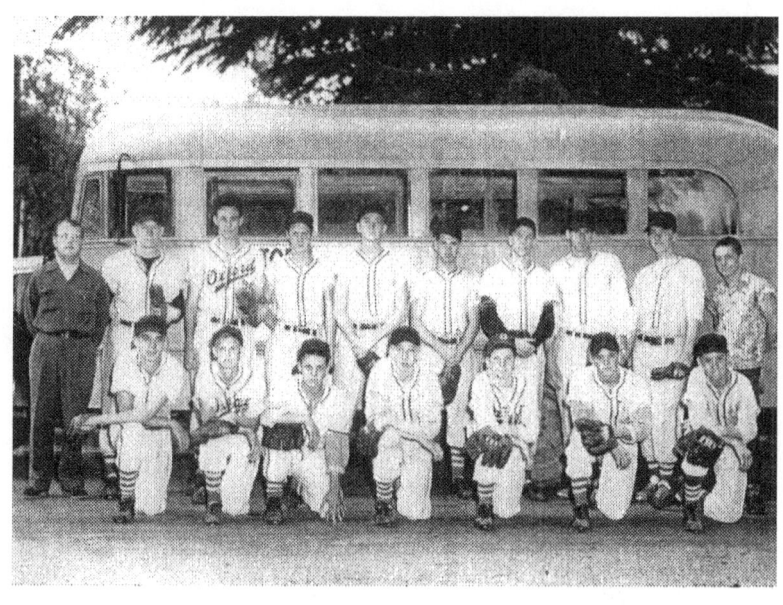

1955 Varsity Baseball Team. Front row: Dalma Evans, Charlie Burton, Bill (.145) Herrington, Troy Regan (Mr. Regan's son), Heman McLendon, Marvin Smith, Jimmy Cox. Back row: Coach "speedy" Talton, Archie (.170) Capps, Charlie Gibbs, Benny Hughes, Red Albertson, Odis Hutchins, Al (.406, with dark sleeves) Provost, Stephen Faucette, Ronald Bullock and Jimmy Frederick. The bus is not a "school" bus, but a "baseball team" bus.

Undoubtedly the biggest mistake any 4-B bully could make was to pick on a 3-B boy's younger brother. Even today that bully's stupidity amazes me.

CHAPTER 72

"Pupils Who Left for Other Reasons"

Alas, E.T. Regan and his Siamese twin child abuser, Reverend A. DeLeon Gray, just refused to admit certain defeat. In November 1956, during my Senior year, Mr. Gray announced one day that there would be a curfew, beginning that same night, and that roll would be called at the end of study hall, that is, at 9:00 p.m. Any boy who missed curfew would be expelled immediately. For good. Forever.

This is a story about trust, and friendship, and the limits some brave boys are willing to go to prove that they are indeed your friends. Those boys didn't let me down because they knew if the tables were turned, I would not let them down either.

An example of just how much Doc's eight-by-ten glossies of my bruised backside stuck in Regan and Gray's throat like a molasses-less peanut butter sandwich, is shown by the Boys' Declamation Contest of 1955. Archie Capps, then a Senior, and I entered the declamation contest that year. I was a lowly Sophomore. However, Little Orphan Al's oratory skills being second only to those of Socrates, I won handily over all the lesser participants. On page 88 of the 1955 high school yearbook, *The Log*, is a picture of Archie, wearing a smirk of envy, and Little Orphan Al, wearing that old winner's smile. Beneath Archie's unsmiling face us printed "Honorable Mention," and everybody knows that that means he didn't win. Beneath Little Orphan Al's grinning face is printed "Winner of Oxford Lodge No. 122 Medal."

At year's end all the awards were given out personally by E.T. Regan, as principal of the school. The son of a bitch refused to present the Oxford Lodge No. 122 Medal. And all my classmates and friends knew exactly why.

Anyway, at the time Mr. Gray called the curfew, Melda had been gone for some time, and I had sniffed out one of the town girls who had some but not all of Melda's qualities, and because I had already promised this town girl I would walk her home after study hall ended, being a man of honor, I kept my word. Well, she and I got all tangled up in the dark of her front porch, and I did not get back to 3-B until well after eleven o'clock. We were playing a game called "stuck pig" and "root hog."

Mrs. Noell, the cottage counselor, was a pretty good friend of mine, and she was waiting up for me with the door of her apartment open. She told me Mr. Regan had checked at 9:00 p.m. and again at 10:00, and knew I had not made curfew. The following day Mr. Gray told me I had to go home. So I packed my clothes, said my farewells to the guys, and got on the bus for Kinston. Stoicism had already by that time in my young life crawled under my skin, so I took this episode in stride just like I've done so the remainder of my life. Get excited? Not me. Or I. After age fourteen I didn't get excited about anything. Stupid pricks thought they were finished with Little Orphan Al. If it were only that easy.

I arrived in Kinston that evening, and the next day enrolled at Grainger High School. No problem. Three days later I had to stop by the principal's office to fill out some transfer forms, and I literally bumped into Red Albertson coming out of the principal's office.

"What the hell are you doing here, Red," I asked in mild shock.

"Well, when the bastards let you go, we boys got to thinking that the best way to get you back was to miss curfew. So four of us did, and old man Gray sent us home. But we won't be away for long."

"Why so?"

"Because the Masons won't stand for it."

Friendship. Can't beat it with a stick. So the following night Dan Cook of the Kinston Masonic Lodge stopped by my home, introduced himself to mama, and asked if I wanted to return to Oxford. The next day the five of us boys returned to Oxford. Another "W" for Little Orphan Al, with some help from my buddies, and another big fat "L" for those two arrogant dickheads.

In helping me, my friends had caused us to lose the last game of the football season. We were scheduled to trounce Chapel Hill High School, like we had trounced most of the teams we played that season. Chapel Hill beat us by a score of 20-0. On page 138 of the 1957 yearbook, *The Log*, is the following statement.

"Playing without the services of four first stringers, including two co-captains, the Red Devils were upset by the Chapel Hill Wildcats by a score of 20-0 at Chapel Hill on November 9th."

I had lived with the majority of these boys for nearly a decade. They knew of me as a person of character, and they knew I would have done the same for them. I was proud of them for the stand they took. And Marvin Smith, Bill Herrington, Red Albertson and Van Edwards' brother Wayne were proud of the stand they took. Friendship. Priceless.

But my "nine lives" were being exhausted, one miserable life at a time. On page seventeen of the Eighty-Fifth Annual Reports of Oxford Orphanage, dated December 31, 1957, are noted the following comments:

Pupils returned to relatives during year 31
Pupils who ran away during year 3
Pupils who left for other reasons 1

In February 1957 I was seventeen and was looking forward to graduation in May. My brother Pete was thirteen and living in 4-B. One Sunday morning as we were dressing to go to (and then skip) church in downtown Oxford, one of my friends from 4-B came upstairs into my dorm room, and informed me that his brother had just beat up my younger brother.

I told my friend to tell his brother, a loudmouthed bully who was every bit my size, to meet me in my dorm room immediately. A few minutes later the bully walked into my room, and I hit him three times in the mouth before he hit the floor. He ended up in the first floor boys' ward at Hicks Memorial Hospital, with a broken nose, black eye and a few really ugly-looking bruises around his mouth. I went by to see him in the hospital, and told him what would happen to him if he ever touched Pete again. He apologized for what he had done.

The following Tuesday morning I was in math class when I was summoned to Mr. Regan's office, where I discovered the two Hounds from Hell, Regan and Gray, seated expectantly at Regan's desk.

Mr. Gray informed me he had spoken to the bully, who confirmed that he had indeed assaulted my kid brother. However, the superintendent said, the bully's relatives had threatened to bring a legal action against the orphanage if I remained at Oxford. Mr. Gray conceded, however, that if he sent me home, the Masons would likely bring me back. You see, Kinston Masons did not really care that much for the Reverend A. DeLeon Gray. Therefore, Mr. Gray pleaded, would I consider leaving voluntarily.

It suddenly came to me that it was time to go, and I could breeze through the last three months of my senior year at Kinston. So I told Mr. Gray I would leave, if it would save the orphanage from any possible legal liability. Mr. Gray thanked me for my cooperation, and I shook hands with both men.

That afternoon I said my farewells to Mrs. Ligon, Mr. Davis, Mr. McSwain, and even shook hands with Mr. Talton, who wished me well. I stopped by the hospital and said my fond farewell to Mrs. Mary Daniel, and asked her if I might have a word with the bully. I very calmly told the boy that if I ever heard from my kid brother, I would return one night and it wouldn't go well for him. He said he understood. He never bothered my kid brother again. That night I said goodbye to my friends, and told them I would see them at their graduation in May.

So this was the reason for that really odd entry on page 17 of the Eighty-fifth Annual Reports of Oxford Orphanage,

Pupils Who Left for Other Reasons 1

The "1" was Little Orphan Al. I was likely the only orphan in ten years who left the orphanage through negotiation, because not only would Dan Cook have brought me back, my brother Doc would have exposed Regan's brutality and Gray's knowledge of it.

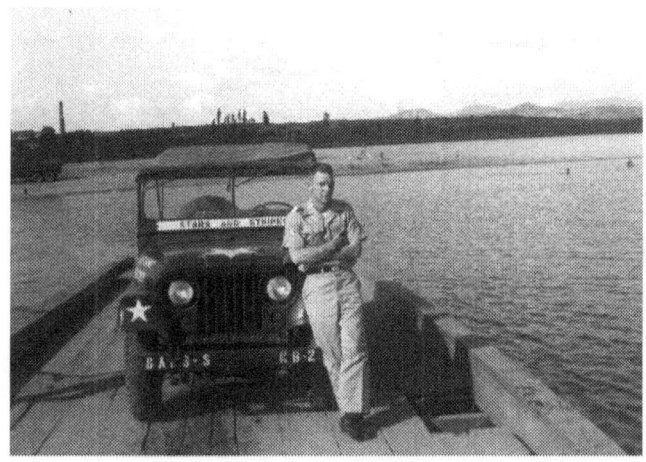

1962. South of Seoul, South Korea. The author crossing the Han River on a vehicle pole barge, on assignment with *The Pacific Stars and Stripes*.

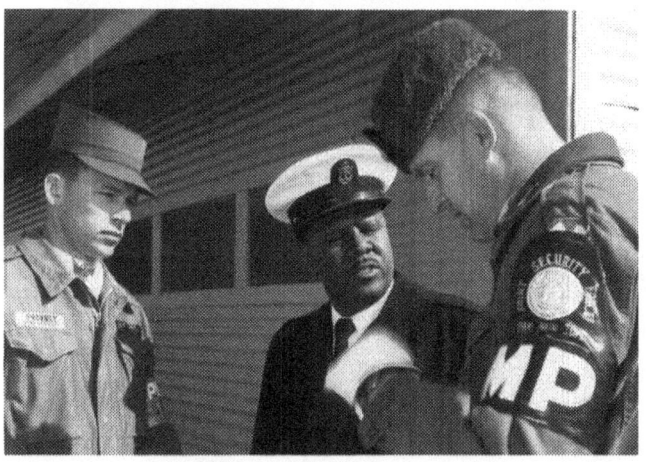

1962. Panmunjom, Korea. Covering the Military Armistice Commission (MAC) meeting for *The Pacific Stars and Stripes*. The author (left) with a U.S. Navy officer and a U.S. Army MP.

CHAPTER 73

On the Occasion of My Departure from "This Damned Place"

With remarkable clarity I recall the early morning of February 15, 1957. Walking briskly through a light albeit freezing rain down the center of the Main Road after declining the offer of a lift to the Oxford bus station by Lucifer's favorite dog E.T. Regan, laden down with a bushel basketful of confusing emotions, I negotiated my final, irrevocable and (non?)nostalgic left turn onto College Street at the Main Gate, never once pausing to glance back at my home of the last decade, terminating one chapter in my young life's journey while simultaneously (and apprehensively?) opening another, hopefully more promising one.

Oxford Orphanage had been for me a heartbreaking, demoralizing, agonizing experience, impossible to describe in simple terms or a few pages of stilted prose. At times I felt as though my young life, far from being simply a normal period of growth and advancement, was on hold, suspended, if you will, as though I were traveling the wrong way on a one-way street, or stuck permanently going up the down-staircase.

But hopefully at this juncture in my journey toward young adulthood and beyond, I finally had the worst behind me. And I realized at that very moment I had become the person I would forever be, that my attitude toward people, my ethics, morals and personality, had been molded by years of living in a place I never was supposed to be, that I had indeed finally survived the aforementioned "goddamn orphanage thing," with my sanity intact and a positive outlook on life that would carry me far in this post-orphanage world.

The "Oxford" experience had left on my life an impression as indelible as a 1947 Black Ford sedan's whitewalls across a 1940's deep piney woods lovers' lane. Fortunately, however, my mind has been astute enough to winnow out the childhood detritus foisted upon me by uncaring, abusive grownups.

The unwelcomed cycle of events through which each timid, apprehensive and guileless seven-year-old orphaned child passed during that seminal period in life known universally as "growing up," was accentuated, at least for the period of time between the ages of seven and fifteen, by the constant daily realization that the hapless youngster was wholly at the mercy of often truculent, detestable, Fascist-trained grownup orphanage staff members. The singular constant tangible intangible notion that pervaded and dominated our youth was FEAR, most assuredly an all-capper, and we children spent our waking hours, or so it seemed, ducking beneath the scudding clouds of quaking disquietude.

Underneath the constantly shifting circumstances of my mistreatment at the hands (literally) of callous and uncaring adults, the intangible notions of honesty, duty and responsibility had become quite difficult to bring to the boil of my understanding, to the extent that eventually I felt forced by circumstances to become the absolute master of guile, cunning and craftiness, that threatened on more than one depressing occasion to cull the time-tested Christian concepts of honesty, duty and responsibility from my psyche. My life at Oxford was characterized by continuing and unwanted vicissitudes inherent in life in a large postwar Southern orphanage, and the direction of my life's fortunes was about as predictable and certain as finding a needle in a stack of identical needles.

However, I simply refused to be swallowed up by the maw of the pervasive abuse and lack of genuine concern for my welfare, and with a great deal of effort, fortunately I survived Oxford Orphanage with my dignity intact.

At no time during my ten-year stay did I ever feel a physical, emotional or spiritual merging of my being with the fiber of the orphanage, nor did I ever get a sense that I "belonged" in "this damned place." My stay in this foreign land, though quite defined in the number of years, was excruciatingly unbounded in effect, and I realized I had been, and would likely forever be, an "outsider" in my relationship with Oxford Orphanage. And that suited me just fine.

Often I am reminded of Dickens' thoughts at age twelve after being sent from home to work for a manufacturer of boot blacking, a circumstance that gave the young lad a sense of abandonment by his family, when he wrote

> "No advice, no counsel, no encouragement, no consolation, no
> support from anyone that I can call to mind, so help me God."

My youthful search for identity, for who I was and what I stood for, for what my place was in my shattered and highly structured world, grew eventually into an adult pragmatism that has been with me for nearly half a century. If there is a singular quality I gained from the experience of my childhood, it is determination to complete any task once started, and to fear no person or situation. And I planned to change my name from Little Orphan Al Milquetoast to Little Orphan Al Determined.

On that rainy, wind-swept departure from Oxford Orphanage, I carried the following tangible items:

1. My treasured Dr. Grabow walnut smoking pipe, that Henry Martin had purchased for me as a "present" for my brother Doc in the Summer of 1953.
2. My cherished and much-used Barlow pocket knife given to me as a present by my brother Bill while I was on vacation in the Summer of 1951.
3. My Bulova men's wristwatch, a "present" to me from the Masons of North Carolina, that I discovered while shamelessly opening already-wrapped Christmas presents in the downstairs Toy Room of the Industrial Building in December 1949.
4. The medium-sized suitcase full of mint-condition funny books, again a "gift" from these same benevolent Masons, accumulated

from numerous already-brightly-wrapped Christmas presents that same December 1949.

5. A large black suitcase crammed full of my clothes plus many more new outfits swiped from the Industrial Building the night before my departure by my friends.

6. Two brand-spanking new twenty dollar bills given to me by my friend Maurice Parham, the orphanage business manager, the afternoon before my departure. The two twenty dollar bills came from Mr. Parham's billfold, not from a desk drawer.

And in addition to the aforementioned corporeal items, I carried with me a heart filled with hope and enough confidence to overflow the dairy's manure wagon.

I had emerged from my laborious ten-year odyssey with my dignity intact, fully prepared to enter my post-orphanage life with pluck, spunk and determination. Along this arduous path I had had the distinct pleasure of developing lifelong friendships. Some wise sage once surmised that we can never understand a person unless we have first walked in his shoes. For ten years I had the oftentimes excruciating and depressing experience of walking in the shoes of hundreds of boys and girls who found themselves in my same or similar situation in life. And I understand. I understand these brothers and sisters and their grief, heartache, disappointment and sense of abandonment. We all shared a common fate.

Along my way to the bus station in downtown Oxford, and not even attempting to control the sudden flood of tears, I consciously resolved to leave behind me this poignantly unhappy chapter of my life, to make my way in this world, to get as much education as possible, to avoid a life of bets, guesses and maybes, to overcome all obstacles, to be a success. From that day forward I would embark upon my own course through life, never looking back, from then on doing it my way, braking and accelerating, but at my own pace, in my own time. My march into my new life was made with a quiet determination. The date was ten years to the day after I first arrived at Oxford Orphanage.

On the advent of my last day at Oxford, I did not get the sense of leaving behind my dozens of "brothers" and "sisters"-we would remain friends for life. But I was severing ties with the part of my life for which no one could ever have prepared me. My departure from Oxford most assuredly occasioned no terribly aching regret on my part. No doubt it created much relief in the homes of Mr. Regan and Mr. Gray, because my brother Doc still possessed "The Pictures."

And as the bus pulled away from the station for the three-hour return to 208 East Bright Street and what I was confident was still The World's Foremost Tobacco Center, fidgeting with not my second grade report card of ten years prior but with my twelfth grade report card, the salient, still unanswerable question continued to elude my sense of the rational, and haunt my soul-Why me?

And somewhere along the North Carolina highway, sitting directly behind the unsuspecting bus driver, prepared to viciously attack him should he attempt to make a U-turn and head back to Oxford, I sensed the past ten years of my life folding into my present. But would it ever? And would my past forever be, and forever control, my future?

But alas, there is no "statute of limitations" on the memories of personal grief and heartache. The subconscious may attempt to suppress these recollections; however, the great storehouse of the mind has recorded them indelibly, retrieving them with a force of will over which we seem powerless to control. Can't erase them from my mind. Can't ignore them. Can't reconcile them with any logical reasoning. They are mine, forever, and will follow me to my gibbet.

In this grand "walking shadow" we call "life," the passage of time will never transform a brick wall into a speed bump, nor convert a glacial crevasse into a mere pothole on the oversized panoramic screen of human experience. To the contrary, physical abuse, neglect and mental suffering, however brief or prolonged, however severe, however motivated, leave impressions on the memory and psyche of small children as indelible as a hydrogen bomb blast on the Eniwetok atoll.

Routine physical abuse suffered in childhood at the hands of bullying and insensitive grownups will never be transformed with the passage of time into harmless-appearing anecdotal humor. Painful childhood experiences should never become glossed over, denied, ignored or excluded from the conscious. My sheer indignation at the pervasive mistreatment we young orphans suffered as guileless, innocent children, at the hands of these human predators, prevented me from repressing such memories, and I believe I am a better person because of this attitude.

Often I analogize my ten years of life at Oxford with the weather. At times it would be sunny and clear. On other occasions there would come a light rain, just enough to water the beautiful flowers. Interspersed among sunny, clear days and pretty flowers, however, were long, foreboding intervals of lighting (striking thrice, and very, very close), booming thunder, and ominous rain clouds dark enough to block out the sun for extended periods of time.

My mistreatment at the hands (literally) of some members of the teachers and staff at the orphanage, and the blatant and pervasive use of indiscriminate and often brutal beatings inflicted upon many of the orphanage children, brought a salient and nagging question to my mind, even at an early age. Were the children of Oxford Orphanage sent there to be nourished, educated and cared for, or simply to be warehoused until they finished high school?

Although I take pride in furthering my vocabulary in this rich and beautiful English language of ours, still at times it has been nigh onto impossible to find the words, ideas and expressions that truly literalize my thoughts and feelings concerning my life at Oxford. Unfortunately my good friend Gene Autry's "Happy Trails" did not run anywhere near Oxford, North Carolina.

Was I looking for peace, or contentment, or happiness at the end of this seemingly never-ending arc of a rainbow colored in shades of tragedy? Subconsciously perhaps, I expected some sort of resolution, or finality, at the end of my journey. But this never came to pass.

My life since Oxford has been filled with accomplishments, occasioned by study and hard work, and for the forty years preceding my return to homecoming in 1997 at age fifty-eight, my previous life was pushed into the background, but never forgotten.

Eternity and infinity are not the same, but neither are these two entities mutually exclusive. At Oxford my perpetually benighted, oppressed youth seemed to last an eternity; my torment at the hands of my despised Nazi concentration camp guards appeared to be infinite indeed.

And a final word about this elusive concept, "home." Home is where the heart is. Nearly every child at Oxford came from a broken home.

Never once did we entertain the thought that Oxford Orphanage was home. Not even close.

Escapees and graduates alike refrain from stating that "Oxford Orphanage was my home." Rather, we 'sylum dogs tend to use the benign expression "Oxford Orphanage is where I grew up." In our mature, experienced minds we are drawing a meaningful distinction between the place we dreamed would exist for a lifetime, and the latitude and longitude surface coordinates where we languished broken-spirited and for the most part unloved throughout the Maker's greatest gift to us all, our childhood.

And if we take a bushel basket and gather up all the clichés, trite remarks and outworn expressions, for example, "it's the luck of the draw," "well that's life," "you gotta play the hand you're dealt," "make the best of a bad situation," et cetera ad infinitum, I still am left with the singular, unanswerable question, namely, Why me?

And in what I expect to be a close footrace, should death finally overtake and consume my immortality, I wish the reader to know that never was I able to answer that question posed by orphans worldwide.

And alas, you will have to be satisfied with this truncated version of my miserable life at Oxford Orphanage. The unabridged version of my story would occupy a space parallel to the first six volumes of the Encyclopedia Britannica, requiring the use of Köchel numbers to maintain order.

In retrospect, in my heart of hearts, if over the years some Masons (and God bless them all for their love and generosity) had taken the time to study the facts before them in the Annual Reports of Oxford Orphanage, sensed that something was greatly amiss here, and carried out an investigation, which was their right and duty, the likes of A. DeLeon Gray, E.T. Regan, Tom Adams, Mamie Baldwin and others would have been fired from their positions at Oxford Orphanage outright, and the lives of hundreds of orphan children would have turned out for the better. But alas, this did not happen.

I am often reminded of a passage from T.S. Eliot's *The Dry Salvages*.
"Lying awake, calculating the future,
Trying to unweave, unwind and unravel,
And piece together the past and the future."

God, it's hard to do! Still, at times of quiet and solemn pause here in the latter years of a long and prosperous adulthood, I sit alone with my past, idly scanning the pages of my dimly-fading memory, reflecting, dissecting and wondering-Why? I don't know. Life is filled with odd occurrences. Some of them really, really odd. Oxford Orphanage was odd.

Was Oxford Orphanage just another detour on my travels down that great interstate called "life?" Or, was my life before and after Oxford Orphanage the detour? Was it fate that carried me on this ten-year odyssey into abuse, heartache, confusion and self-discovery?

Enough of this. I have about had it up to here in the matter of Oxford Orphanage and its influence on my life. I trust the reader has gained something from my *Reflections*, and that he or she was able to place himself or herself in my shoes for a brief time.

Assuming that the greatest of all levelers, the unforgiving Law of Averages, makes no special allowances for old 'sylum dogs, my license on this life likely will expire sometime within the next two decades, and Jehovah has informed me, with the appropriate apologies, that unfortunately He cannot renew the entitlement, nor even grant an extension. Not even for Little Orphan Al.

But that's okay. I understand. At least the All-Powerful has allowed me to complete with good health and dignity what I refer to as The Full Circle, and for this consideration I am in His debt.

My daddy was buried in Maplewood Cemetery in Kinston on February 11, 1946. Mama was buried beside my daddy on March 1, 1962. All four of my beloved grandparents are buried in Maplewood Cemetery. I intend to purchase a plot as close to my parents as possible, and my children have promised me that should my wife of thirty-five years precede me in death, they will honor my wishes in this regard.

Try as I might over the years, I cannot bring myself to believe in the afterlife, in any conceptual form. However, it is my desire to be in death as close as possible to the two kind and dear persons who are responsible for my life on this earth. And should I be mistaken concerning the existence of the hereafter, I want to be close enough to tell these two dear beings just how much they mean to me, and how much I love them.

At this crossroads of my life, more of my soul (and body) rests at the bottom of the hourglass of time than at the top. "The Moving Finger writes; and, having writ, moves on. And all your piety and wit will not change a single line."

And I still love my daddy. And I still wonder Why?

EPILOGUE

Life After Oxford

As you have seen, I did indeed (barely) survive the bloody decade-long "detour" in my life, that nine-miles-high speed bump that was Oxford Orphanage. I'll be brief. If you don't like this book, tear out the last six or seven pages, return it to the bookstore as "defective," and trade it in for a book entitled, appropriately for you, "How to Appreciate Good Literature." I won't be offended. So long as I don't find out what you did to my book.

Anyway, when I got off the bus at Kinston, and walked the eight city blocks home, Dan Cook of the Kinston Masonic Lodge was deep into a conversation with mama, both of them sipping Dr. Peppers. I was envious. A few years before my departure from Oxford, mama had married a successful photographer, and they had moved into his home on Caswell Street, right next door to Ersul Sowers' aunt. Ersul's aunt and mama used to travel together to visit us kids one Sunday each month, and we enjoyed some nice Sunday afternoon picnics together.

Dan Cook had already heard what had occurred at Oxford. He asked me if I wanted to return to Oxford. I thanked him graciously, but said no, I could make it at home for the next three months. Mr. Cook then asked if I would come live with him, his wife Becky and their three daughters until I graduated high school. He complained that he had never had a son, so at least he could discover what it was like to have a son. I was honored, and spent three wonderful months with a loving Masonic family.

I earned a letter in baseball as the team's second pitcher, got tagged with the nickname "Einstein," and discovered that two of the Sophomore girls had tongues just about as long as Melda's. On graduation night, the high school principal had me stand up in the auditorium, and expressed his regret that I could not have spent the last four years at Wheat Swamp High School. I was deeply honored. Mama and her husband and Mr. Cook and his family all shared the moment. I cried. Mama cried. The two Sophomore girls cried.

After spending the early Summer term at East Carolina College in Greenville, I told mama I wanted to leave home to see more of the world. Mama cried. I cried. And after we stopped crying, I packed all my belongings into my 1951 two-door Chevrolet Power Glide, and headed south. I started to head north, but the humiliation suffered by my ancestors between 1860 and 1877 still stuck in my craw, so south it was. To hell with the North. Southerners may talk a little funny at times, but we are a proud people. And we have long memories.

I drove down through South Carolina, but didn't even stop for gas. Too many poor people and too damn hot for me. Desolate state. So I drove on down through Savannah, Georgia. Could have sworn I was on the set of *Gone with the Wind*, you know, the scene where they show all those hundreds of colored people picking cotton. But people were friendly. The girls had big tits, bouncing butts and were very pretty. Even some of the white girls. Not being in a great hurry to get anywhere, I inquired of a wizened old colored man who seemed to be permanently bent at the waist, dragging what must have been two hundred pounds of cotton in an open tow sack, if I could help them pick cotton awhile. So I stooped over and picked cotton with about twenty stooped-over colored men, women and children for about an hour. You can bet your cotton-picking life I'll never pick cotton again.

In those days there were no "fast food" eating places, so before continuing my journey southward, I stopped by a grocery store outside Savannah. As I approached the store, I reached out to push open one of the two large glass swinging doors, when suddenly I heard a loud noise, like metal contacting metal, and both large glass doors popped open and just stayed in the open position, quivering, like they couldn't make up their minds whether to stay open, or close again. Being a little spooked, I slowly backed away, and the doors closed again, on their own.

Scared hell out of me, it did. Now that's progress, I thought. Doors that open and close without touching them. And being an inquisitive 'sylum dog, I must have walked in and out of that grocery store a dozen or more times, until the manager picked up the phone like he was going to call the Savannah cops or something. So at age eighteen I experienced my first ever automatic door opener. Simply amazing.

Next thing you know, I thought, some genius is going to find a way to send a rocket to the goddamn moon or somewhere. But what fool would want to do that, I wondered. Probably the same fool who invented the automatic grocery door opener, when there was absolutely no good reason under God's bright sun to have such an invention. Then, on October 4, 1957, damned if "Sputnik" didn't become a household word throughout the world. We were in another time entirely; the "simple" life was gone forever. And I wondered aloud at the time if Sputnik was equipped with automatic grocery door openers.

But first, to continue with my journey of discovery and enlightenment, where I met my first ever "foreigners."

So I headed farther south, and ended up in Miami, Florida. Visited the University of Miami in Coral Gables, and stopped by the cafeteria for dinner. Nearly every student had a big old hawk nose, even the girls. And it seemed like to me that every other one of them was named "Youse." What's "youse," I asked the lone white student. They use that when they should be saying "You all," he tells me. Oh, I say, then why don't they just say "You all?" Don't know, he says. And they all talk so damn fast, like they were going to run out of breath before they run out of words or something.

Where they from, I ask the lone white student. New York, was the reply. They Americans, I asked. Don't know, he says. Jews. From New York. Talk fast. Even the girls have big noses. Can't say a sentence without using "youse" at least three times. May or may not be Americans. Really odd people, these Jews. I'd have to write home to mama about this.

Lone White Boy seemed nice enough. Didn't talk too fast. Friendly. Helpful. Like he was from North Carolina or somewhere in that neck of the woods. Where you from, I ask. From Georgia, he says. Whereabouts in Georgia, I ask. At-Lanta, he says. That anywhere near Atlanta, I ask. Close enough, he says. So here I was, caught smackdab betwixt "youse" and "At-lanta." Time to go. You like Georgia, I ask White Boy. Yeah, he replies. Short on words, he was. You like South Carolina, I ask. Naw, he says, too damn hot and too many poor people. Who would want to live in South Carolina? Perceptive fellow, American White Boy was.

Then it was unanimous. It was Georgia. I said "so long" to Lone White Boy in a Swarm of Fast-talking Jews, got the hell out of Little New York as fast as I could, and pointed the whitewalls of my Chevy northward.

Mr. Cook was a civilian flight instructor, and his company trained pilots for foreign governments. At about the time of my high school graduation, Mr. Cook and his family moved to the company's location in Moultrie, in South Georgia. I helped out during the move, driving one of the rental trucks. So following my narrow escape from South New York, I stopped by Moultrie and spent some time with Dan, Becky and the girls.

I applied and was accepted to Berry College, a four-year liberal arts college situated outside Rome, Georgia, about sixty miles northeast of At-Lanta. I double-majored in Physics and Mathematics. I was elected President of my Freshman Class, Treasurer of my Sophomore Class, first Secretary, then Vice President and finally President of the Men's Student Government. I rewrote the Berry College Men's Handbook, and at the end of my Junior year became the first ever recipient of the Jesse Pritchett Parish Student Leadership Award, presented to the one student at Berry College who had demonstrated the greatest leadership abilities of any student on campus. I was honored, and while at Berry College became good friends with Dr. John R. Bertrand, President of the college. My no-nonsense, kick-ass attitude developed as a youngster in the orphanage was already paying big dividends.

In June 1958 I had just completed my first year at Berry College. Mr. Cook had started building his dream home on a large one hundred acre lake east of Moultrie. I worked with the carpenters every day, and Mr. Cook came to help out when his work schedule ended at the flight school.

On July 4, 1958, as we were working on the roof of the new home, Mr. Cook suffered a heart attack, and died two hours later. We took his body back to Kinston for burial. Mr. Cook was only forty years old when he died. He was a good Mason, a good friend, and I still miss him today. If only Dan Cook had been Superintendent of Oxford Orphanage . . .

Following graduation from Berry College in May 1961, I enlisted in the U.S. Army. After completing Basic Infantry Training at Fort Jackson, South Carolina, and Advanced Artillery Training at Ft. Still, Oklahoma, I was sent to Korea with a thousand other vomiting, seasick soldiers on a troopship for twenty-eight days.

Mama had suffered a stroke during my last year in college, and one afternoon while the ship was midway across the Sea of Japan bound for Inchon, South Korea, the ship's captain summoned me to his quarters. He informed me that the previous day, mama had died in a hospital in Kinston. I cried. The captain cried with me. I thanked him.

Mama was only fifty-five years old when she died. During the sixteen years between my daddy's death in February 1946, and her death in February 1962, I rarely ever saw mama smile. Even today this knowledge causes me great pain.

Once we landed in South Korea, I wrangled a job as the youngest reporter and only feature writer on the *Pacific Stars and Stripes*, a daily newspaper that was distributed to more than 35,000 soldiers in South Korea. I was assigned my own jeep, and allowed to roam freely throughout South Korea, writing about anything of a civilian or military nature that interested me. In addition, it was my assignment as the lone feature writer, to cover all the Military Armistice Commission meetings at Panmunjom, in the Demilitarized Zone between North and South Korea. It was a lot of responsibility, and I did a good job.

Following a tour of duty in Korea, I was accepted into the Defense Language Institute, located in Monterey, California, where I studied the Korean language six hours a day, five days a week, for a year. I graduated first in my class of thirty students.

After completing the months-long course in Army intelligence at the U.S. Army Intelligence Center at Ft. Holabird, Maryland, I returned to Korea as the youngest prisoner interrogator, stationed at the U.S.

Army Intelligence compound in Seoul. We interrogated captured North Korean communist espionage agents who had failed in their attempt to infiltrate South Korea, usually along the irregular coastline. The majority of the captured agents cooperated with us, but if one did not cooperate, we called a special unit of the South Korean Army, and they took him away and put him "in his place." Then we couldn't shut him up.

In December 1965 I received an Honorable Discharge from the U.S. Army, and in September 1967 was accepted into the University of Houston College of Optometry. I graduated in May 1972 with a doctorate in Optometry, and began a private Optometry practice outside Ft. Lauderdale, Florida.

In 1977 I was accepted into the Nova Southeastern University College of Law, and in 1980 graduated with a Juris Doctor degree. I took and passed the Florida Bar examination and the Georgia Bar examination in 1980, and have practiced Law and Optometry outside Atlanta since 1984.

My wife Evelyn is an electrical engineer and attorney. We have been married since 1967, and have raised four wonderful and talented children. Our sons Bret and Drew are in their fourth year of Optometry School. My daughter Karen, the only one of my children ever sent home from sixth grade for fighting, now teaches math and science to sixth graders in middle school in the Los Angeles area. My oldest son Derek and his wife are both realtors and restaurant owners in the Atlanta area. We have two delightful grandchildren, Daniel, named for my daddy, Benjamin Daniel Provost, and Kristen.

Well, that's my life in a nutshell. After about age fourteen, it has been a good life. Any demons I had not conquered by that age, I left lying with a tobacco stick on Miss Gracie's farm outside Oxford, North Carolina. May God bless orphans everywhere, especially 'sylum dogs.

www.ingramcontent.com/pod-product-compliance
Lightning Source LLC
Chambersburg PA
CBHW031809170526
45157CB00001B/16